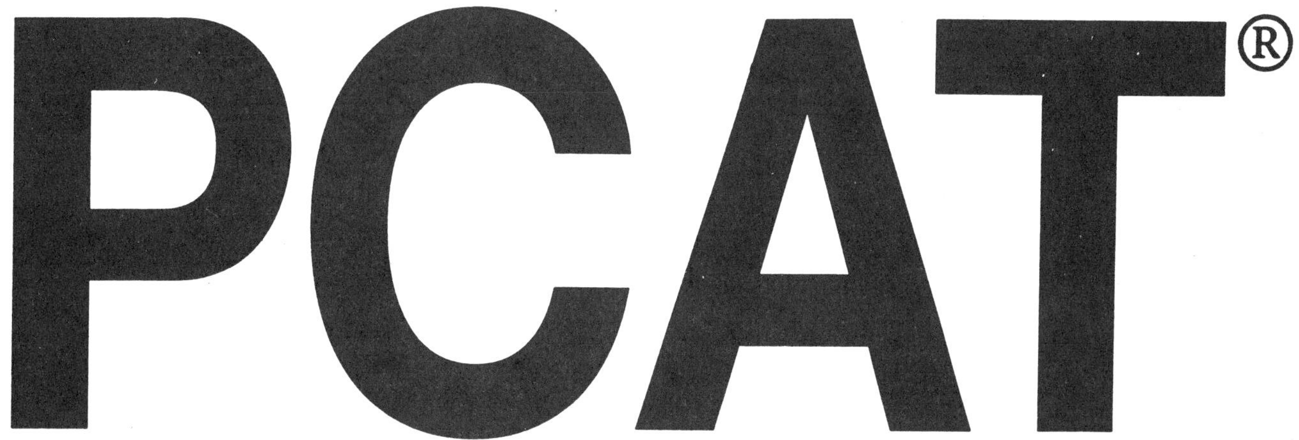

COMPLETE PREPARATION FOR THE PHARMACY COLLEGE ADMISSION TEST™

2000 Edition

THE SCIENCE OF REVIEW™

AFTAB S. HASSAN, Ph.D.

Contributing Authors
LEON ANDERSON, JR., D.M.D.
RUTH E. LOWE GORDON, B.S.
FRANK KESSLER, M.A.
EMILY MEYER NAEGELI, M.A.
JEFFREY D. ZUBKOWSKI, Ph.D.

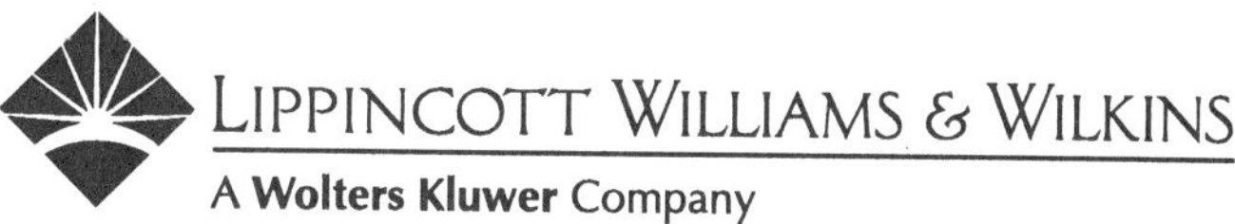

Philadelphia • Baltimore • New York • London
Buenos Aires • Hong Kong • Sydney • Tokyo

351 West Camden Street
Baltimore, Maryland 21201-2436 USA

227 East Washington Square
Philadelphia, PA 19106

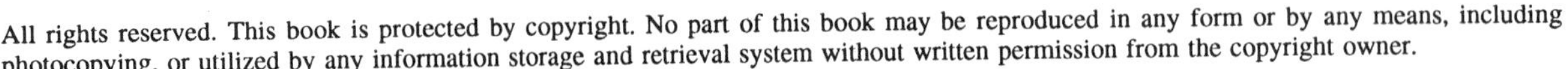

Printed in the United States of America

ISBN: 0-683-30781-9

99 00 01 02 03
2 3 4 5 6 7 8 9 10

CONTENTS

Chapter 5: Developing Quantitative Reasoning and Ability

Chapter 6: Preparing for PCAT Chemistry

Part III: Test Taking Skills and Sample PCAT

Chapter 7: Test-Taking Skills

Chapter 8: Pharmacy College Admission Test: Model Examination

Appendix A: Scope of Examinations

LIST OF FIGURES

LIST OF TABLES

PREFACE

Welcome to the 1999 edition of *Complete Preparation for the Pharmacy College Admission Test*. The concepts and skills included here correlate with the latest model of the Pharmacy College Admission Test, according to The Psychological Corporation's PCAT preparation materials. Practice questions and exercises simulate the admission test's format, and terminology of the Pharmacy College Admission Test is used throughout the book.

Complete Preparation for the Pharmacy College Admission Test is organized to facilitate your PCAT preparation. Presented in three parts, the book first introduces PCAT study skills; then science content review concepts; and, finally, the test-taking experience itself in the form of test-taking strategies and a sample examination. In this way, the guide provides the synthesis of knowledge and skills needed for high performance on the test.

- In the first part of the guide, chapter 1 includes information for students preparing for the Pharmacy College Admission Test. It contains study skills information, time management suggestions, and memorization techniques.

  Chapters 2, 3 and 5 consist of skills development materials for verbal ability, reading comprehension, and quantitative reasoning. Each of the skills development sections includes sample questions to help you judge how much time you will need to prepare for taking the exam.

  The skills development material in chapters 2, 3 and 5 begin with verbal ability development. A thorough treatment to develop reading comprehension and quantitative abilities is given in chapters 3 and 5. This section requires daily practice. Some students underestimate the reading skills level required for a major admission test like the PCAT and over-estimate the skills they have acquired. A lengthy section on math is provided in the quantitative reasoning chapter because mathematics skills may have suffered from underutilization. Practice will bring them back up to the level required for the exam.

  On the second part of the guide, required science knowledge is outlined in chapters 4 and 6. These chapters summarize the basic concepts required for the PCAT in biology, general chemistry, and organic chemistry. Each section is followed by PCAT-type test questions. Discussion of answers is also included for further review and self-assessment to aid you in discovering your individual strengths and weaknesses. Use your science textbooks for a comprehensive review.

  The third part of *Complete Preparation for the Pharmacy College Admission Test* provides test-taking skills and a sample test. Chapter 7 tells how the test is scored and describes strategies to use on the test day. This includes strategies to help you attain the best possible scores on the PCAT.

  Chapter 8 is a sample PCAT provided for practice and evaluation. You will know you are ready for the test when you have developed a strong science knowledge base, good reading and math skills, and efficient speed and time management practices.

An appendix is included to help you focus on specific exam topics. It provides a detailed outline keyed to each topic and shows an itemized distribution of content. This information is based on The Psychological Corporation's testing program reports.

How To Use This Guide

The science content review and skills materials included in this guide are presented according to the PCAT content outlines. When you review the sciences (chapters 4 and 6), begin with the concepts that were not covered in your college curriculum, or the ones you failed to master because of time constraints.

The following 5-step model is recommended for learning science concepts:

1. define or describe,
2. give examples,
3. apply equations, formulas, or drawings,
4. compare and contrast, and
5. apply the concept to problem solving, using questions and vocabulary/skills checklists in your review.

Recommended study skills are given in chapters 1, 2, 3 and 5, the first part of this guide. Following the science content chapters, test-taking strategies for the PCAT are given in chapter 7 because both skills and content review material should be mastered fully before taking the test. It will help you to review efficiently and improve your performance on the actual test if you prepare for the examination using the skills chapters before reviewing PCAT science concepts.

Your best overall strategy is to learn from all the sections as thoroughly as you can. Practice your skills and your performance will improve. Remember that the skills and concepts provided in this guide will aid you in achieving good scores, regardless of changes in test format. Organized preparation using the guide also will help you get ready for pharmacy school.

ABOUT THE AUTHORS

Leon Anderson, Jr., D.M.D., Assistant Professor of Restorative Dentistry, University of Mississippi School of Dentistry. Bachelor and Master of Science degrees in Biology from Jackson State University and Doctor of Pharmacy Medicine from the University of Mississippi School of Dentistry. He is presently the attending dentist at the University of Mississippi Medical Center in restorative dentistry and also the director of minority student affairs. Dr. Anderson served in the Jackson Public School System as a teacher of Biology for a number of years. He has years of teaching experience and up-to-date knowledge concerning health care and the educational needs of students interested in the health professions. He is the author of numerous publications and abstracts and serves on the Medical and Pharmacy School Admissions Committee at the University of Mississippi.

Ruth E. Lowe Gordon, B.S., Assistant Director/Education Specialist, Office of Minority Student Affairs, University of Mississippi Medical Center. Bachelor of Science Degree in Mathematics and Science from Alabama State University. She has carried out graduate study work at the University of Illinois. Ms. Gordon has been a mathematics teacher in the United States, Ghana, and Scotland. She has worked with premedical and predental training programs and has considerable knowledge and familiarity with pre-professional, paraprofessional, and professional science education in the medical school environment. She has developed and implemented Medical College Admission Test (MCAT) and other preprofessional health preparation workshops at undergraduate schools.

Aftab S. Hassan, Ph.D., Doctorate Water Resources and Hydraulics, Columbia Pacific University (UCLA Program); doctoral scientist in Ocean, Coastal and Environmental Engineering, George Washington University. Dr. Hassan is an educational specialist in the sciences and has strongly supported active learning and problem based teaching through his extensive teaching experience. Dr. Hassan also specializes in hydrodynamics, pollutant transport and coastal engineering. He was formerly affiliated with George Washington University School of Engineering and Applied Science, and with Georgetown University, Department of Community and Family Medicine. He has been actively involved in mcAT and DAT teaching for students at Georgetown University, Washington, D.C., and provides active learning workshops for approximately twenty other schools across the U.S. He has taught, tutored and advised premedical and engineering students for over twenty-two years.

Frank Kessler, M.A., History, Eastern Michigan University. Formerly, Assistant Professor in history at Virginia State University, Petersburg. Mr. Kessler entered graduate studies program in American history at the University of North Carolina. He is currently reading instructor at the Academic Learning Skills Center, University of North Carolina, Chapel Hill.

Emily Meyer Naegeli, M.A., Art Historian. Bachelor degrees in English and Art History from Vanderbilt University and Master of Arts degree in Art History form Northwestern University. She is currently involved in the appraisal, cataloging and research of several private collections. Mrs. Naegeli is also serving on the Board of the Center for American Archeology. While at Block Gallery, Northwestern University, she worked as an exhibit and catalog researcher, and as a lecturer on Chinese ceramics at an exhibition in Chicago. As an avocation, she indulges in her lifelong love of word origins, puzzles, and intellectual challenges.

Jeffrey D. Zubkowski, Ph.D., Associate Professor of Chemistry, Jackson State University. Bachelor of Science in Chemistry from the University of Pittsburgh, and Doctor of Philosophy in Chemistry from Indiana University. He is an Associate Professor of Chemistry at Jackson State University. Dr. Zubkowski was a postdoctoral fellow at the University of Toronto, Ontario, Canada, and is author or coauthor of a number of scientific publications.

ABOUT THE SCIENCE OF REVIEW

Williams & Wilkins is a world-wide leader in medical publishing, offering thousands of publications to keep medical students and professionals informed, educated, and prepared throughout their careers. With the purchase of your first Science of Review product, you join a long tradition of excellence. We are the experts in presenting medical information. No other test preparation company has this focus or expertise. Simply put, we know what you need for success on the MCAT, throughout your years in medical school, and in your medical career.

ACKNOWLEDGMENTS

Complete Preparation for the Pharmacy College Admission Test, formerly known as *The Betz Guide,* is written to help students understand the level of skills and knowledge required for high performance on the PCAT. In this new volume, directed to prepare students for the Pharmacy College Admission Test, the work of the original authors was augmented by the collaborative efforts of Aftab Hassan, Frank Kessler, and Emily Naegeli.

Frank Whitehouse, Jr., M.D., Associate Professor, Department of Microbiology and Immunology, Medical School, University of Michigan, helped with the final edit of this work, correlating it with the latest available information on the Pharmacy College Admission Test. His efforts in the final phase of this edition were greatly appreciated by the authors of the text.

Peter A. S. Smith, Ph.D., Professor Emeritus of Chemistry, Department of Chemistry, University of Michigan, helped in the review of content and test items by concentrating on the general and organic chemistry chapter. His critical analysis was very helpful.

We also acknowledge the expert assistance rendered by Holly Wagner, in bringing this work to life by her technical assistance in preparing the manuscript, and Sandra Michael for the many hours and special care taken in typesetting and preparing the final version of this book.

PART I

SKILLS DEVELOPMENT FOR THE PHARMACY COLLEGE ADMISSION TEST

Chapter 1:

Introduction to PCAT Study Skills

1.0 THE PHARMACY COLLEGE ADMISSION TEST

The Pharmacy College Admission Test (PCAT) evaluates the level of your knowledge in biology, general chemistry, and organic chemistry. It also measures your skills in reading comprehension, quantitative ability, and verbal ability.

The PCAT accentuates the importance of developing good reading ability, data interpretation, and scientific reasoning skills. These are skills that take time to master and are difficult to develop in a month or two of preparation. For this reason, what you did in college and high school may have already prepared you for the PCAT (and the pharmacy profession). If you feel your reading/study/interpretation skills are relatively weak and your school or college offers a remedial course, take it. Select courses that demand interpretive and inferential reading, such as literature, logic and history. Science courses will also help you to understand and apply principles and to interpret data.

Read beyond your classroom assigned texts, particularly newspapers, news magazines, and scientific journals. Although the PCAT content has been largely covered in your course work, remember that the PCAT stresses test items linked to pharmacy preparation and education, perhaps to a greater degree than your classwork. When you read, force yourself to draw conclusions, interpret graphs and charts, predict trends in data, and assay the limitations and errors presented in data or opinions expressed. When studying biology correlate what you have learned in chemistry or even physics (although physics is not tested on the PCAT). When reading an article, check the data and conclusions against other texts. As humans, we understand and learn best using complex webs of skills and knowledge not in isolated pieces.

The study habits and skills you develop to reach your goal of a pharmacy degree will last a lifetime. They will help you achieve a high level of performance on the PCAT, in pharmacy school, and as a practicing professional. This chapter describes different parts of the PCAT, study skills to prepare for the PCAT, and applied reasoning skills required to do well on the PCAT.

What is the Pharmacy College Admission Test? When is the PCAT Administered?

The PCAT testing program is conducted by The Psychological Corporation. The Psychological Corporation works with the American Association of Colleges of Pharmacy to assure that the PCAT content outline reflects current requirements for pharmacy school admissions. Examinations are given three times yearly in October or November, February, and April at many testing centers in the United States and in foreign countries. It is advisable for students to take the exam during the spring of the year before applying to pharmacy school.

How do I Register to Take the Exam?

Registration materials are available at no charge for the three annual administrations of the PCAT. The registration booklet contains all the information needed to register for the exam and a small sample of PCAT items. You may obtain this information by contacting your health professions or prepharmacy advisor; or by writing to:

Pharmacy College Admission Test (PCAT)
The Psychological Corporation
555 Academic Court
San Antonio, Texas 78204-2498
1-800-622-3231 or FAX 210-921-8861

In case you need counseling specific to your goals call us at Betz Publishing Company (Call toll free at 1-800-634-4365, 24 hours a day, seven days a week) or write to us. We will help you get pharmacy related books (admission requirements and test taking for the PCAT).

What does the Pharmacy College Admission Test Cover?

In the chart below, the first five sections named are listed in the order in which they appear in the PCAT. Beginning in 1994, the five sections may appear in a different order. The actual content of the PCAT, as well as time guidelines, proctoring, and monitoring of the test, is managed by The Psychological Corporation. Usually, toward the end of the exam, one section may be used for field testing of new items and is NOT graded to determine your PCAT scores.

TABLE 1: PCAT Schedule

Examination Section	**Number of Questions**	**Maximum Time (Minutes)**	**Average (Seconds / item)**
Verbal Ability - Antonyms (25) - Analogies (25)	50	30	(36 secs/item)
Biology	50	30	(36 secs/item)
Reading Comprehension	45	45	(60 secs/item)
——— *Break* ———	—	30	—
Quantitative Ability	65	45	42 secs/item)
Chemistry	60	30	(30 secs/item)
Reading Comprehension	45	45	(60 secs/item)

Usually the examination begins at 8:30 A.M. and lasts until 1:50 P.M. The number of test items and allotted time for each of the examination sections is indicated in the above chart and may vary depending on the coding of the exam, site for testing and other testing parameters. On the test day, the time given for each subtest will be printed on the test booklet. You are also instructed to have only #2 lead pencils with you in the testing room.

What Types of Questions are Covered on the Exam?

The PCAT is an achievement test that uses standard multiple-choice questions with one best answer for each question. The science content consists of subject matter covered by first-year courses in biology, general chemistry, and organic chemistry. Biology and chemistry are tested separately, and separate subscores are given for each science section; therefore, it is important that you pace yourself. Performing mathematical calculations at a fast pace is important for the general and organic chemistry sections. Understanding medical terminology is helpful for the science sections, and is also good information for Reading Comprehension.

The Reading Comprehension section consists of four to six (short or long) reading passages, each containing a variable number of items. The passages are typical of new descriptive information that might be read in the first year of pharmacy school. One must read, comprehend, and apply the material to answer the questions based on connecting details in the passage.

The Verbal Ability section measures your nontechnical word knowledge. Analogies and antonyms are used to measure your general verbal ability and knowledge of words used in unfamiliar contexts. Usually there are 25 analogies and 25 antonyms in the section. Understanding medical terminology is <u>not</u> required on this part of the test.

The Biology section measures your basic and applied knowledge of general biology and human biology (basic anatomy and physiology). In this section you will be asked to recall and apply fundamental concepts and principles in solving word problems using biology contexts.

The Chemistry section measures your understanding of inorganic (general) chemistry and organic chemistry. This part of the test is more difficult to complete because most chemistry problems require math calculations to solve them. The exam will test your recall of important principles and concepts, as well as application of those concepts to biological systems, e.g. vertebrate systems. The chemistry section places greater emphasis on inorganic chemistry items and reduced emphasis on organic chemistry. Usually about 90% of the items are inorganic chemistry items and 10% of them are organic or bioorganic chemistry items.

The Quantitative Reasoning test measures the ability to reason with numbers, manipulate numerical relationships, and solve quantitative word problems.

How do I Prepare for the PCAT?

To prepare for the Pharmacy College Admission Test, you may select self-managed preparation, and/or commercial or college preparation courses, depending on individual needs. In any case, you must organize your study. Initially, it is important to identify the subject areas where you lack competency. It is advantageous to continue identifying your weak and strong areas throughout your study, using the following means: 1) review old examinations, 2) self-administer sample PCAT examinations, 3) review the topics and skills in this book, *Pharmacy College Admission Test: The Betz Guide,* and 4) practice test items using biology and chemistry software in an active format. Call us for details!

First, begin by studying your weakest subjects. This will help raise your competency level in weaker areas to that of your stronger ones. Next, study weak and strong subjects together, emphasizing the topics you need to strengthen in each. The special skills and content review topics need for each exam section are given in chapters 2 through 6.

You are more likely to prepare successfully if you have an organized approach to your study. Self-motivation is an important factor in success. Keep a clear goal always in mind and achieve it through concentrated preparation. Preparation alternatives are shown below.

Self-managed study. Self-managed study involves an organized study plan that you design and use along with notes, texts, and preparation materials specific to the PCAT. The cost of this method is relatively low. Self-managed preparation may be more difficult, but it will yield the best results when well planned and diligently pursued. A major factor in the advantage of self-managed study is the development of a disciplined approach that will also serve you well in pharmacy school. It is important that you keep complete class notes, course outlines, and access to textbooks, as well as Pharmacy College Admission Test materials, to use as references and guides.

Other advantages of self-managed study include having the use of a guide such as *The Betz Guide*, which provides study protocols and practice with PCAT-type problems. Your class notes and the text books you already own help to link your classwork to PCAT preparation and make this method very economical. (For more information, refer also to the Betz PCAT Packages described on the inside back cover of this guide. Use the prepaid postcards or call 1-800-634-4365 for more information.

Preparatory Programs Sponsored by a College or University. Cost of this method is minimal to intermediate and there are few disadvantages. The advantages include the possible involvement of professors who regularly teach at the university, a familiar environment and teaching staff, and the teaching staff's awareness of each student's weak and strong areas. The opportunity to participate in group study sessions is also frequently very helpful. A major disadvantage is that attendance may lapse.

Commercial Preparation. A major disadvantage of commercial preparation courses is expense and a "fixed" content taught in a passive format. Research has shown mixed results regarding their effectiveness. Some advantages include the chance to meet other pharmacy school applicants and the opportunity to obtain condensed course materials or notes pertinent to the PCAT. Better attendance may result because of the expense. You should ask questions about the materials.

How is the PCAT Scored?

Each section of the pharmacy college admission testing program yields a raw score that is the sum total of your correct answers. The raw score is converted to a standard score so test takers can compare their performance on one subtest with another (such as comparing Reading Comprehension with Quantitative Ability) and across different administrations of the PCAT (winter versus spring). Chapter 7 provides more insight into scoring formulas.

How are the Scores Reported?

Test scores for the PCAT are reported to pharmacy schools in terms of standard scores and percentile ranks. Percentile ranks compare a candidate's performance on each section with a norm group consisting of applicants to schools of pharmacy from across the U.S. Scores from the most recent attempt, and the total number of times you took the PCAT, will be reported.

How are Scores Used?

Through the use of standard scores it is possible to compare the performance of one applicant with the performance of all applicants on any or all of the measures included in the PCAT. The conversion of raw scores to standard scores is based on the underlying ability defined by test items. Obtain a copy of the "Pharmacy School Admission Requirements" book by calling Betz Publishing Company, Inc.

The Role of the PCAT in the Admissions Process

The PCAT is a standardized test designed to measure the cognitive skills and scientific knowledge that are important for pharmacy education. As objective measures, PCAT scores can be included in the student profile of GPA, recommendations, and personal interview. Some schools may require other equivalent tests, such as CLEP or achievement tests, in addition to, or instead of, the PCAT. Carefully check the admissions requirements of the schools to which you expect to apply using the "Pharmacy School Admission Requirements" guide.

Pharmacy College Admission Test: The Betz Guide

Pharmacy College Admission Test: The Betz Guide contains specific information on each subtest of the Pharmacy College Admission Test. It describes the topics covered by the test in details that focus on pharmacy school requirements. In addition, to further inform you in advance of the exam, a sample practice test similar in form and content to the actual PCAT is given in chapter 8.

This guide is designed to stimulate self-managed study for the PCAT. Read and review the basic principles that precede each subtest. The sample test questions will familiarize you with the actual examination because the practice questions are similar to those found in the PCAT.

The authors and editors of this book offer no promises or guarantees as to your performance on the PCAT. The value you will derive from the use of this book as a study aid is directly related to the amount and quality of time you invest in review. The important point in preparing to take any examination is to have a definite plan in mind before you begin.

1.1 STUDY SKILLS FOR PCAT PREPARATION

It is important to emphasize that the best background for taking the PCAT is good preparation in high school and college, including reading comprehension, solving algebra word problems, and working with geometry. A well-planned review can improve your performance on the test. PCAT preparation time is an opportunity to master currently deficient skills and concepts. Good skills and a solid knowledge of science concepts will provide the solid foundation you need as a pharmacy student and a practicing pharmacist. A positive attitude toward test preparation is helpful.

Some general and specific study strategies are provided below and can be applied to all portions of the test. Suggestions for managing your preparation time immediately before the test and for the test-day itself appear in chapter 7.

1.1.1 Make a Schedule

Create a realistic, well-planned schedule that provides appropriate time to study the natural science subjects. If you don't like a specific subject, plan to study the subject *first.* Find the reasons that keep you from studying that subject (for instance, the material is too difficult, you don't have good books, you don't conceptualize the subject, etc.). You *need* that subject to do well on the PCAT, whether you like it or not. Make a schedule for each day with checklists called "Things *To Do* Today" and "Things *Done* Today." Before going to bed, check off what you finished. Make sure that things scheduled but not reviewed one day are reviewed the next day. This should help you gauge how realistically you have planned your time. See Fig. 1.1 for sample checklists and retain these daily checklists until the PCAT is over. They will serve as memos during your preparation.

Make a study schedule for each day. Block out available time for PCAT self-managed study and list as precisely as you can what you plan to study in each session. Link your lecture or laboratory class time wherever possible to your PCAT preparation. Review while you study for class. The two activities can be mutually beneficial. (Remember that many questions in the organic chemistry subtest will integrate laboratory experience with the lecture material, e.g., the NMR spectroscopy labs.

THINGS TO DO TODAY

1. Read TIME magazine article on biofeedback instruments.
2. Learn probability concepts.
3. What are orthographic projections? Do library research.
4. Review carboxylic acids and their stereochemistry.
5. Learn the differences between virus, virion, bacteriophage, and bacteria.
6. Take GRE test for reading Comprehension.

THINGS DONE TODAY

1. Read TIME magazine article in a hurry; didn't understand it.
2. Learned probability concepts.
3. Found two references on orthographic projections and 3-D drawings.
4. Took + graded GRE test for reading comp.
5. Did some probability problems.
6. skipped 4+5 on Things To Do Today list due to lack of time, interest, + resources.

Fig. 1.1 — Scheduling with daily checklists

Even if the time is theoretically available, do not schedule a six-hour PCAT preparation day. Four to six hours of study time with quick breaks is enough. If you have still more free time, practice reading comprehension, and scientific reasoning and logic problems. Work more on improving verbal abilities by reviewing antonyms, synonyms, analogies, and by improving your general vocabulary. Spend time in preparing a list of words you don't know and recording them in a daily diary.

Of all the areas you will be tested on, reading comprehension will probably be the slowest to improve. Foregoing television during your PCAT preparation time will free up more time for reading.

Lastly, do not schedule study time later than 11:00 p.m., even though you may consider yourself to be a "night person." You learn best when you are fresh, and, of course, the PCAT is not given at night.

1.1.2 Develop a Disciplined Approach

The science subtests consist of 50 items in biology and 60 items in chemistry (inorganic and organic). You must be as disciplined in <u>taking</u> these tests as you will need to be in studying for them. For example, if you don't like organic chemistry, you may procrastinate before that section of the test, spending more time in biology than is appropriate, a situation that does not necessarily guarantee a high biology score but which may cause you to rush through general or organic chemistry. Test-taking discipline begins with good study habits.

1.1.3 Use Test Items Efficiently and Effectively

When practicing test items, work on only a small number of items, such as one reading passage with follow-up questions or ten independent test items at one time. To improve, you need to analyze your errors in order to remember the reasoning you used as you worked the problems. Record your errors in a daily diary.

To analyze your errors, go to the answer key first. Understand why the answer is correct and explain it satisfactorily to yourself. Use the answer analysis section only as a last resort and to check yourself after you can explain the answer in the key. Only after you understand why the keyed response is correct should you check your reasoning against the answer analysis section.

Review on a regular basis the written record of your errors; call it your "error journal." Use the outline found in the *Pharmacy College Admission Test: The Betz Guide* and mark (√) the appropriate topic. Errors can be classified in a number of ways. For example, specific content errors (e.g., genetics problems in biology), as well as specific question format errors (e.g., multiple choice), can give you trouble. Your record of errors will help you use your time most efficiently, since you will know where you most need to review or to develop more successful strategies for answering the questions. For a full listing and explanation of these classifications, refer to chapter 3, section 3.3.5.

As you work problems, note where the test emphasis lies. Once again the outline in the *Pharmacy College Admission Test: The Betz Guide* will help. For example, you may find that genetics is an important topic, so time spent on reviewing Mendelian genetics and applying the Hardy-Weinberg principle will repay the effort; conversely, you do not need to take a course just so you can answer a single obscure question from a topic that may only appear once.

1.1.4 Prepare for the Skills Areas Tested on the PCAT

Short daily practice in reading, and quantitative and scientific reasoning, is relatively better than infrequent and ill-planned blocks of sustained practice. Plan to spend 30 to 45 minutes daily on skills development, possibly alternating your practice for the Reading Comprehension, Quantitative Ability, and Verbal Ability sections of the test. Plan to spend more time on the skills that are the most difficult to master.

If you have forgotten the basic math skills used in quantitative reasoning, you need to schedule additional time for basic math review. For speed, it is good to practice how to estimate a reasonable answer. **If you usually work with a calculator, stop using it while you are preparing for the PCAT; calculators are not allowed.**

For additional practice items in basic math, obtain copies of scholastic aptitude tests (SAT) from Educational Testing Service (Princeton, New Jersey), which publishes them in book form.

Verbal ability described as a problem-solving skill may be a new idea to you. If so, try the following method of working with vocabulary words. When you make an error on the practice material for the Verbal Ability test, create another item that exactly parallels the one that gave you trouble. Use a college thesaurus to find similar and opposite words, don't waste too much time fishing for words in a dictionary.

The most basic way to improve reading is to read more and pick out the underlying assumptions, hypotheses, inferences, and conclusions in what you read. In addition to practicing test items, read daily at least one of the following periodicals: *Time, The New York Times* (especially the Tuesday edition that regularly has a science and education section), *Discover, USA Today, Science,* and pharmacy journals such as the *Journal of the American Pharmacy Association.* After you read an article, summarize it. One way to do this is to explain the author's main points to a friend. You can form a reading group to discuss articles; or write a five-minute critical summary. Collect lists of antonyms and analogies.

Try working test items for the Reading Comprehension, Quantitative Ability, and Verbal Ability portions of the test as though they are warm-up exercises. Or use skills practice as a break from your science review.

1.1.5 Review the Sciences: Biology and Chemistry

Once you know your skill levels in reading comprehension, quantitative reasoning, and verbal ability and can gauge how much time you need to develop these skills further, you are ready to begin your science review in biology, general chemistry, and organic chemistry.

Review at least *one* topic in each of the three science subject areas every day—even if you spend the bulk of your study time on only *one* topic. You need to put this basic information into your long-term memory. The best long-term memory development technique is constant review. Do not set a schedule that reserves a week for biology, a week for general chemistry, and a week for organic chemistry. Do not schedule any single day devoted to only one subject.

In general, most of us like to work on what we do best; we tend to review what we already know. In preparing for the PCAT, you need to develop strategies to correct these habits. Keep in mind the following suggestions as you plan your science subject review for the PCAT. Study your *least* favorite subject first. If you schedule a four-hour block of time for your PCAT preparation on a given day, divide the time as follows: older content review, new skills review, new content review, and older skills review. This is the most efficient review pattern. Then divide the four hours between content review and skills development. If you have scheduled three months for your PCAT preparation, keep in mind that you will be tested on what you review at the beginning of your preparation as well as on what you review immediately before the test; therefore, spend some time each day staying current with the material you reviewed earlier as well as studying any new material.

1.1.6 Anticipate PCAT-Type Questions: Conceptual Learning

When you study or read, try to formulate PCAT-type questions and possible responses. For example, for each test item and the corresponding responses, think about what is false, or the exception, as well as what is true. This is especially important when the text provides a concept and one or two examples. The examples are important for understanding, but not really for rote memorization because the test maker is unlikely to use those precise examples in a test item. Rather, the test maker will check to see if you can understand "new" examples by applying your understanding of examples you have been given in textbooks and/or in class notes. The entire PCAT review can be grouped into "single concepts." Each concept can be learned using its five analytical components (see Fig. 1.2).

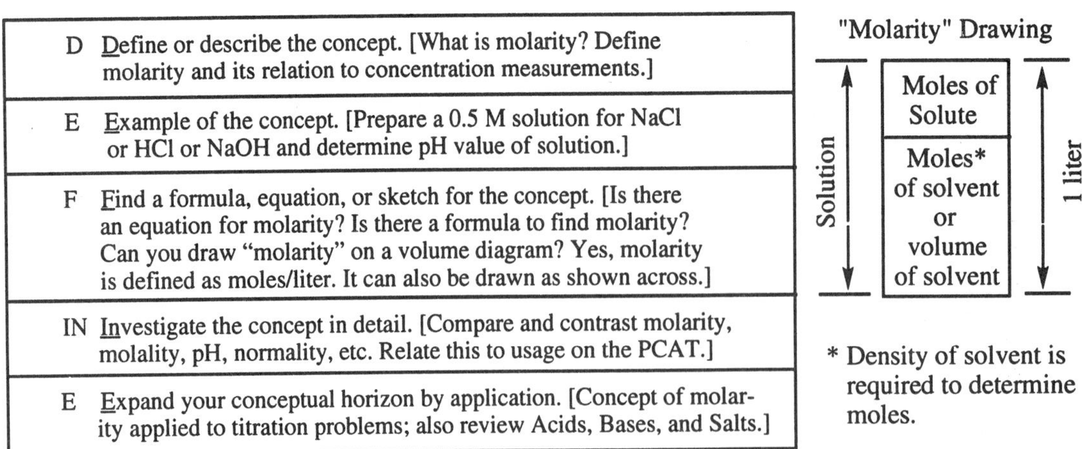

Fig. 1.2 — Components of a PCAT Concept: D - E - F - I N - E

1.1.7 Look for Error Patterns

In an ideal multiple-choice item, errors are spread evenly across all the distractors (the incorrect responses or words that catch a test-taker's attention. This means that each distracter ideally represents a typical error. To complicate things further, each of us has patterns of errors that we continue to repeat unless an intervention strategy is introduced.

When you make an error, pay attention to whether you react by saying: "I always have trouble with Boyle's law," followed with a rationalization such as, "It's not that I don't know it, it's just that the wording of the test item threw me." We sometimes confuse "recognition" with "knowing" or "understanding." You should understand a concept well enough to answer it correctly in whatever form it appears. If you cannot explain a concept clearly to someone who knows it well, and who can therefore check your reasoning and accuracy, you really do not know it. Use graphic or visual skills to reinforce and remember each concept that caused an error.

The first step in correcting error patterns is to recognize when they occur. The second step is to develop a mnemonic or memory device that you can apply each time you do an item in the category you have identified. For example, it may help you to remember Boyle's law by thinking of your car. As you step on the accelerator, the piston is pushed down; as the volume decreases, the pressure increases. You can even draw a picture as a reminder. If you need to use a mnemonic, you must apply it every time the topic appears. Patterns of error tend to be well developed, and they do not lend themselves to correction by rote memorization alone.

1.1.8 Develop Your Concentration

To test your problem-solving abilities, the PCAT requires a full morning of concentrated problem solving that includes knowledge and reasoning. You need to work on applying yourself without a break for an entire morning. Without practice, concentrating on problem solving can be unexpectedly difficult. During the test the difficult aspects of the test increase while your concentration may decrease. To increase your concentration, learn to study with awareness. Work with a clock in front of you. Notice the time you begin and the time you would normally take a break, which can be both *conscious* and *unconscious*. Getting coffee is an example of a conscious break; reading a page or more without knowing what you have read constitutes an unconscious break.

The next step to improving your concentration is to legitimize your breaks. It is important that you take conscious breaks. Give yourself permission to stop when you cannot concentrate on problems. Remember that without permission, your brain will take a break anyway, only you won't always be aware of what you missed. If you can only concentrate for 15 minutes at a time, then 15 minutes is the base-line from which you will build.

The third step is to build your concentration slowly. If you begin at 15 minutes, work up to 20 minutes, then 25 minutes, and so on, until you can work without losing concentration for two full hours.

The fourth step is to be self-aware. Which subjects are hardest for you to concentrate on? What time of day do you concentrate best? When is your concentration worst? Does the food you eat affect your concentration? How about background noise or the lack of it? Does stress in school or your job affect your concentration? Does your working place or study area affect your concentration?

Concentration requires both endurance and discipline to correct for variables. It helps to limit the time you plan to work. Avoid open-ended study sessions, the kind where you say, "I'm going to work on this organic chemistry until I've finished it, all night if I must." Open-ended study sessions encourage daydreaming. Instead, say to yourself, "I have exactly one and one-half hours to finish this organic chemistry. If it isn't finished by then, too bad." Then stop. Limitless sessions encourage a lack of focus; limiting the time you spend on specific material encourages you to manage your time and concentrate harder.

1.1.9 Find a Study Partner

Explaining difficult material to someone else is a good way to check your understanding of what you read. Find a study partner who is strong in your weak subjects and weak in your strong subjects. If your study partner is having difficulty, you can act as listener. It is the job of the critical listener to make sure that what the speaker says is accurate, complete, precise, and to the point. Working with someone provides feedback and is less punitive than waiting to test your knowledge on exam day. It is important to understand that the weaker student in a given topic *cannot* serve as a critical listener for the stronger student in that topic. The weaker student should use a textbook, class notes, or course outlines to evaluate the partner's level of understanding.

1.1.10 Develop Your Short-Term Memory

Short-term memory is also useful. Short-term memory items are forgotten as soon as you finish using them. Do not waste time memorizing short-term information three months before the test. Seldom-used equations or a chart comparing smooth, skeletal, and cardiac muscles are examples of short-term memory tasks. When working with items that require short-term memory information, solve the problem with the information in front of you. During the last few days of your study time just before taking the PCAT, commit to memory what you have identified as short-term memory tasks. And on the test day itself, take a few minutes just after the exam begins to write out some of those short-term memory items so you have them for your use without having to concentrate retaining them.

1.1.11 Develop Your Long-Term Memory

Compared with students from other countries, the ability of American students to memorize information is relatively weak. This is partly because Americans rely heavily on the written word to build information and the information base cumulatively or a little at a time. Thus the science courses you took before college were supposed to build a foundation for those you took in college. Now both are supposed to provide a foundation for pharmacy school.

Very little attention is given to developing memory in school. Some students acquire useful strategies accidentally or by trial and error, but in general there is no formal instruction or guidance to help you, although reading several texts for comparison can help boost your understanding and your memory.

In a cumulative information model of how our memory works, there is an assumed distinction between long-term memory and short-term memory. An example of short-term memory is when you make a doctor's appointment. After the appointment, you "erase" the date and time. Similarly, when you attempt to memorize materials for tomorrow's test without conceptualizing them, they tend to be stored in your short-term memory. Immediately after the test the memory of these new materials is erased just as the doctor's appointment was erased. While almost everyone has experienced this, the point to remember is that rote memorization alone is a short-term memory technique.

Long-term memory, on the other hand, is based on an understanding of what is read or learned. Thus you tend to retain information you understand, such as the biology you took in high school, because the understanding formed the foundation for subsequent learning. But you probably handled those areas in high school biology that you didn't understand by using rote memorization. This helped you pass the tests, but did not create a strong foundation for subsequent learning. A better approach to learning biology is to use the PCAT conceptual learning model presented in section 1.1.6. When you understand what you are learning the information is retained. The best way to check your understanding is to explain the topic to someone who knows enough about it to act as a critical listener.

While it is also true that we remember best what we enjoy, we also tend to like what we understand. When someone says "I never liked mathematics," they are really saying "I never fully understood mathematics." Their lack of understanding may be caused by poor teaching or a bad classroom experience. Math, science, and Shakespeare are topics too large and important to dismiss by saying, "I never liked it."

If understanding a topic contributes to liking it, then liking it contributes to how long you retain it. If you think you don't like a subject, pretend that you do. That is, look for reasons to find it interesting and remember that you need it for the PCAT. Connect it in some way with other subjects that you like. Every time you say to yourself, "I don't like this," you make learning more difficult.

Understanding information also works in favor of your long-term memory because it allows you to build a complex web of information. The hardest task is memorizing a list of discrete and unconnected statements or items. The more connections you make, the easier it is to memorize. Teach yourself to look for connections or pathways to enhance your ability to learn.

Long-term memory is also enhanced by increasing the different ways in which you can absorb and express the information you are learning. You probably already know what this is about.

When you particularly like a course in school, you tend to discuss it; in talking about it, you reinforce what you learned, clarify your conceptual understanding, and increase the precision of your use of details. Although you may have done this unconsciously in the past, use it consciously now to enhance your learning. If you read difficult information in a textbook, can you express that information in a simpler way in a letter to your grandmother? Can you explain it to a friend over lunch?

Immediate review is also important for long-term memory. Research shows that unless you review what you have read or heard before you go to sleep at night, you will forget more than 90 percent of it twenty-four hours later. High school is structured to take advantage of this because most classes are held each day. But when you go to college, classes are held less frequently. To improve your retention, you need to review your class notes every night before bed, or tell a friend about your class at dinner. If you are preparing for the PCAT, the same principle applies. Unless you review what you did that day, you will not remember it. You will still know those topics that you understood and learned to like, but your study time for the PCAT will be wasted unless you build immediate review time into your schedule. The charts in Fig. 1.1 suggest you make lists of "Things To Do Today" and "Things Done Today." Prepare a journal for periodic review called "Things Learned" and review this journal with your study partner.

Finally, practice contributes to long-term memory. Your chemistry teacher knows much about chemistry and has a remarkable amount of information to discuss the subject without referring to notes or books. This is partly because your chemistry teacher works with chemistry every day both in lecture and the lab. If your teacher stopped teaching chemistry for a while, some information would fade over time. While preparing for the PCAT, work with various subject areas every day and apply them in solving complex problems.

1.1.12 Explore Active Learning of Scientific Concepts

Ideally, most of your learning will be long-term. As an example, learning the circulatory system is a long-term memory task. It requires you to understand what happens at each step as the blood enters and leaves various chambers in the heart. As you talk about it, explaining it to your study partner, you will be storing it in your long-term memory. Drawing a flow diagram (another mode of expression) as you explain it will also help. Go to a grocery store and purchase animal organs, such as heart and kidneys. Hold each organ under a water faucet in your kitchen or bathroom and fill it up with water. Feel and observe the shape, size, and texture of the organ and various parts of the organ by cutting it and observing water flow through each organ, thus making a model for blood or fluid circulation. This will help improve or strengthen your visual skills, which is an aid to long-term memory.

When you visit a drugstore and look at the labels of prescription and non prescription drugs, try to remember chemical names, symbols, and units of measurement for chemical compounds. This will give you real-life exposure to chemicals and a basic preparation in stoichiometry. For example, what are the ingredients in aspirin? Can you draw the molecules of the ingredients? *Repetition and conceptual drawing are also keys to long-term learning.* They will help you retain the details of a topic and understand related concepts. Include drawings and observations to improve your long-term memory of biology concepts in your classwork and review materials. Organic chemistry may be difficult, but buying plastic model molecules and observing changes in structure by changing atoms or groups is a useful tool. This way, you can actually *observe* and *remember* what kinds of mistakes you make in organic chemistry. Three-dimensional perception can also be improved with these organic molecular structures. Organic chemistry concepts can then become a part of your long-term memory.

1.2 PROBLEM SOLVING SKILLS FOR PCAT PREPARATION

The reasoning approaches described below will help you to review scientific topics from different and more challenging directions. Go through the exercises and examples to identify various patterns in reasoning. These reasoning patterns will help you become a better problem solver.

DIAGRAMMING SKILLS

Venn or association diagrams help you to improve your concentration and to focus on science concepts. They help you think about the difference between *some* and *all*, and about *what is not* as well as *what is*. In a way, a Venn diagram is a visual representation of an outline. Circles, ovals, or squares may be used to construct Venn diagrams.

Example: The statement "All roses are red" can be diagrammed as follows:

– things that are red
– roses (all red)
– things that are red but are not roses

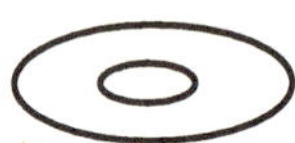

In a Venn or association diagram, a circle entirely contained within another circle means that all the members of the inner group belong in the outer group as well. In the above diagram representing "All roses are red," the inner circle denotes *roses* (and all of them are red) and the outer circle denotes *things that are red.* (Note: Look only at the **given relationship** in the statement; for the purpose of this diagram it does not matter that in real life not all roses are red.)

Example: The statement "*Some* roses are red" can be diagrammed as follows:

– roses
– red things

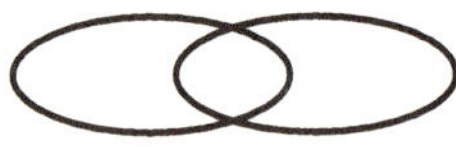

If you look at the intersecting lines of the ovals above, you can see the relationship between red things and roses, only some of which are red. But if you look at the spaces rather than the lines, you see the relationships between three categories:

– roses that are not red (the space on the left)
– *some* roses that are red (the space in the middle)
– red things that are not roses (the space on the right)

Example: The statement "*No* roses are red" can also be diagrammed as follows:

– roses (none of which are red)
– red things (which include no roses)

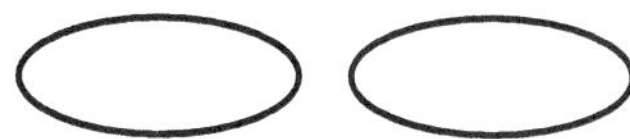

Exercise 1: Make a Venn diagram to illustrate the relationship between the following:

- – mothers
- – daughters
- – grandmothers
- – aunts

(This is not an easy relationship to diagram. As a hint, start with mothers and daughters only, and remember that any circle that is contained within another circle means that *all* its members belong to both groups. When you have that relationship represented by Venn diagrams, add a circle for grandmother. Then add aunts.)

When you have completed your drawing, turn to the solution in section 1.3 and compare your drawing with the one shown.

What has this to do with PCAT preparation? Consider the following narrative reprinted from Betz Publishing Company's book, *A Complete Preparation for the MCAT.*

SAMPLE READING COMPREHENSION PASSAGE

CARBOHYDRATES

"Carbohydrates have the general formula $C_n(H_2O)_m$ where n and m are whole numbers. Monosaccharides are the basic units of carbohydrates. They are classified by the number of carbons they contain, i.e., hexoses (C_6), pentoses (C_5), etc. Hexoses and pentoses exist in predominantly ring forms called pyranoses (six membered rings) or furanoses (five membered rings) in equilibrium with the open-chain forms. Ring forms are hemiacetals; open-chain forms are polyhydroxyl aldehydes. In the ring forms, a (alpha) or b (beta) anomers are possible. The pyranoses exist in the stable chair conformation with most, if not all, of the hydroxyls in equatorial positions. When two monosaccharides differ by the configuration of one hydroxyl group, they are called epimers. If n is the number of asymmetric carbons, then 2^n is the number of optical isomers (based on open chain).

Hexoses usually have n = 4 and pentoses usually have n = 3. Sugars are given a relative configuration on the basis of the orientation of the next to last carbon's hydroxyl group as compared to D-glyceraldehyde. Most naturally occurring sugars have the D configuration. A ketose is a carbohydrate with a ketone group; an aldose has an aldehyde group.

Monosaccharides bond together to form disaccharides. Thc ncw bond is callcd a glycosidic bond and is between the hemiacetal carbon and an hydroxyl group of the other sugar; water is released when the bond is formed. Hydrolysis (breaking) of the bond requires water. The glycosidic bond is an acetal grouping. Sucrose (common sugar) is made of glucose and fructose. Lactose (milk sugar) is made of galactose and glucose. Maltose (a-1,4 bond made of two glucose units and is an hydrolysis product of starch or glycogen. Cellobiose (b-1,4 bond) is also made of two glucoses, and it is the breakdown product of the cellulose.

Polysaccharides are many monosaccharides joined by glycosidic bonds; they may be branched also. Starch (plant energy storage), glycogen (animal short-term energy storage), and cellulose (plant structural component) are all made from glucose. Cellulose has b-1,4 bonds not found in the other two. Starch and glycogen both have a-1,4 bonds but differ in the frequency and position of branch points (a-1,6 bond).

Insulin is a polymer of fructose."

Exercise 2: Using the passage above, draw an association diagram using the following words : carbohydrates, monosaccharides, disaccharides, starch, glucose, polysaccharides, fructose, sucrose, lactose, maltose, cellobiose, glycogen, and cellulose.

Your association diagram:

When finished turn to section 1.3 and check to see if your association diagram reflects the same relationships as the one shown.

Exercise 3: More practice diagrams. The more you work these problems the more proficient you will become. In working them, first decide what information belongs in the diagram to help you remember the concept, then be as careful and precise as possible. Check especially what each *space* represents.

(a) Draw a Venn diagram illustrating the characteristics of eukaryotic cells and prokaryotic cells.
(b) Draw Venn diagrams that illustrate the relationship between isomers, stereoisomers, and enantiomers.
(c) Draw Venn diagrams to illustrate the relationship between diasteromers and meso compounds.

Remember, problem areas present opportunities for learning. Use your textbook or other resource to clarify any word or term that is difficult for you.

REASONING SKILLS

A conscious awareness of reasoning skills can improve your understanding of the material you study and result in improved test performance. As you read the section that follows, think about what you are reading. Continue to refer to it during your review, consciously applying the different forms of reasoning described.

1. Analytical Reasoning

Analysis involves breaking something down into its component parts. This is as true of chemical analysis as it is of textual analysis. Taking notes in class is one way to use analytical reasoning in your academic life. A good note taker is able to select out the main points (the primary information) and the supporting details, and, at the same time, indicate by means of an outline the relationship between the two. Underlining is also a tool for analyzing text. The good student selectively underlines key words. At the same time, he or she makes notes in the margin or uses numbers to indicate the relationship of one piece of information to another and especially how both relate to the whole. Analysis identifies significant terms (often nouns) or pieces of information, but the work is incomplete unless the relationship of the part to the whole also is recognized—and this is where you use reasoning.

If analysis involves identifying key nouns as indicators of primary and secondary information, reasoning often requires a focus on words that the careless or hurried reader can overlook. These are qualifying words such as *always, some, for example, most likely, probably, however, consequently, as a result of, or* (as distinguished from *and*), etc. These words are the traffic lights and road signs for reading. As you work practice test items, circle these qualifying words and think about what they are telling you—how to proceed, what to look for, which of your stored information is relevant, which is irrelevant, etc.

To strengthen your analytical skills, we recommend Whimbey and Lochhead's *Problem Solving and Comprehension*, which may be ordered from Betz Publishing Company.

2. Synthetic Reasoning

Learning is incomplete unless analysis is followed by synthesis. Can you summarize the main points read in a textbook? Can you write in complete sentences the notes you wrote in class? Can you explain to a classmate what was covered in class? Can you clearly explain a concept such as entropy, to someone in your family who may not understand it? All these things require you to synthesize what you've learned. Synthesis is thus the test or proof of your learning. In addition, you are expected to synthesize facts from various subjects to construct new possibilities, e.g., the way that human physiology may be seen in light of what you have learned in physics, chemistry, biology, math, reading, visualization, and common sense. In memorizing concepts, try to link the key words together. Thus, the words synapse, axon, neuron, dendrite, effector organ, and neurotransmitter belong *together* and should be associated in memory to provide an interrelated web of information. For practice, make a list of words to memorize the pancreatic duct. Then check the accuracy of your list in your biology book.

3. Associative/Analogical Reasoning

Associative reasoning is also a tool recommended for improving memory by remembering similar or analogical situations. For example, it is easier to remember a difficult list if you associate the items on the list with something you know very well, such as the rooms in your house. Another example is to associate the action of driving a car with Boyle's law. In Boyle's law, pressure is inversely proportional to volume. When you push on the accelerator, you are decreasing the volume and increasing the pressure in the piston. Conversely, when you let up on the accelerator, the volume in the piston increases and the pressure decreases. Find other examples for Boyle's law.

Analogical reasoning uses associations in a particular way. To better understand a concept, an unknown is compared to something known. You can use associative reasoning to transfer concepts from one subject to another, as in learning biology principles within a chemistry framework. For example, does the movement of blood inside veins and arteries relate to the concept of chemical structure of hemoglobin in organic chemistry? Explain. Can you make an analogy between biological cells and chemical cells? Explain.

Understanding by analogy is often a creative tool used by scientists and developed through years of practice. It is not by accident that the discovery of the structure of DNA was presented in a dream as a visual analogy of two snakes coiled around each other.

4. **Comparative Reasoning**

Associative reasoning leads naturally to comparison/contrast. We tend to compare things that are similar in some ways and dissimilar in others. That is, no one bothers to compare an orange and a truck. But textbooks do present comparisons and contrasts between smooth muscles and skeletal muscles, or between afferent and efferent nerves. When reading how two things are different, remember that they are being contrasted because they also have similarities. To memorize comparison/contrast information, you also need to organize it in a way that will enable you to separate in your mind the things being compared. It is easy to confuse the functions of the liver with those of the spleen, for example, as every test maker knows.

Comparison/contrast test items are often very difficult to answer correctly, partly because students tend to read textbooks passively without doing the active work that would enable them to anticipate comparison/contrast questions. Avoid this by constructing a comparison/contrast chart or table whenever a textbook compares and contrasts. For example, look at the table of similarities and differences between liquids, solids, and gases; or eukaryotic and prokaryotic cells.

For the following comparison/contrast exercises, think up aspects that are or are not shared and make a yes/no list for each. Then check your list against information in Betz Publishing Company's book, *A Complete Preparation for the MCAT*, or other reference or textbooks.

(a) Electrolytic, galvanic, and concentration cells
(b) Heterozygous and homozygous genes
(c) Period and group for the atomic table
(d) Entropy and enthalpy

5. **Intuitive Reasoning**

Creative use of the imagination to solve problems is a subject rarely mentioned in the classroom because we know neither how to teach it nor how to test it. Basically, creative imagination makes an intuitive leap (usually unasked for and instantaneous) that was not logically apparent. Thus, a doctor might have a preliminary diagnosis that is then systematically and carefully checked with further questions, examination, tests, etc. The scientist who discovered the way stars age did so by making an intuitive connection between stars and aging humans.

If you would like to develop your creativity further, you might work some of the exercises in Edwards' *Drawing On the Right Side of the Brain*. Meanwhile, Vitale's *Unicorns are Real: A Right-Brained Approach to Learning* also includes information about individual learning styles.

6. Visual Reasoning

There is experimental evidence that very young infants can reason visually—well before they have acquired language. Although the ability to reason visually is the key to solving many science problems, some students find they have neglected their visual reasoning skills.

Picture a first-floor apartment and a sixth-floor apartment in the same building. Which apartment is likely to have better water pressure in the shower? Why? Which apartment is likely to have the better bathtub drainage? Why? How could you improve water pressure or drainage?

Now try some more exercises:

(a) Visualize the Kreb's Cycle. Can you explain in one sentence what causes the cycle to work?
(b) Draw the molecules of epimers and anomers to help you conceptualize them in your mind.

As you work other science problems, notice how many require visual reasoning skills. Visual reasoning skills are directly tied to your perceptual abilities. Perceptual ability can be developed both directly and indirectly. Direct observation of mechanisms or processes makes you reinforce pictures in your memory. Drawing small scale, freehand sketches or views of large scale objects (e.g., bioreactors, houses, trains, and trailers) makes you develop visual insight and also learn to simplify details. Indirect observation is more or less imagining mechanisms, molecules, or systems, such as drawing a sketch to illustrate words or concepts such as antigen-antibody interactions, pressure, molecular arrangement of chemicals in a cup of coffee, path of a bolus of food through the digestive system, bee's extraction of nectar from a flower, etc. Direct and indirect observation leads to improved perception.

7. Logical Reasoning

Because it is concerned with proof, logical reasoning is a way of thinking that is associated with the development of science and scientific methods. Logical reasoning provides a systematic means of testing or proving a hypothesis or conclusion. Conclusions come in three degrees of certainty: hypothesis, conclusion suggested, and conclusion confirmed. Conclusions can be valid or invalid.

There are many books available that provide the formal rules of logic and exercises to practice them. We recommend that you consult them to improve your logical reasoning ability. A recommended text is S. Morris Engel's *With Good Reason: An Introduction to Informal Fallacies.*

8. Quantitative Reasoning

An improvement in quantitative reasoning depends primarily on the ability to estimate a reasonable answer before calculating it. Unfortunately, much skill in this area has been lost as a result of using calculators. (Calculators are not allowed while taking the PCAT, so begin now to practice estimating reasonable answers.)

Quantitative reasoning is involved when you quickly and precisely carry out mathematical operations in your head. For example, what is 41 times 41? Quantitative reasoning is also used to translate words to numbers and numbers to words. For example, looking only at a graph or chart in a newspaper, can you tell what the accompanying story is about? Conversely, can you read the article and picture the graph or chart?

9. Proportional Reasoning

Proportional reasoning may be used to solve problems in biology and chemistry, such as flow of blood in arteries or veins of varying diameters, acid-base concentrations, etc. Proportional reasoning is also used to measure changes in one variable relative to another, as in problems applying Boyle's law. Both flow and concentration problems often require you to use proportional reasoning. In the PCAT quantitative ability section, questions about population tables or charts can also require proportional reasoning.

Proportional reasoning is often aided by visualization or the ability to picture the elements of a problem (see Visual Reasoning, item 6 above). Schematic drawings in the margin sometimes are helpful.

Although you are now ready to go on to chapter 2, refer to this study skills chapter from time to time to reinforce your good study habits and determine which of these study skills is most useful to you.

1.3 SOLUTIONS

Exercise 1: In the left-hand drawing, the outer circle is "daughters" because all mothers are daughters, but daughters are not necessarily all mothers. The space between the two circles thus becomes "daughters who are not mothers."

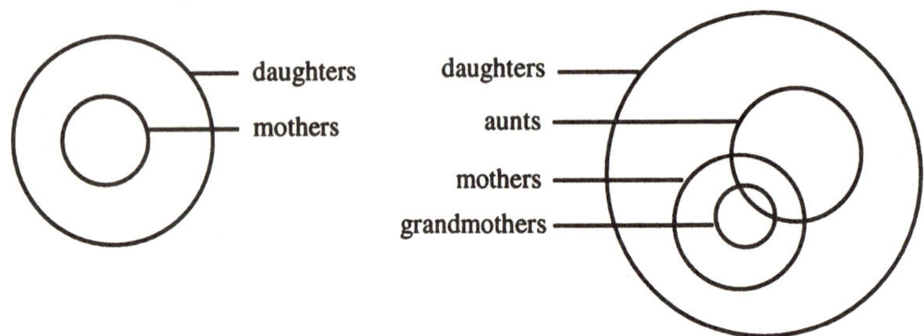

Exercise 2:

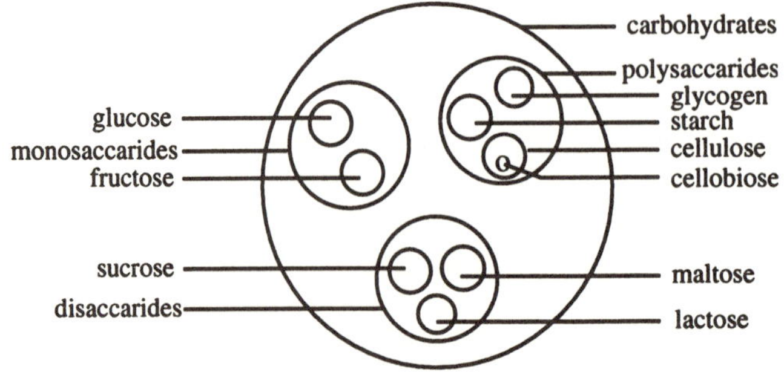

1.4 REFERENCES

Atkinson, Rhonda H., and Debbie G. Longman. *Reading Enhancement and Development* (St. Paul, Minn.: West Publishing, 1992).

Harris, Albert J., and Edward R. Sipay. *How to Increase Reading Ability* (White Plains, N.Y.: Longman, 1985).

Miller, L. L. *Increasing Reading Efficiency* (Fort Worth, Tex.: Holt Rinehart & Winston, 1984).

Psychological Corporation, The. *The Pharmacy College Admission Test* (candidate information booklet), latest ed. (San Antonio, Tex.)

Quinn, Shirley, and Susan Irvings. *Active Reading in the Arts and Sciences*, 2nd ed. (Boston: Allyn and Bacon, 1991).

Whimbey, Arthur, and Jack Lochhead. *Problem Solving and Comprehension* (Hillsdale, N.J.: Lawrence Erlbaum Assoc., 1991).

Chapter 2

Developing Verbal Ability

2.0 INTRODUCTION

2.1 WHAT VERBAL ABILITY MEASURES

It is generally acknowledged that good verbal skills are important for success in the field of pharmacy. Good communication depends in large part on your ability to express yourself clearly and precisely, and to understand others precisely. Such precision depends on your vocabulary. Antonym, synonym, and analogy questions measure your vocabulary and your ability to analyze. The kinds of analyses required for verbal ability questions include matching similar and opposite concepts, forming conclusions about relationships, and categorizing ideas, structures, and concepts.

2.1.1 Types of Questions Encountered

- ***Antonyms*** are words opposite, or nearly opposite, in meaning. Antonym questions require you to choose the one word, from a list of four choices, which means the opposite of the given, capitalized word.

- ***Synonyms*** are words that have the same, or nearly the same, meaning. You will need to know precise definitions and shades of meaning. From a list of four possible answers, synonym questions require you to choose the one word that means most nearly the same thing as the given, capitalized word.

- ***Analogies*** are sets of word pairs that describe a similar, or analogous, relationship. You will be asked to choose, from a list of four, the one word that best completes the second pair of the analogy. The answer you choose to complete the question pair must represent the relationship most similar to that of the given pair.

2.1.2 Time Allotment

You have a limited amount of time to answer each question. Analogy questions generally take longer to solve than antonym or synonym questions. In addition to a working knowledge of the dictionary definitions of the words encountered, in analogy questions you are also required to extrapolate a relationship between these words. Since each question will score the same value, you should spend less time on the relatively easy questions, thereby saving time for the more difficult ones. Use your test booklet to mark the "short-cuts" that eliminate potential answers quickly for you (e.g., cross out incorrect choices or divide an unfamiliar word into its prefix, suffix and root).

Master the following strategies to solve analogies, antonyms or synonyms well in advance of your exam. This will enable you to work on increasing your speed. Vocabulary building works best in frequent small increments, perhaps ten words at a time. It is better to concentrate on expanding your working knowledge of the multiple meanings of words you already than to memorize lists of unknown words.

2.2 ANTONYMS

2.2.1 Definition

Antonyms are words **opposite in meaning** from each other (*high* is the antonym of *low, empty* is the antonym of *full*). Antonym questions consist of a given word (capitalized), followed by four answer choices. Look carefully at each word, paying attention to spelling, roots, prefixes, suffixes, and parts of speech.

2.2.2 Steps for Solving Antonyms

Step 1. Look for the ***opposite word*** *to answer antonym questions.*

Since many words do not have an exact opposite, look for the word **most nearly opposite** in meaning.

Step 2. Look for the word that fits as the ***best answer*** *to the given word.*

Several choices may seem to be answer words, but only one will be the best right answer.

Step 3. Place the capitalized word ***in context.***

Think of a sentence or phrase in which you might use the word. Even if you are not sure of its exact definition, you will have a sense of its meaning if you can use the word in a sentence. If you cannot think of a sentence immediately, keep going. There are other steps to help you recognize the given word.

Step 4. Search for ***more than one meaning,*** *especially in verbs and nouns.*

Keep in mind that many words have more than one meaning, as you write out context phrases and consider as many variations as possible. Occasionally, a word can even have opposite meanings, depending on context. *Sanguine*, for example, can mean either murderous or optimistic. Use a good thesaurus (not a dictionary) to find words with similar meaning (synonyms).

Step 5. Look for ***shades of meaning.***

Many words in the English language differ only slightly from each other because English is such a rich language. Context phrases can help you sort out the best uses of the given word.

Step 6. Create your own antonym ***before looking*** *at the choices provided.*

You can then look for the answer word most similar in meaning to your own antonym. If none of the answers provided matches the antonym you selected, think of alternate meanings and contexts suggested by the answer list; then return to step 3 above and compose new phrases.

Step 7. Know the ***prefix, root, and suffix*** *of the given word.*

Read each answer choice carefully, considering the spelling and part of speech. Many words are confusing (*ingenuous* and *ingenious*, for example), and one letter makes a big difference.

2.2.3 Tips for Solving Antonyms

- **Read all choices** carefully. Note spelling, part of speech, and word components (prefix, root, and suffix).

- Eliminate words with **no clear opposite** (e.g., pregnant, warmth, roadway).

- Identify the **synonym** of the given word. Almost always, one of the answer choices is a synonym. Use it to help you clarify the meaning and shades of meaning of the given word.

2.2.4 When You Don't Know the Given Word or an Answer Choice

- **"Sound it out"**. Circle the prefix, root, and suffix. Use the clues you gain from your knowledge of those elements to make a good guess. If the prefix is negative (mal-, dis-, non-), look for a positive (bene-, eu-, -ful) element in the answer list.

- If you can identify the word's elements, but cannot remember what they mean, think of **a word you know with the same prefix or root** as the given word.

- Don't be misled by the apparent **difficulty or easiness** of a question. Sometimes a complicated given word has an easy word for an antonym, and sometimes simple words are confusing. Remember to read carefully and consider alternate meanings.

Example: Solve an antonym question when the given word and several choices are unknown.

IRREFRAGABILITY

A. expulsion
B. equivocality
C. incontestability
D. fragrant

"Sound out" the word: ir - re - frag - abil - ity (break it into components)

Although you may not know this word, you can begin to decode it. The suffixes indicate that it is a noun, having to do with a quality or a characteristic. The prefix ir- is negative. (If you are unsure about that, think of other words with the ir- prefix whose meaning you do know: irresponsible, irregular, irresistible.) The prefix re- means again. The root, frag-, appears in such words as fragment, meaning broken part. You can now approximate the meaning: "not-again-break-able-ness," or something like permanence, reliability, or decisiveness. Its opposite might be uncertainty or vagueness. "The irrefragability of Alice's research conclusions," or "the irrefragability of the evidence," are context phrases that may come to mind.

If a first reading of the answer list does not yield a definite choice, eliminate any that do not have real opposites, like fragrant. (Fragrant may also be dismissed because, while it looks like it contains the root frag-, it has nothing to do with the meanings you have deduced from the components.) Incontestability appears to be a synonym of the meaning derived from the given word's components and can therefore be eliminated. It also has a negative prefix, in-, and is therefore unlikely to be the antonym of a word with a negative prefix. Of the remaining two choices, expulsion can be eliminated (even if you don't know what it means) because it has a negative prefix, ex-, and because it is not a noun having to do with a quality, as demanded by the suffixes of irrefragability. The only remaining choice is equivocality, meaning vagueness, imprecision, or uncertainty. You may, of course, have deduced its meaning from equi- (same) and vocal- (voice), if you did not already know it.

You can see how, by following the suggested steps and tips, it is possible to solve the puzzles that antonym questions can pose even when you are presented with unknown words.

It is, of course, faster and easier when you know all the words. It is strongly recommended that you work on improving your vocabulary skills, no matter how little time you may have between now and the test date.

2.3 SYNONYMS

2.3.1 Definition

Synonyms are words that have **similar meanings**. You will be asked to find the word or phrase that is most nearly similar in meaning to the word in capital letters. Like the antonym question, synonym questions are primarily a measure of your vocabulary. The broader the scope of your word knowledge, the better your chance of answering the questions correctly. Memorizing lists of words without understanding their meanings (in many cases, multiple meanings) will not ensure a higher score on your test. Though you may not be familiar with all of the meanings of the words you will encounter, you will recognize most of the words. Many of the synonyms will require you to distinguish fine shades of meaning. Despite this, synonyms will generally be easier to decipher than will antonyms because many words do not have exact opposites. Some tips and rules for solving synonym questions follow.

2.3.2 Steps for Solving Synonyms

In general, the steps for solving synonym questions are the same as those used for antonyms. You are to select the word or phrase that is the closest, *most similar* to the given phrase. Remember, your answer must be the best available choice. Some questions may seem to have several possible answers, but there is only one whose meaning *most closely matches* the given word. (Flaming, warm, tepid, and hot are all related terms, but only one is similar to cozy.)

2.3.3 Tips for Solving Synonyms

Follow the tips and suggestions outlined in the antonym section when you are looking for clues to solving synonym questions. Read all choices carefully, eliminating the ones whose meanings are clearly opposite from the capitalized word (e.g., positive versus negative meaning). Don't be misled by easy words; do try to visualize the word. Almost always one of the choices is an *antonym* of the given word. Use this word to help you clarify the meaning, and shades of meaning, of the given word.

2.3.4 When You Don't Know the Given Word or an Answer Choice

Again, use the techniques you developed for solving unknown words in antonym questions: sound out the word, associate the word with one containing a similar prefix or suffix, look at the root word and visualize other words that use this same root.

2.4 ANALOGIES

2.4.1 Definition

Analogies are sets of word pairs that describe a similar, or analogous, relationship. Analogy questions measure your ability to visualize a relationship between a pair of words, to distinguish the correct meaning of each word in this context, and to recognize a similar or parallel relationship.

2.4.2 Types of Analogies

Most analogies fall into one of two word types:

NOUN : NOUN pairs such as LEAF : TREE or ICE : RAIN, or

NOUN : ADJECTIVE pairs such as SANDPAPER : ROUGH or OVEN : HOT.

Occasionally verbs will also be included in analogies such as COW : MOO or BIRD : MOLT, and some are ADJECTIVE : ADJECTIVE pairs such as HAPPY : SAD or HAIRY: BALD.

2.4.3 Common Relationships Used in Analogies

Analogies can be classified into certain common relationship types. Learning to recognize these basic relationships will help you place the word pairings found in analogies into a more manageable form. These are the most common relationships found in analogies and are provided as guidelines for analogical thinking. Other types of relationships are possible, and sometimes categories can overlap. Practice using and recognizing the following relationship pairings until you are comfortable with each category.

1. CHARACTERISTIC

   Relationships in which one of the words in the pair describes a characteristic of the other. For example:

   diamond : hard (A diamond can be described as being hard.)
   owl : wise (An owl is said to be wise. Note: the characteristic can be fictional.)
   sharp : knife (A knife may be described as being sharp. Note: the order of the pair can be reversed.)

2. TYPE OR KIND

   Relationships in which one term is a type of the other. For example:

   salmon : fish (A salmon is a type of fish.)
   maze : puzzle (A maze is a kind of puzzle.)
   shell : home (A shell is a type of home or shelter. Note: some words can be used as either nouns or verbs. Compare the words in the answer selections to determine usage.)

3. DEGREE

Relationship in which one word in the pair shows a decrease or increase in action, quality, etc. For example:

drizzle : downpour	(A drizzle is a light shower, while a downpour is a heavy rain.)
ecstatic : content	(Ecstatic means overjoyed, while content with its accent on the last syllable denotes a milder state of pleasure.)
nibble : devour	(To nibble is to eat sparingly, while to devour is to consume ravenously.)

4. PART TO WHOLE

Relationship in which one word in the pair is a part or component of the other term. For example:

sentence : paragraph	(A sentence is a part of a paragraph.)
comb : teeth	(Teeth are part of a comb. Note: the order of the words may be reversed in your statement of the relationship.)
purple : blue	(The color blue is a component of the color purple. Note: do not be misled by associations based on similarity. Some relationships require more analysis.)

5. PURPOSE OR FUNCTION

Relationship in which one word in the pair is a function of, or has a use for, the other word. For example:

garage : car	(A garage is a place to store a car.)
pen : write	(A pen is used to write.)
towel : dry	(A towel is used to dry things.)

6. SEQUENCE

A relationship based on order of events, state of being, etc. For example:

acorn : oak	(An acorn is the beginning state of an oak tree. Note: SEQUENCE relationships can easily be confused with TYPE OR KIND relationships. Read all answer choices to determine the relationship.)
dawn : dusk	(Dawn marks the beginning of the day, while dusk comes at the end.)
crawl : walk	(A baby learns to crawl before it learns to walk.)

7. CAUSE AND EFFECT

Relationship in which one term gives either the cause or the effect of the other. For example:

crime : punishment	(A crime may lead to punishment.)
height : dizziness	(Height can cause dizziness.)
scar : cut	(A scar is caused by a cut.)

8. TOOL OR INSTRUMENT

Relationship in which one word functions as a tool for another word. For example:

scalpel : surgeon (A scalpel is a tool for a surgeon.)
voice : ventriloquist (A ventriloquist uses her voice to perform.)
score : musician (A score is a tool for a musician.)

9. ANTONYMS

Relationship in which one word is the opposite, or nearly the opposite, of the other in the pair. For example:

laugh : cry (The state of emotion that brings forth laughter is generally opposite to the one that causes crying.)
high : low (High is the opposite of low.)
prefix : suffix (Prefixes and suffixes are used at opposite ends of a word.)

10. SYNONYMS

Relationships in which the two words of the pair have similar, or nearly the same, meaning. For example:

stray : wander (To stray means to wander.)
abundant : plentiful (Something that is abundant is in large supply, which means the same as plentiful.)
forgery : counterfeit (Both forgery and counterfeit describe something that is not genuine.)

11. ASSOCIATION

Relationship in which one word describes something associated with the other. For example:

red : anger (The color red is sometimes associated with the emotion of anger.)
shamrock : luck (A shamrock is associated with good luck.)
robin : spring (The arrival of robins is associated with the arrival of spring. Note: again, word order may be reversed in the pair.)

12. NONSEMANTIC

Relationship in which one word in the pair is related to the other word in the pair by something other than its meaning: sound, spelling, grammar, form, etc. For example:

see : sea (These words are homophones, which are pronounced alike despite different meanings.)
eat : tea (Eat and tea are anagrams; their letters are rearranged.)
sit : sat (Sit is prcscnt tcnsc, whilc sat is past tcnsc.)

2.4.4 Steps for Solving Analogies

Step 1. In a sentence, state the relationship between the words in the capitalized pair.

To solve an analogy question, state the relationship of the capitalized pair of words in a simple sentence. Your ability to recognize the proper relationship depends upon your ability to define each word. Consider a variant meaning or context of the word if you cannot construct a simple sentence illustrating the relationship of this pair.

For example:

PHRASE : SENTENCE :: PARAGRAPH :
A. essay
B. structure
C. theme
D. grammar

Look at the relationship between the capitalized pair of words, and try to describe it in a short sentence. Try to visualize how the first word phrase interacts with the second word sentence. What does a phrase do in or to a sentence? Which of the common relationship forms does this question seem to use? Is a phrase a degree, type, cause and effect, tool, or part-to-whole of a sentence?

"*A phrase is part of a sentence.*" This states the PART TO WHOLE nature of the relationship of these words.

Look at the third capitalized word, then substitute it and each of the answer choices in turn in your sentence. Which of the answer choices could the word paragraph be part of?

A. A paragraph is part of an essay? Yes, an essay is a short literary composition.
B. A paragraph is part of a structure? No, a structure is the configuration of a composition of elements.
C. A paragraph is part of a theme? No, a theme is a topic of discourse or discussion.
D. A paragraph is part of a grammar? No, grammar is the system of language rules.

Only choice A, essay, correctly fits the relationship. If you eliminated all the answers, then you need to formulate a more specific relationship between the capitalized word pair and try again to state the relationship in a new sentence.

Step 2. Check the order of relationship between the capitalized word pair.

It is essential that you use the same order of relationship found in the capitalized word pair when you are looking for the answer choice to pair with the third capitalized word. PART TO WHOLE relationships are not the same as WHOLE TO PART relationships. CAUSE AND EFFECT relationships are not the same as EFFECT AND CAUSE relationships. Such mistakes occur especially when analogy questions are read hurriedly.

For example:

MONTH : YEAR :: MINUTE :
A. second
B. hour
C. season
D. time

This is a SEQUENCE/TIME analogy. *"A month is shorter span of time than a year."* In choice A, a second is a shorter span of time than a minute, but the direction of the relationship stated in the capitalized word pair is now reversed, so this answer is not correct. In choice B, an hour is a longer length of time than to a minute, so this is the correct answer. Choice C season and D time are associated, but do not measure time and can thus be eliminated.

Step 3. Decode when you do not know all the words.

The strategy for decoding is to eliminate clearly incorrect choices and to decipher meanings that will allow you to analyze and arrive at the correct relationship pair.

Since the parts of speech in the correct pair must match those in the given pair, you may be able to eliminate one or more answer choices. Look carefully at each word you do not know, and determine as much as possible by separating it into its elements (prefix, root, and suffix). Think of contexts suggested by each answer choice; see if that helps you to understand the analogy. If you feel you have enough information, you may choose to guess. If you are spending too much time, then skip the question and return only if you have time later.

For example:

ROCK : IMMUTABLE :: WATER :
A. stagnant
B. turbulent
C. rapid
D. contaminate

Suppose you do not know the word immutable. You can immediately eliminate contaminate because it is the wrong part of speech. The other words are all adverbs and therefore may be correct. You will only be able to describe the relationship of the given pair if you can decode the meaning of the second term. Break it into components: im - mut - able. The prefix im- usually means not, without, or opposing. The suffix -able means something that can be done. The root, mut-, is encountered in other words you may know: mutant and commute, among others. If you dissect those words as well, you can easily arrive at the meaning of mut-, which is to change or move. You can now construct a relationship sentence: "*Rocks are unchangeable or immutable.*" This is a CHARACTERISTIC relationship.

Because you must also know the meanings of all the answer choices, you could apply the same process to choice B turbulent to arrive at the correct answer. Note: this example also illustrates that you need to know antonyms and synonyms in order to solve analogies. When confronted with antonyms and synonyms, keep in mind that the best available answer may not be as obvious as hot/cold or gentle/kind.

Step 4. Do not confuse similar relationships.

For example:

MILK : YOGURT :: GRAPES :
A. raisins
B. fruit
C. champagne
D. fermentation

This is a CAUSE AND EFFECT analogy. "*Yogurt is the effect of fermentation on milk.*" The correct answer is choice C champagne. "*Champagne is the effect of fermentation on grapes.*" In choice A, raisins are also the product of grapes, but this is a different CAUSE AND EFFECT relationship; raisins are the effect of dehydration on grapes. Choice B fruit could work only if this analogy represented a TYPE OR KIND question. Choice D fermentation names the process that creates yogurt from milk, but does not form a relationship with the third word grapes.

Step 5. Be aware of multiple meanings.

BEAR : REJECT :: SHOULDER:
A. carry
B. shun
C. border
D. bone

In this example each of the words have multiple meanings that are quite varied in definition. For example, the word bear used as a verb could mean to support, to produce, to endure, to display, to press or to turn. From reading the complete analogy one can deduce that here the word bear is defined as a verb meaning to support or maintain. Reject is defined as a verb meaning to refuse. So the analogy relationship between the capitalized word pair can be expressed as an ANTONYM: "*To bear is the opposite of to reject.*" Likewise, the word shoulder is defined as a verb meaning to assume or undertake. So the antonym of shoulder would be choice B shun.

Step 6. Read all choices carefully.

Even if you think you have identified the correct answer, examine all the answer words carefully to ensure that you are not overlooking a better choice. Test each answer in the relationship sentence you construct to avoid careless mistakes.

For example:

PEANUT : SHELL :: APPLE :
A. core
B. pare
C. crop
D. plant

Unless you examine each answer carefully you might miss the correct relationship, which is:

You *shell a peanut* to remove its skin, you *pare an apple* to remove its skin. Choice A core means to remove the central part; choice B pare means to cut away skin; choice C crop can be defined as a verb meaning to reap; choice D plant can mean to put into the ground to grow.

2.5 BASIC WORD ELEMENTS

The only test insurance you can obtain is thorough mastery of the English language. If you know the most commonly used prefixes and suffixes, you can combine them with your knowledge of root words to decipher the meaning of many unfamiliar words. You will also find that roots are easier to identify and interpret if you know prefixes and suffixes well.

Study the lists in section 2.5.1.1. Make up your own examples and prepare flash cards. Add to the lists as you find other prefixes, suffixes and roots you need to learn or review. Try to visualize the meaning of the word and add your own personal symbol or sketch to make the word more memorable. Identify with a [+] or [-] whether the word has positive or negative connotations. This knowledge is especially helpful for solving antonym and synonym questions. Utilize mnemonic and memory aids such as rhymes, word associations and visual images. Personify adjectives by attributing their characteristics to familiar persons or objects to help you remember meanings.

2.5.1 Prefixes

A **prefix** is a word element added before the root to change or modify its meaning. Prefixes are abundant and are often combined with other prefixes (hyperinflation, disinclined, unrepresented, antidiscrimination, and superimpose, among others) to create the rich vocabulary of the English language. Many prefixes and suffixes come to English from other languages. Prefixes greatly enrich our language by denoting very specific shades of meaning and allowing us vivid representation of concepts. Knowing prefixes thoroughly is essential to performing well on all verbal portions of your test.

Prefixes pose some special challenges.

- Some have several, occasionally opposite, meanings (in- sometimes means not; as in invalid; in- can also mean very, as in infuriate; it can also mean in or on; furthermore, it changes its form to il-, im-, or ir-, depending on the root!)

- Prefixes that look identical can have different meanings, depending on their origin (a- in apart means away from; a- in amoral means without; a- in atop means on).

- Combined prefixes require you to decode each element and analyze their effects on each other.

Some resources list prefixes according to the language of origin, noting that Latin prefixes are often attached to Latin roots, Greek prefixes to Greek roots, and so on. Because there are so many exceptions, the list below is loosely organized according to function or general effect, rather than according to origin. The general meaning of each prefix is given with examples.

2.5.1.1 POSITIVE, ADDING, INTENSIFYING PREFIXES

ad, ac, af, ag, al, an, ap, ar, as, at	to, toward, very	admit, accrue, afford, allude, appear, assent, attuned
arch	chief	archbishop, architect
be	around, about, away, very	beset, beloved, bemused
bene	good, well	benefactor, benediction
com, co, col, con, cor	with, together, very	combine, cooperate, collude, convene, corrupt
en, em	in, within, among	enable, empathy
eu	good, well, beautiful	euphemism, eulogy
extra	beyond, outside	extrovert, extracurricular
hyper	excessive, over	hyperactive, hyperbole
in, il, im, ir	very (see negatives)	impress, illuminate, inform, irradiate
over	over, excessively	overestimate
per	thorough	permeate, pernicious
pro	for, before, favoring	progress, profuse, provide
super, supra	over, above	superimpose, supervise
sur	beyond, above, extra	surfeit, surtax, surtitle
syn, sym, syl, sys	together	synchronize, symbiosis, systematic
ultra	beyond, excessively	ultramodern, ultraviolet

2.5.1.2 NEGATIVE, DETRACTING, REMOVING PREFIXES

ad, abs, a	from, off, away	abduct, avert, abstain
an, a	without	anarchy, amoral
anti	against, opposite	antidote, antithesis
apo	from, away	apology
cata	down, away	catalysis, catastrophe
contra, contro, counter	against	contradict, contraceptive, countermand
de	down, away from	devalue, decrease
dis, di, dif	not, apart	discord, divest, diffuse
ex, e, ef	out, off, from	export, elude, efface
for	away, off, from	forego, forbid, forgive
hypo	under, beneath	hypnosis, hypodermic
in, ig, il, im, ir	not, opposing	incorrect, illegal, ignoble, immature, irrational
mal, male	bad, badly	malnutrition, malefactor
mis	wrong, poorly	misfire, misconstrue
non	not	nonsense
ob, oc, of, op	against	object, oppose, offend, occlude
se	apart, away	seclude
sub, suc, suf, sug	under	subsist, succumb, suffice, suggest
un	not	unfit

2.5.1.3 DIRECTION, POSITION, LOCATION, ORDER:

ambi	both	ambivalent, ambidextrous
amphi	around, both	amphitheater, amphibian
ana	back, through, against	anagram, anachronism

ante, anti, pre	before, previous	antecedent, anticipate, presuppose
circum, peri	around	circumvent, periphery
dia	through, across	diagnose, diameter
epi	on, over, outside	epicenter, epidermis
fore	before, previous	foreword
inter, intra	between, among	interject, intramural
meta	change of, over	metamorphosis, metaphysics
over	above, beyond	overcast, overnight
para	beside, beyond	paranormal, paramedic, paraphrase
per	through	perforate
peri	around, near	periscope, perimeter
post	after	postpone, postmortem
pre	before	precede
re	back, again	recede, regroup, respond
retro	back, backward	retrospective, retrograde, retroactive
trans	across, beyond, through	translate, transmit, translucent
sub	under	subcutaneous, subbasement
super	above	superscript

2.5.1.4 NUMBERS, FRACTIONS

demi, hemi, semi	half	demigod, demitasse, hemisphere, semiconscious, semicircle
poly, multi	many	polygon, polymorphous, multitude
mono, uni	one	monotheism, unity
bi, di	two, twice	bipolar, bisect, dimeter
tri	three	triumvirate, tricycle
quadr, tetra	four	quadruped, tetrahedron
quint, quinque, penta	five	quintuplets, pentagram
sex, hexa	six	sextet, hexagon
sept, hepta	seven	September, heptameter
oct, octa, octo	eight	octopus, octagon
nona, nonem, ennea	nine	November, ennead
dec, deca	ten	decimate, decalogue, deciliter
duodec, dodeca	twelve	duodecimo, dodecahedron
cent, hecto	hundred	century, hectograph
milli	thousand	millipede, millennium

2.5.2 Suffixes

A **suffix** is a part of a word that follows the root of the word. Suffixes indicate conditions, attitudes, objects of a verb, actions, and places. The part of speech is determined by a suffix (in a combination, the final suffix) of a word. Note: some suffixes can form more than one part of speech; check context when in doubt.

A basic list of suffixes, organized by function in determining a word's part of speech (rather than by etymology) is provided below. It is not exhaustive; you may wish to add others as you encounter them in reference works and general reading. Note: some suffixes can form more than one part of speech.

2.5.2.1 NOUN SUFFIXES (an act or quality of, a state or condition, one who, a result or product of, rank or status of.

age	state, place, process	lineage, patronage
al	pertaining to doing	denial
an, ian	belonging to, concerned with	human, magician
ance, ancy ence, ency, cy	act, state, condition	dalliance, truancy, emergence, fluency, accuracy
ant, ent	doing, showing, agency	servant, agent, pendant
ar	marked by, pertaining to	regular
ard, art	one doing	braggart, wizard
ary	belonging to, showing	adversary
ate	office or function	magistrate, delegate
ation	act or state of, result	education, maturation
cle, cule, let	little	icicle, molecule, platelet
cy	state	democracy
dom	state, rank, condition	kingdom,
er, or	doer, actor, maker	climber, advisor
ery	action, skill, state	surgery, robbery
ese	of, relating to, language	governmentese
ess, ette	feminine	actress, suffragette
et	diminutive	midget
hood	state, condition	womanhood, statehood
ic	caused by, showing	comic
ice	act, state, quality	novice
id	marked by, showing	putrid
ile, il	marked by, showing,	juvenile, civil
ine	marked by, dealing with	serpentine, marine
ion	action, state, result	commission, condition
ism	act, manner, state, belief	atheism, purism
ist	practitioner, doer, believer	anarchist, socialist
ite	native, citizen, or member	suburbanite, socialite
ition	action, state, result	abolition
ity, ty	state of being, quality	fluidity, honesty
ive	tending to, belonging	incentive
ment	result, means, action	commencement, adornment
mony	resulting state, condition	acrimony, matrimony
ness	quality, state	loneliness, meekness
oid	something like	anthropoid
ory	a place of, serving for	repository
ry	condition, practice	chivalry
ship	condition, office, skill	friendship, craftsmanship
sion, tion	act or state of	exclusion, fruition
t, th	act, state, quality	height, flight, warmth
tude	that which is, quality	plentitude, fortitude
ure	act, result, state, rank	overture, censure
y	result, action, quality	perjury, augury

2.5.2.2 VERB SUFFIXES (to make, do)

ate	become, form, make, treat	create, animate
en	become, cause to be	enliven, fasten
esce	grow, continue, become	effervesce, coalesce
fy	make, cause	beautify, solidify
ish	do, make, perform	furnish, embellish
ize	make, cause to be, treat with	familiarize, polarize

2.5.2.3 MODIFIERS: ADJECTIVES AND ADVERBS (like capable of being, pertaining to, resembling, belonging to, causing, excessively)

Adjective Suffixes

able, ible	able, fit, likely	doable, edible
acious, aceous	having the quality of	capacious, herbaceous
al	belonging to, characteristic	familial, practical
an	belonging to	human
ant	showing	jubilant
ar	pertaining to	lunar, solar
ary	belonging to, showing	fragmentary
en	made of, like	silken, golden
ent	doing, showing, agent	evident, fluent
escent	beginning, becoming	effervescent
ese	of a place, style, language	Portuguese
esque	like, in the style of	romanesque
fic	making, causing	beatific
ful	full of, marked by	doleful, grateful
ian	pertaining to	mammalian
ic	dealing with, showing	prolific
id	marked by, showing	acrid
ile, il	marked by, showing	fragile
ine	marked by, dealing with	sanguine
ish	rather, suggesting, like	impish, boyish
ist	practicing, characteristic of	feminist
ite	showing, marked by	favorite
ive	tending to, relating to	effective
less	lacking, without	helpless, guileless
ly	like	friendly
ory	pertaining to	compensatory
ose	marked by, given to	comatose
ous, ious	marked by, given to, full of	amorous, sagacious
some	showing, tending to	loathsome
ward	in the direction of	eastward
y	showing, suggesting	throaty

Adverb Suffixes

ly	in the manner of	quickly, dryly
ward	in the direction of	forward

Note that adverbial suffixes are often used in combination with others: artfully (ful + ly), comically (ic + al + ly).

2.5.3 Roots

A **root** is a core word element embellished with prefixes, suffixes, or both. Learn as many roots as you can. The more you know, the easier it will be to decode unfamiliar words. The following list of roots includes meanings and examples.

ag, act	to do	act, agent, inactive
cap, capt, cep, cip	to take	capture, anticipate, perception
cad, cas	to fall	cadence, casual
ced, cess	to yield, to go	proceed, accession
cid, cis	to cut, kill	incisive, homicide
cred, credit	to believe	discredit, credible
curr, curs	to run	cursory, incursion
da, don	to give	data, mandate
dic, dict	to say	indictment, prediction
duc, duct	to lead	abduct, induction
fac, fic, fec, fect	to make or do	infect, factory, fiction, perfection
fer, lat	to bring or carry	translate, infer
graph, gram	writing	telegraph, epigram, grammar
leg, lect	to choose, read	select, eligible
mitt, miss	to send	missile, emissary, admittance
mori, mort	to die	immortal, moribund, mortality
pon, posit	to place	expose, proponent, positive
port, portat	to carry	import, portable, transport
scrib, script	to write	inscribe, circumscript
sequi, secut	to follow	sequel, consecutive
spec, spect	to look at	inspect, spectacular
tang, tact	to touch	contact, tangent
ten, tent	to hold	tenure, tenacious
veni, vent	to come	convene, prevent
anthrop	man, mankind	anthropology
auto	self	automobile, autobiography
bibli	book	Bible, bibliophile
bio	life	biosphere, biology
chrom	color	chromosome, chromatography
chron	time	anachronism
cosm	world	cosmic
crac, crat	power, rule	democracy, autocracy, bureaucracy
cycl	wheel, circle	bicycle, encyclical
dem	people	demographic
dox, doct	belief	orthodox
erg	work, power	energy, ergometric
gen	kind, race	genetics
hetero	other, different	heterophile
homo	same	homogenized
metr, meter	measure	thermometer

2.6 RECOMMENDED READING AND OTHER SUGGESTIONS FOR IMPROVING VOCABULARY

The best way to ensure that you will do well on the test is to increase your knowledge of words. However limited your time may be, you can improve your vocabulary by spending just a few minutes a day.

Your local public or school library has a wealth of resources to help you build word knowledge. Familiarize yourself with the call numbers for books on language, such as vocabulary building, in the library you use. (Consult with the reference librarian for related headings.)

Also look in the reference room for books to use while at the library. Seek out books that provide clear explanations in a format that is useful for you as a learning tool. Look through the table of contents for the organization of the book. Stay away from lengthy lists of unusual words and those that merely list uncommon words and uses.

Read good books all kinds, newspapers (especially *The Wall Street Journal* and *The New York Times*), and magazines (*Science*, and *Scientific American).* Make it a habit to look up words and confirm your knowledge of new and alternate meanings. Play with words: Scrabble, Anagrams, Boggle, crossword puzzles and other word games can be fun, even if you have never been enthusiastic about them before.

You can even use word games for group study. Scrabble, for example, can be played by alternate rules. To increase its usefulness as a learning tool, play with all the tiles exposed; all players participate at each turn with the goal of forming the best available word. Try scoring each word and aiming for a high combined total; or concentrate on prefixes and award extra points. Ask players to provide synonyms and antonyms for each word formed. The possibilities for enjoyment and learning are endless.

You need to *know* the words used in the questions in order to make the analyses necessary for answering verbal questions of all types. You may sometimes think that this test is the only time you will ever need these words, or that the selections in the sample questions are esoteric and useless for your future. If so, you may be surprised to learn that the words listed on the next page appeared on three consecutive weekdays in either *The Wall Street Journal* or *The New York Times*. Whatever career you choose, you will need to communicate clearly, accurately, and effectively.

Most of these words are probably in your recognition vocabulary. But can you define them out of context? If not, look them up, learn them, think of current uses and specific contexts such as economics, social sciences, politics, the arts. Make them a part of your working vocabulary.

WORD LIST FOR ADDITIONAL PRACTICE

abrogate
acclaim
allege
anemometer
animosity
atrocities
augment
austere
barometer
besieged
bioaccumulate
boom
bureaucratic
cache
cavalierly
comprehensive
consolidation
conspicuous
contingent
counteroffensive
culminate
curb
cyclical
debenture
decry
deploy
disconsolately
dominant
downturn
emblematic
embroil
expediency
extraneous
flagrant
founder
gouging
homily
hygrometer
hyperbole
impetuous
incursion
index
intractable
intransigent
lionize
lobby
mandate
myopia
nondescript
obviate
pantheon
parliament
partisan
phenomenon
precarious
prototype
ramification
referendum
reignite
relinquish
retarding
shore up
skeptical
slowdown
slump
solidarity
sovereignty
stopgap
subsidize
sumptuous
surge
surrogate
augment
thwart
tribunal
wake
waning
yen

The vocabulary skills you have perfected in analyzing antonyms, synonyms and analogies will provide a solid background for developing your verbal reasoning skills, which will be discussed in the next chapter. Increasing your ability to solve a variety of verbal analytical questions will sharpen other analytical skills. As you test your reasoning and problem solving abilities, keep a list of the new words you encounter and continue to review them to build an effective vocabulary.

2.7 SAMPLE PCAT ITEMS

2.7.1 Antonyms

1. UNDULATE
   - A. straight
   - B. beyond question
   - C. excessive
   - D. feathered

2. DIVEST
   - A. dress
   - B. inspire
   - C. assemble
   - D. converge

3. CONGRUENT
   - A. coincide
   - B. diverge
   - C. guess
   - D. empty

4. VACILLATE
   - A. fill
   - B. intelligent
   - C. resolute
   - D. inoculate

5. DANK
   - A. dry
   - B. tight
   - C. light
   - D. cowardly

6. PRETENSION
   - A. sincere
   - B. a rightful claim
   - C. timid
   - D. agreeable

7. LUCID
   - A. unclear
   - B. angelic
   - C. flawed
   - D. discerning

8. PETITE
   - A. large
   - B. lacking oil
   - C. stubborn
   - D. small

9. EXEMPLARY
   - A. flawless
   - B. reprehensible
   - C. imitated
   - D. excusable

10. PARADIGM
    - A. model
    - B. elliptic
    - C. illustrative
    - D. non-standard

11. ZEAL
    - A. diligence
    - B. apathy
    - C. culmination
    - D. passion

12. ALTRUISM
    - A. egoism
    - B. concern
    - C. oblique
    - D. selflessness

13. HARASS
    - A. disturb
    - B. forbid
    - C. flee
    - D. comfort

14. MOROSE
    - A. enervated
    - B. shout
    - C. sullen
    - D. elated

15. PHLEGMATIC
- **A.** gloomy
- **B.** excitable
- **C.** sluggish
- **D.** bloody

16. SCRUPLE
- **A.** comprehensible
- **B.** careful
- **C.** unethical
- **D.** erect

17. PLAUDITS
- **A.** disapproval
- **B.** planetary
- **C.** approbation
- **D.** invalid

18. ACCOST
- **A.** flee
- **B.** agree
- **C.** fight
- **D.** solicit

19. CRAVE
- **A.** require
- **B.** abhor
- **C.** yearn
- **D.** dispute

20. WINNOW
- **A.** dispense
- **B.** analyze
- **C.** calm
- **D.** gather

21. CHIDE
- **A.** impel
- **B.** goad
- **C.** compliment
- **D.** scold

22. PROVOCATION
- **A.** job
- **B.** calming
- **C.** incite
- **D.** irritate

23. ALIENATE
- **A.** befriend
- **B.** isolate
- **C.** indifferent
- **D.** naturalized

24. MOLLIFY
- **A.** calm
- **B.** soothe
- **C.** mystify
- **D.** inflame

25. FRIVOLOUS
- **A.** unnecessary
- **B.** essential
- **C.** trivial
- **D.** flip

26. ENCROACH
- **A.** impede
- **B.** avoid
- **C.** retreat
- **D.** intrude

27. INANE
- **A.** insubstantial
- **B.** sane
- **C.** lifeless
- **D.** meaningful

28. WANTON
- **A.** cruel
- **B.** extravagant
- **C.** chaste
- **D.** squander

29. RUSE
- **A.** pretense
- **B.** truth
- **C.** confabulation
- **D.** artifice

30. FINITE
- **A.** terminal
- **B.** final
- **C.** limited
- **D.** endless

31. PROVINCIAL
- **A.** cosmopolitan
- **B.** urban
- **C.** serious
- **D.** unworldly

32. FRUGAL
- **A.** stingy
- **B.** profligate
- **C.** abstemious
- **D.** thrifty

33. FASTIDIOUS
- **A.** careful
- **B.** slovenly
- **C.** particular
- **D.** fatuous

34. SANGUINE
- **A.** pessimistic
- **B.** confident
- **C.** dry
- **D.** unclean

35. VIVACIOUS
- **A.** lively
- **B.** energetic
- **C.** dour
- **D.** healthful

2.7.2 Analogies

36. PRESCRIBE : ASSIGN :: PROSCRIBE :
- **A.** invite
- **B.** banish
- **C.** mollify
- **D.** stimulate

37. POPPY : OPIATE :: FOXGLOVE :
- **A.** tranquilizer
- **B.** narcotic
- **C.** stimulant
- **D.** carcinogen

38. ARSENIC : PEACH PITS :: CYANIDE :
- **A.** persimmon
- **B.** mint
- **C.** morel
- **D.** hemlock

39. KNUCKLE : DIGIT :: WRIST :
- **A.** muscle
- **B.** elbow
- **C.** arm
- **D.** leg

40. PEN : PAPER :: CHALK :
- **A.** slate
- **B.** point
- **C.** ink
- **D.** paper

41. BRONZE : PATINA :: SILVER :
- **A.** tarnish
- **B.** luster
- **C.** alloy
- **D.** burnish

42. ARCHITECT:BLUEPRINT::GARDENER:
- **A.** weed
- **B.** flowers
- **C.** hoe
- **D.** plant

43. FOIBLE : VICE :: APTITUDE :
- **A.** penchant
- **B.** forte
- **C.** vocation
- **D.** paucity

44. RARIFIED : MOUNTAIN :: DANK :
- **A.** delta
- **B.** mesa
- **C.** jungle
- **D.** desert

45. ISLAND : CONTINENT :: MOON :
- **A.** sun
- **B.** earth
- **C.** galaxy
- **D.** planet

46. CANYON : MESA :: GORGE :
- A. plateau
- B. tundra
- C. steppe
- D. declivity

47. VARIEGATED : SOLID::CHAMELEON:
- A. skunk
- B. zebra
- C. elephant
- D. leopard

48. PEEL : EXCORIATE :: SHAVE :
- A. depilate
- B. pare
- C. desiccate
- D. escape

49. SPHERE:CIRCUMFERENCE:: HYPOTENUSE:
- A. pentagram
- B. radius
- C. triangle
- D. theory

50. CAVE : PETROGLYPH :: BOOK :
- A. ossification
- B. pagination
- C. phobia
- D. autograph

51. SPARK : FLAME :: IMPUDENCE :
- A. provocation
- B. mollification
- C. announcement
- D. insurgence

52. DILEMMA : PREDICAMENT::ENIGMA:
- A. perfidy
- B. perplexity
- C. perseverance
- D. perdition

53. REPUDIATE : RESCIND :: PRECLUDE :
- A. engender
- B. relegate
- C. inhibit
- D. embroil

54. PORTENTOUS:POMPOUS::PENCHANT:
- A. perfidy
- B. pejorative
- C. profusion
- D. propensity

55. PLATITUDE : BROMIDE :: APHORISM :
- A. chisel
- B. clip
- C. saw
- D. gaffe

56. SEMANTIC: SEMINAR :: SEMAPHORE :
- A. signal
- B. seminal
- C. lasting
- D. code

57. PETROLEUM : PLASTIC :: CLAY :
- A. pitch
- B. amalgam
- C. porcelain
- D. dirt

58. CAFETERIA : EPICUREAN :: COMIC BOOK :
- A. humorist
- B. lampoon
- C. pseudonym
- D. bibliophile

59. INTEMPERATE:TUNDRA :: BUCOLIC :
- A. polar
- B. bovine
- C. prairie
- D. urbane

60. PUPIL : IRIS :: SUN :
- A. solar system
- B. planet
- C. star
- D. flower

61. ISTHMUS : CONTINENT :: LIGAMENT :
- A. muscle
- B. corpuscle
- C. epidermis
- D. emolient

62. LEITMOTIF:WAGNER::POINTILLISM :
A. Monet
B. Pollock
C. Seurat
D. Picadilly

63. LAMBENT : CANDLE :: REDOLENT :
A. alms
B. rose
C. scent
D. hybrid

64. KINETIC : MOVEMENT :: EPICENE :
A. gastronomy
B. geology
C. gender
D. germination

65. CUNEIFORM : HIEROGLYPH :: PICTOGRAPH:
A. photograph
B. epigram
C. ephitaph
D. ideograph

66. INTERIM : INTERMINABLE :: ACUTE :
A. chronic
B. obtuse
C. grave
D. dull

67. GOAT : SATYR :: HORSE :
A. harpy
B. sphinx
C. centaur
D. siren

68. EYE : BLINK :: LIPS :
A. whistle
B. yawn
C. snarl
D. kiss

69. IMMIGRATE:EMIGRATE::VICARIOUS :
A. viscous
B. heretical
C. direct
D. visceral

70. POISON : ANTIDOTE::AFFECT :
A. affected
B. antimatter
C. drug
D. effectual

71. PHEROMONE : COLOGNE :: LEATHER :
A. vinyl
B. wool
C. chamois
D. carapace

72. LUNG : BREATHE :: METRONOME :
A. osculate
B. oscillate
C. osculant
D. oscitant

73. EPISTEMOLOGY : KNOWLEDGE: ONTOLOGY :
A. logic
B. ethics
C. being
D. conduct

74. ICONOCLAST:AMULET::MISOGYNIST:
A. warfare
B. laughter
C. tattoo
D. harem

75. PHILANTHROPIST : PARSIMONIOUS :: CYNIC :
A. facetious
B. desultory
C. gullible
D. edacious

2.8 ANSWER KEY

Antonyms

1. A straight
2. A dress
3. B diverge
4. C resolute
5. A dry
6. B a rightful claim
7. A unclear
8. A large
9. B reprehensible
10. D non-standard
11. B apathy
12. A egoism
13. D comfort
14. D elated
15. B excitable
16. C unethical
17. A disapproval
18. A flee
19. B abhor
20. D gather
21. C compliment
22. B calming
23. A befriend
24. D inflame
25. B essential
26. C retreat
27. D meaningful
28. C chaste
29. B truth
30. D endless
31. A cosmopolitan
32. B profligate
33. B slovenly
34. A pessimistic
35. C dour

Analogies

36. B banish
37. C stimulant
38. D hemlock
39. C arm
40. A slate
41. A tarnish
42. C hoe
43. B forte
44. C jungle
45. D planet
46. A plateau
47. C elephant
48. B pare
49. C triangle
50. D autograph
51. A provocation
52. B perplexity
53. C inhibit
54. D propensity
55. C saw
56. B seminal
57. C porcelain
58. D bibliophile
59. C prairie
60. A solar system
61. A muscle
62. C Seurat
63. B rose
64. C gender
65. D ideograph
66. A chronic
67. C centaur
68. B yawn
69. C direct
70. D effectual
71. A vinyl
72. B oscillate
73. C being
74. D harem
75. C gullible

2.9 REFERENCES

Bader, William, et al. *MAT: Miller Analogies Test* (Englewood Cliffs, N.J.: Prentice Hall, 1988).

DeVries, Mary A. *The Complete Word Book* (Englewood Cliffs, N.J.: Prentice Hall, 1991).

Morse-Cluley, Elizabeth, and Richard Read. *Webster's New World Power Vocabulary* (New York: Simon & Schuster, 1988).

Random House Thesaurus, College Edition [organized alphabetically], 1984, and Roget's International Thesaurus [organized by topic], 1977. A good thesaurus is an indispensable tool for improving vocabulary.

Schur, Norman W. *The 1,000 Most Challenging Words* (New York: Ballantine Books, 1988).

Schur, Norman W. *Practical English: 1,000 Most Effective Words* (New York: Ballantine Books, 1983).

The Random House Dictionary, 1987. Used as the authoritative reference for this guide. See also *American Heritage Dictionary of the English Language, New College Edition*, 1982, and *Webster's New World Dictionary of American English, Third College Edition*, 1988.

Whimbey, Arthur, and Jack Lochhead. *Problem Solving and Comprehension* (Hillside, N.J.: Lawrence Erlbaum Associates, 1991). (Available from Betz Publishing Co.)

Chapter 3
Reading Comprehension Skills

3.0 INTRODUCTION TO READING COMPREHENSION IN THE PCAT

According to the Psychological Corporation, the PCAT Reading Comprehension test measures three major skills areas. These are given as the ability "to comprehend, analyze, and interpret...." It is designed to test your reading ability through multiple-choice questions. Reading comprehension passages are selected from scientific books and journals. The selections are typical of materials encountered in the first year of pharmacy school. No prior knowledge of the science topic is required for the Reading Comprehension test.

The Reading Comprehension test consists of five or six passages. Each passage is either short (200-600 words) or long (700-950 words) followed by a varying number of questions (ranging from four to twelve). These questions test the comprehension skills and analytical skills required to understand ideas and concepts developed in the passage.

3.1 PCAT READING COMPREHENSION SKILLS

Special reading skills may be developed and new skills learned to prepare for the Reading Comprehension examination of the Pharmacy College Admission Test. You will need at least an hour a day to develop these skills and it is useful to know what they are before attempting to master them.

As shown in the following outline, the major skills areas have been expanded into practice topics that are explained in greater detail in the text of this chapter. With the practice they afford, these expanded topics will permit you to master the major skills more completely.

PCAT READING COMPREHENSION SKILLS (3.1)

I. COMPREHENSION OF "NEW" INFORMATION (3.2)
   A. Source Material for "New" Information (3.2.1)
   B. Reading (3.2.2)
      — understanding new words
      — scanning and correlating
      — developing speed and rhythm
   C. Organizing (3.2.3)
      — marking techniques
      — timing
      — developing quick charts (mind mapping)
   D. Analyzing (3.2.4)
      — reading test items with choices
      — eliminating wrong answers; choosing the *best* answer
      — question analysis strategy

E. Remembering (3.2.5)
  - reasoning and diagramming
  - vocabulary, building
  - extraction of information

II. COMPREHENSION OF "CURRENT" INFORMATION (3.3)
  A. Definition (3.3.1)
  B. Applying Logic to Comprehension (3.3.2)
  C. Interpretation of Scientific Information (3.3.3)
  D. Reading Comprehension Questions (3.3.4)
  E. Errors in Reading and How to Avoid Them (3.3.5)

3.2 COMPREHENSION OF "NEW" INFORMATION

New information includes pharmacy research reports, magazine articles, and even newspapers such as *The New York Times.* These sources of new information are easy to obtain if you visit your school library. Sometimes, new information is provided in your textbook or during lectures by the professor. The PCAT tests your abilities to read, organize, and analyze "new" information as you encounter it. "New" means previously unseen, unrehearsed, and representing information at first glance. "New" does *not* mean unknown, unfamiliar, or information never heard before. You may or may not have prior knowledge of the topic presented.

3.2.1 Source Material for "New" Information

Following is a suggested list of sources to read on a regular basis. These sources will provide you with "new" information passages.

1. *The New York Times* (daily newspaper)
2. *Scientific American* (monthly magazine)
3. *Discover* (monthly magazine)
4. *American Scientist by Sigma Xi* (bimonthly magazine)
5. *The New England Journal of Medicine* (weekly journal)
6. *Encyclopedia Britannica* (latest edition)
7. *American Pharmacy*
8. *American Journal of Hospital Pharmacy*
9. *Journal of the American Medical Association*
10. *USA Today*

3.2.2 Reading

Reading ability, a difficult concept to define, depends on the difficulty of the passage, your concentration level at the time you read it, your interest in the subject matter of the passage, your speed in reading and understanding the text, and, finally, your retention of various parts of the passage to make connections.

The difficulty of the passage results from unfamiliar vocabulary (author's word choice) and minute details of content. Construct a vocabulary notebook and record on a daily basis the new words you encounter. Vocabulary expansion on a short-term basis is possible with constant review. A larger vocabulary will also enhance your verbal ability review.

Use analytical reasoning while you read. Covered below in section 3.3.2, "Applying Logic to Comprehension," analytical reasoning will make you more critically inclined when reading various types of complex and detailed information. Analytical reasoning involves breaking a complex passage into short, understandable pieces. When reading a passage requiring conceptual understanding, break the sentences into short understandable phrases.

For the PCAT, reading passages should be encountered as typical comprehension exercises using reading ability skills, which include understanding new words, scanning and correlating, and developing speed and rhythm. Before elaborating on these skills, attempt the following sample PCAT passage. This passage is similar in format and style to PCAT passages used in previous examinations.

Exercise 1: Comprehension of Material from Pharmacy Journals

Use the following reading techniques during this exercise:

1. Skim the passage first—approximately 30 seconds. Find the main topic covered.
2. Correlate the questions to get clues (do not read the responses or choices).
3. Correlate—take about two to four minutes to read the passage and develop connections among various parts (use light underlining or highlighting).
4. Answer the questions, consulting the passage as necessary.

Sample Passage
Reading Comprehension Test

Connective Tissue:
General Characteristics and Functions

Connective tissue allows movement and provides support. In this tissue there is an abundance of inter-cellular material called matrix, which is variable in type and amount and is one of the main sources of difference between the types of connective tissue. It consists of various fibers embedded in a ground substance.

Loose Connective Tissue. The fibers of loose connective tissue are not tightly woven. The tissue, filling spaces between and penetrating into the organs, is of three types: areolar, adipose, and reticular.

Areolar Tissue. The most widely distributed connective tissue is pliable and crossed by many delicate threads; yet, the tissue resists tearing and is somewhat elastic. Areolar tissue contains fibroblasts, histiocytes (macrophages), leukocytes, and mast cells.

Fibroblasts are small, flattened, somewhat irregular cells with large nuclei and reduced cytoplasm. The term fibroblast refers to the ability of a cell to form fibrils. Fibroblasts are active in repair of injury. It is generally believed that suprarenal steroids inhibit and growth hormones stimulate fibroblastic activity. **Histiocytes** are phagocytic cells similar to leukocytes in blood; however, they perform phagocytic activity outside the vascular system. The histiocyte is irregular in shape and contains cytoplasmic granules. The cell is often stationary (or "fixed"). **Mast cells,** located adjacent to small blood vessels, are round or polygonal in shape and possess a cytoplasm filled with meta-chromatic granules. Mast cells function in the manufacture of heparin (an anticoagulant) and histamine (an inflammatory substance responsible for changes in allergic tissue). Depression in mast cell activity results from the administration of cortisol to patients. Areolar tissue is the basic supporting substance around organs, muscles, blood vessels, and nerves forming the delicate membranes around the brain and spinal cord and comprising the superficial fascia, or sheet of connective tissue, found deep in the skin.

Adipose Tissue. Adipose tissue is specialized areolar tissue with fat-containing cells. The fat or lipid cell, like other cells, has a nucleus, endoplasmic reticulum, cell membrane, mitochondria, and one or more fat droplets. Adipose tissue acts as a firm yet resilient packing around and between organs, bundles of muscle fibers, nerves, and supporting blood vessels. Since fat is a poor conductor of heat, adipose tissue protects the body from excessive heat loss or excessive rises in temperature.

Reticular Tissue. Reticular fibers consist of finely branching fibrils taking a silver stain as observed under the microscope. The primary cell of the reticular fiber is the reticular cell. Reticular fibers form the framework of the liver, lymphoid organs, and bone marrow.

Dense Connective Tissue. Dense connective tissue is composed of closely arranged tough collagenous and elastic fiber. It can be classified according to the arrangement of the fibers and the proportion of elastin and collagen present. Examples of dense connective tissue having a regular arrangement of fibers are tendons, aponeuroses, and ligaments. Examples of dense connective tissue having an irregular arrangement of fibers are fasciae, capsules, and muscle sheaths.

Specialized Connective Tissue

Cartilage. Cartilage has a firm matrix consisting of protein and mucopolysaccharides. Cells of cartilage, called **chondrocytes**, are large and rounded with spherical nuclei. Collagenous and elastic fibers are embedded in the matrix, increasing the elastic and resistive properties of this tissue. The three types of cartilage are hyaline, fibrous, and elastic.

In utero, **hyaline cartilage**, the precursor of much of the skeletal system, is translucent with a clear matrix caused by abundant collagenous fibers (not visible as such) and cells scattered throughout the matrix. Hyaline cartilage is gradually replaced by bone in many parts of the body through the process of ossification; however, some remains as a covering on the articular surfaces. The hyaline costal cartilages attach the anterior ends of the upper seven pairs of ribs to the sternum. The trachea and bronchi are kept open by incomplete rings of surrounding hyaline cartilage. This type of cartilage is also found in the nose.

Fibrous cartilage contains dense masses of unbranching, collagenous fibers lying in the matrix. Cells of fibrous cartilage are present in rows between bundles of the matrix. Fibrocartilage is dense and resistant to stretching; it is less flexible and less resilient than hyaline cartilage. Fibrous cartilage, interposed between the vertebrae in the spinal column, is also present in the symphysis pubis, permitting a minimal range of movement.

Elastic cartilage, which is more resilient than either the hyaline or the fibrous type because of a predominance of elastic fibers impregnated in its ground substance, is found in the auricle of the external ear, the auditory tube, the epiglottis, and portions of the larynx.

Bone is a firm tissue formed by impregnation of the intercellular material with inorganic salts. It is living tissue supplied by blood vessels and nerves and is constantly being remodeled. The two common types are **compact**, forming the dense outer layer, and **cancellous**, forming the inner lighter tissue of the shaft of a long bone.

The **dentin** of teeth is closely related to bone. The crown of the tooth is covered by enamel, the hardest substance in the body. Enamel is secreted onto the dentin by the epithelial cells of the enamel organ before the teeth are extruded through the gums. Dentin resembles bone but is harder and denser.

Blood and Hematopoietic Tissue. Marrow is the blood-forming (hematopoietic) tissue located in the shafts of bones. The red blood cells (erythrocytes) and most white blood cells (leukocytes) originate in the capillary sinusoids of bone marrow. Some leukocytes are formed in the lymphoid organs. Blood is a fluid tissue circulating through the body, carrying nutrients to cells, and removing waste products.

Lymphoid tissue is found in the lymph nodes, thymus, spleen, tonsils, and adenoids. The germinal centers of lymph tissue produce plasma cells and lymphocytes. Lymphoid tissue function in antibody production.

Connective tissues perform many functions, including support and nourishment for other tissues, packing material in the spaces between organs, and defense for the body by digestion and absorption of foreign material.

Reticuloendothelial system. Connective tissue cells, carrying on the process of phagocytosis, are frequently referred to as the reticuloendothelial system. The cells ingest solid particles similar to the manner in which an amoeba takes in nourishment. Three types of phagocytic cells belong to this classification: reticuloendothelial cells lining the liver (Kupffer's cells), spleen, and bone marrow; macrophages, termed tissue histiocytes or "resting-wandering" cells; and microglia, located in the central nervous system. The reticuloendothelial system is a strong line of defense against infection.

Synovial Membranes. Synovial membranes line the cavities of the freely moving joints and form tendon sheaths and bursae.

1. Which of the following is not a type of areolar connective tissue?
   A. Histiocytes
   B. Plasma cells
   C. Leukocytes
   D. Fibroblasts

2. The connective tissue forming the framework for the liver is classified as
   A. loose connective tissue.
   B. synovial membranes.
   C. fibrous cartilage.
   D. areolar tissue.

3. Mast cells function in the production of
   A. histamine.
   B. cortisol.
   C. **1** and **2** only.
   D. all of the above.

4. Which of the following is not a function of specialized connective tissue?
   A. Producing plasma cells and lymphocytes
   B. Phagocytosis
   C. Protecting the body from an excessive increase or decrease in temperature
   D. Producing blood cells

5. Which of the following terms does not apply to any connective tissue?
   A. Squamous
   B. Areolar
   C. Reticular
   D. Lymphoid

6. Which of the following is not a characteristic of the reticuloendothelial system?
   A. Microglia cells
   B. Macrophages
   C. Serve as framework for bone marrow and liver
   D. Defense against infection

7. Which of the following type(s) of tissue is largely characterized by the nature of material that lies between the cells?
   A. Connective tissue
   B. Smooth muscle tissue
   C. Nervous tissue
   D. Pseudostratified tissue

8. The most widely distributed connective tissue is
   A. dense connective tissue.
   B. adipose connective tissue.
   C. areolar connective tissue.
   D. specialized connective tissue.

9. The type of connective tissue that acts as a precursor to much of the skeletal system is
   A. hyaline cartilage.
   B. fibrous cartilage.
   C. elastic cartilage.
   D. synovial membrane.

10. Cartilage cells are called
    A. histiocytes.
    B. erythrocytes.
    C. chondrocytes.
    D. mast cells.

1. Control passage as it branches from the intro paragraph — Keep looking for differences in structure (S) and function (F).

2. Develop a mental layout of passage as it expands in content.

Approx. 500 words

Connective Tissue: General Characteristics and Functions

Connective tissue allows movement and provides support. In this tissue there is an abundance of intercellular material called matrix, which is variable in type and amount and is one of the main sources of difference between the types of connective tissue. It consists of various fibers embedded in a ground substance.

Loose Connective Tissue

The fibers of loose connective tissue are not tightly woven. The tissue, filling spaces between and penetrating into the organs, is of three types: areolar, adipose, and reticular.

Areolar Tissue. The most widely distributed connective tissue is pliable and crossed by many delicate threads; yet, the tissue resists tearing and is somewhat elastic. Areolar tissue contains fibroblasts, histiocytes (macrophages), leukocytes, and mast cells.

Fibroblasts are small, flattened, somewhat irregular cells with large nuclei and reduced cytoplasm. The term fibroblast refers to the ability of a cell to form fibrils. Fibroblasts are active in repair of injury. It is generally believed that suprarenal steroids inhibit and growth hormones stimulate fibroblastic activity. **Histiocytes** are phagocytic cells similar to leukocytes in blood; however, they perform phagocytic activity outside the vascular system. The histiocyte is irregular in shape and contains cytoplasmic granules. The cell is often stationary (or "fixed"). Mast cells, located adjacent to small blood vessels, are round or polygonal in shape and possess a cytoplasm filled with metachromatic granules. Mast cells function in the manufacture of heparin (an anticoagulant) and histamine (an inflammatory substance responsible for changes in allergic tissue). Depression in mast cell activity results from the administration of cortisol to patients. Areolar tissue is the basic supporting substance around organs, muscles, blood vessels, and nerves forming the delicate membranes around the brain and spinal cord and comprising the superficial fascia, or sheet of connective tissue, found deep in the skin.

Adipose Tissue. Adipose tissue is specialized areolar tissue with fat-containing cells. The fat or lipid cell, like other cells, has a nucleus, endoplasmic reticulum, cell membrane, mitochondria, and one or more fat droplets. Adipose tissue acts as a firm yet resilient packing around and between organs, bundles of muscle fibers, nerves, and supporting blood vessels. Since fat is a poor conductor of heat, adipose tissue protects the body from excessive heat loss or excessive rises in temperature.

Reticular Tissue. Reticular fibers consist of finely branching fibrils taking a silver stain as observed under the microscope. The primary cell of the reticular fiber is the reticular cell. Reticular fibers form the framework of the liver, lymphoid organs, and bone marrow.

Dense Connective Tissue

Dense connective tissue is composed of closely arranged tough collagenous and elastic fiber. It can be classified according to the arrangement of the fibers and the proportion of elastin and collagen present. Examples of dense connective tissue having a regular arrangement of fibers are tendons, aponeuroses, and ligaments. Examples of dense connective tissue having an irregular arrangement of fibers are fasciae, capsules, and muscle sheaths.

Specialized Connective Tissue

Cartilage. Cartilage has a firm matrix consisting of protein and mucopolysaccharides. Cells of cartilage, called chondrocytes, are large and rounded with spherical nuclei. Collagenous and elastic fibers are embedded in the matrix, increasing the elastic and resistive properties of this tissue. The three types of cartilage are hyaline, fibrous, and elastic.

In utero, hyaline cartilage, the precursor of much of the skeletal system, is translucent with a clear matrix caused by abundant collagenous fibers (not visible as such) and cells scattered throughout the matrix. Hyaline cartilage is gradually replaced by bone in many parts of the body through the process of ossification; however, some remains as a covering on the articular surfaces. The hyaline costal cartilages attach the anterior ends of the upper seven pairs of ribs to the sternum. The trachea and bronchi are kept open by incomplete rings of surrounding hyaline cartilage. This type of cartilage is also found in the nose.

Fibrous cartilage contains dense masses of unbranching, collagenous fibers lying in the matrix. Cells of fibrous cartilage are present in rows between bundles of the matrix. Fibrocartilage is dense and resistant to stretching; it is less flexible and less resilient than hyaline cartilage. Fibrous cartilage, interposed between the vertebrae in the spinal column, is also present in the symphysis pubis, permitting a minimal range of movement.

Elastic cartilage, which is more resilient than either the hyaline or the fibrous type because of a predominance of elastic fibers impregnated in its ground substance, is found in the auricle of the external ear, the auditory tube, the epiglottis, and portions of the larynx.

Bone is a firm tissue formed by impregnation of the intercellular material with inorganic salts. It is

remember elasticity and springs from Physics (are density and elasticity related?)

dense outer layer (next page)

living tissue supplied by blood vessels and nerves and is constantly being remodeled. The two common types are **compact**, forming the dense outer layer, and **cancellous**, forming the inner lighter tissue of the shaft of a long bone.

The **dentin** of teeth is closely related to bone. The crown of the tooth is covered by enamel, the hardest substance in the body. Enamel is secreted onto the dentin by the epithelial cells of the enamel organ before the teeth are extruded through the gums. Dentin resembles bone but is harder and denser.

Blood and Hematopoietic Tissue. Marrow is the blood-forming (hematopoietic) tissue located in the shafts of bones. The red blood cells (erythrocytes) and most white blood cells (leukocytes) originate in the capillary sinusoids of bone marrow. Some leukocytes are formed in the lymphoid organs. Blood is a fluid tissue circulating through the body, carrying nutrients to cells, and removing waste products.

Lymphoid tissue is found in the lymph nodes, thymus, spleen, tonsils, and adenoids. The germinal centers of lymph tissue produce plasma cells and lymphocytes. Lymphoid tissue function in antibody production.

Connective tissues perform many functions, including support and nourishment for other tissues, packing material in the spaces between organs, and defense for the body by digestion and absorption of foreign material.

Reticuloendothelial system. Connective tissue cells, carrying on the process of phagocytosis, are frequently referred to as the reticuloendothelial system. The cells ingest solid particles similar to the manner in which an amoeba takes in nourishment. Three types of phagocytic cells belong to this classification: reticuloendothelial cells lining the liver (Kupffer's cells), spleen, and bone marrow; macrophages, termed tissue histiocytes or "resting-wandering" cells; and microglia, located in the central nervous system. The reticuloendothelial system is a strong line of defense against infection.

Synovial Membranes. Synovial membranes line the cavities of the freely moving joints and form tendon sheaths and bursae.

What is most difficult in this passage? ⇒ classification of tissues, bones, cartilage, and other anatomical features, e.g., types of cells.

Fig. 3.1 — Marked-up Passage

ANSWERS TO EXERCISE 1
(All answers are found within the passage.)

1. **(B)** Paragraph two under loose connective tissue. Topic: areolar tissue.

2. **(A)** Paragraph six under loose connective tissue. Topic: reticular tissue.

3. **(C)** Paragraph three under loose connective tissue. Topic: areolar tissue.

4. **(C)** The functions of specialized connective tissues are found under that heading. As explained under the topic adipose tissue, response **4** is a function of this type of connective tissue.

5. **(A)** This is covered adequately in the passage.

6. **(C)** Found under the topic Reticuloendothelial System.

7. **(A)** Paragraph one under connective tissue.

8. **(C)** Found under the topic areolar tissue.

9. **(A)** Found under the topic specialized connective tissue. Topic: cartilage.

10. **(C)** Found under the topic specialized connective tissue. Topic: cartilage.

3.2.3 Organizing

Good organization is required for success on the PCAT Reading Comprehension test. The elements of a good organizing system several techniques to help you locate information quickly. These techniques include underlining, circling, using brackets and parentheses, and drawing mind maps in sufficient detail. Mind maps are quick charts that trace your thoughts when reading a passage.

Exercise 2: Passage Marking and Mapping

How many correct answers did you get in Exercise 1 (section 3.2.2)? If you had fewer than five correct answers, begin here to reinforce your skills in passage analysis. Try to answer the following questions about the passage; then proceed to the marking and mapping suggestions presented below.

a. How long (in words) is the passage?
b. How much time did you spend reading the passage?
c. What is the main idea conveyed in the passage?
d. Did you make scratch notes (highlight, underline, etc.) as you extracted information from the passage?
e. Do you remember 20 vocabulary words (difficult ones) or terms? (Do not look at the passage again!)
f. Are you ready to write a short summary of the passage?
g. Which parts of the passage were the hardest?
h. Did you find any irrelevant information in the passage?

MARKING: After you finish answering all the above questions, look at the marked-up passage (fig. 3.1). The marks include underlining, circles, and other relevant marks that illustrate active reading. As you read the passage, you should have marked it actively to highlight important points. Questions **a** through **h** above may be answered at this stage. Use the following hints to check your answers. To answer question **a** above, count the average number of words per line and multiply by the number of lines in the passage. The connective tissue passage is approximately one and one-half typed pages and about five hundred words long. The answer to question **b** will vary according to your insights into the subject matter of the passage, your underlining, notes taken, and other factors. For this kind of information, reading should take about five minutes (no more). On the actual PCAT you are given approximately 45 minutes to answer 45 test items. An average student would read the passages and work the 45 items in the approximate times shown below:

TABLE 2: Suggested Time Distribution for Reading Comprehension in the PCAT

Two Models Showing Arrangement of Passages in Reading Comprehension

Model I (5 passages, 45 items)					Model II (6 passages, 45 items)				
Passage I (long)	+	12 items	=	8 min	Passage I (long)	+	10 items	=	7 min
Passage II (short)	+	4 items	=	3 min	Passage II (short)	+	5 items	=	3 min
Passage III (short)	+	6 items	=	4 min	Passage III (long)	+	11 items	=	7 min
Passage IV (long)	+	12 items	=	8 min	Passage IV (short)	+	4 items	=	3 min
Passage V (long)	+	11 items	=	7 min	Passage V (long)	+	11 items	=	7 min
		Total	=	30 min	Passage VI (short)	+	4 items	=	3 min
							Total	=	30 min

Note: The remaining 15 minutes should be used to review and reexamine your marked answer sheet and to read specific details in each passage.

This time distribution chart assumes that all passages and items are of equal difficulty and length. Allocate time for passage reading at half the item reading and answering time. Return to items that are difficult or readdress any part of a passage that may have confused you. You will save time by noting important terms as you encounter them in the passage.

MAPPING: To answer question **c**, refer to the Mind Map given below. The Mind Map shows that the passage relates structure, function, and examples of various types of connective tissue. A mind map helps you make the right connections to various parts of a passage if you have forgotten any term or definition used there. The purpose of question **d** is to make sure you highlighted or underlined the passage for very fine details. Use long arrows or leaders to connect various ideas or thoughts in the passage. For example, look at the arrows connecting the use of words such as “fibroblasts” and “histiocytes.” The mind map helps you to manage the details of the passage right from the start and it traces major ideas as you scan or read them. It is a useful tool for developing a layout for the entire passage. Mind maps are useful for either long passages or for complex/detail-oriented passages.

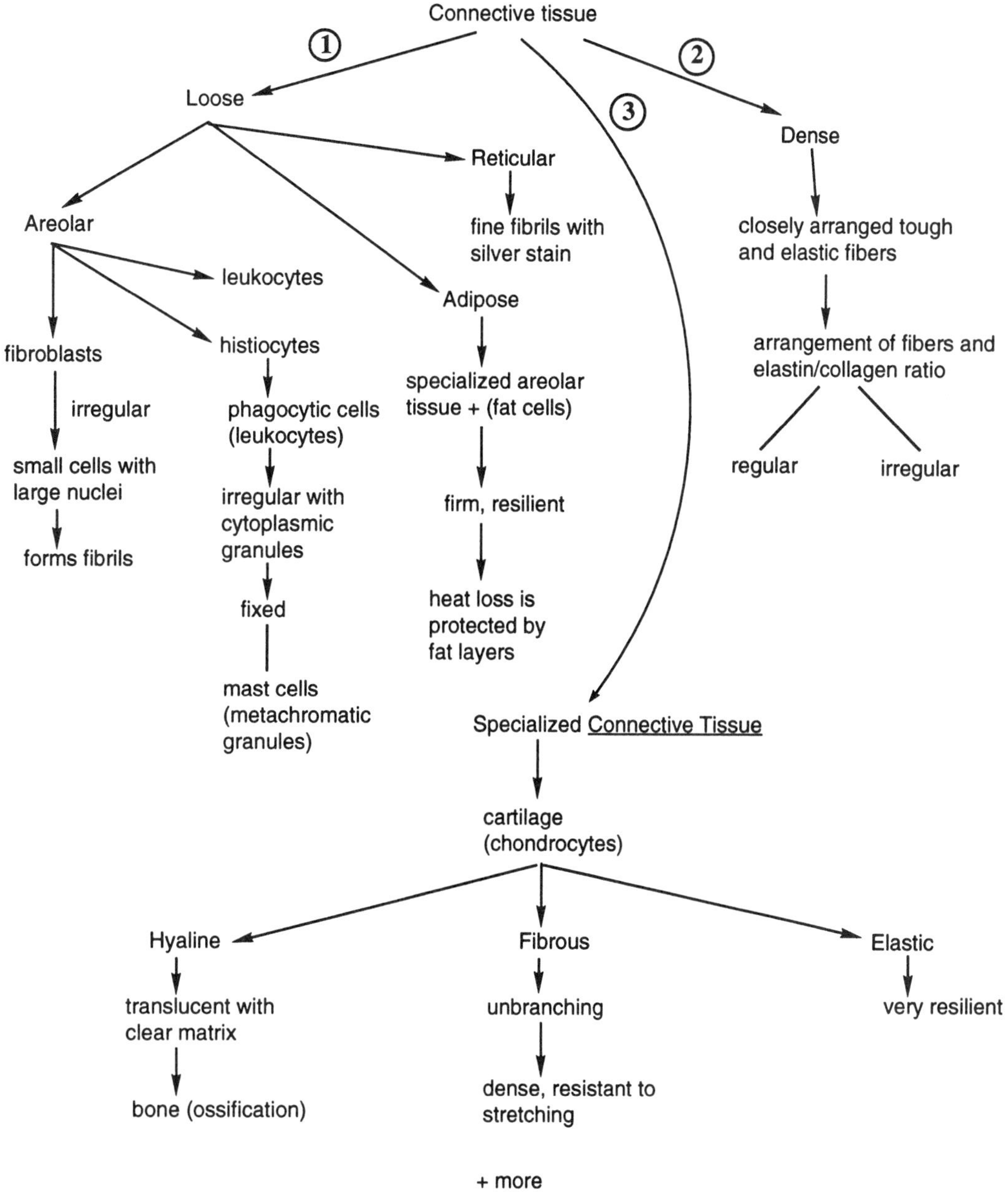

Fig. 3.2 — Mind Map

A mind map, like the one illustrated here, traces and records your ideas as your eyes travel through a reading passage. Mind maps are very useful for extracting basic detail and rearranging it for later use. Mind maps should produce a schematic chart of your observations as you read a passage. Construct mind maps for every article you read. After a while, you will be able to draw such maps quickly and accurately. The mind map shown here was made from the earlier connective tissue reading passage. Mind maps also lead and connect you to the right segment or paragraph when you answer the questions at the end of active reading.

To answer question **e**, use the mind map in fig. 3.3 to find the twenty vocabulary words, which could include the following: loose tissue, dense tissue, areolar, adipose, reticular, fibroblasts, fibrils, histiocytes, cytoplasmic granules, mast-cells, metachromatic granules, hyaline, ossification, cartilage, chondrocytes, fibrous cartilage, elastic cartilage, elastin/collagen ratio, phagocytic cells, leukocytes, resilient, and so on. Record in a notebook all the new words added to your vocabulary. Referring again to the mind map to answer question **f**, write a brief summary (one or two paragraphs) based on the marked up connective tissue passage (fig. 3.1). This summary more or less repeats important ideas in the passage and writing it will improve your short-term memory.

In response to questions **g** and **h**, by marking the passage you have located hidden information there. Look at the use of the word "where?" in the marked-up passage that asks, "Where is that kind of connective tissue found in the body?" The key word is "where?" because the introduction does not stress it. Irrelevant information is usually limited in such passages (textbook or encyclopedia information). Information you do not use to answer questions is unused information, but do not consider it irrelevant.

Your reading ability should now improve—you have learned to scan information, mark a passage, correlate information using a mind map, and increase your working vocabulary. You have also taken steps to develop your speed, which is based on developing a rhythm while you work that allows you to integrate all the above skills. Such rhythm comes from practice and a heightened interest in improving your reading ability. You should now answer questions more confidently.

3.2.4 Analyzing

This section relates to developing your analyzing skills to read test questions and the corresponding choices or responses. It shows you how to eliminate bad answers and how to choose the *best* answer not just a good one.

The conventional multiple-choice question is composed of a stem and a set of four answer choices. Multiple-choice items appear to be made in much the same way on tests from high school-level SATs right through the national pharmacy professional exams. The test maker puts a correct answer in one of the slots. Then the trickiest, hardest wrong answer is added. This most difficult wrong answer tends to be very close to the right answer—which is why we call it the "almost-right" answer. The test maker knows that the closer the almost-right answer is to the correct answer, the more difficulty you will have distinguishing one from the other. For example, if the question stem says, "All of the following are functions of the liver EXCEPT," the exception might be a function of the spleen, one that the test maker knows that students tend to ascribe to the liver. In many cases, thinking of difficult, almost-right answers is hard work, so the test maker tends to fill in the remaining letters with relatively easy-to-eliminate wrong answers.

Because there tends to be at least two seemingly right answers, the test taker who leaps for a single answer can easily be misled. For example, under the pressure of the real PCAT, you might be tempted to choose the first answer choice that seems correct, but it may turn out to be the almost-right answer, or what the test makers call "the most likely distracter." You need to read *all* the answer choices. If you do not see at least two possibly correct responses (that is, if you don't see what the test maker thought was difficult) you are probably in trouble.

"What if I know the answer? Shouldn't I just mark the answer sheet and keep going?"

The PCAT eliminates contestants by posing a large variety of questions around a limited basic content. Taking the PCAT is therefore more like running a marathon than a sprint. When running a sprint, the contestant simply runs as fast as possible from starting gun to finish line. In running a marathon, on the other hand, the contestant develops an overall plan well in advance with appropriate strategies for each part of the race. The runner then practices those strategies so that performance in the actual race is deliberate yet automatic. In preparing for and in taking the PCAT, you will do best if you have an overall plan and well-practiced specific strategies for reading comprehension. When you have decided on a strategy for answering multiple-choice questions, for example, it is less time-consuming and less risky to use that strategy consistently rather than sometimes using it and sometimes not. Remember that "consistently" means "every time" or "without exception." (It is also a word that sometimes appears in test questions, the meaning of "consistently" must be distinguished from "trend.")

When working with multiple-choice questions, we recommend that you use the following strategies consistently until they become habit:

1. Eliminate clearly wrong answers by putting a slash mark (/) through the identifying number.
2. Once you have identified at least two "right" answers, SLOW DOWN to make the best possible choice.

A word of warning: in many ways much of a student's classroom training runs counter to the deliberate, careful strategies suggested here for best performance on multiple-choice items. From junior high school on, many students have competed not only for the right answer, but for getting it faster. This focus on speed encourages students to rely on rote memory and intuitive leaps rather than rewarding those who carefully work their way to the correct answer. To benefit from these recommendations, you will need to practice deliberate strategies consistently until they are automatic.

But if the answer choices require so much thought, how can you find enough time in the reading subtest deliberately to select the right answer? We recommend that you learn to use the question analysis strategy below.

QUESTION ANALYSIS STRATEGY

For most readers, even good ones, recall is insufficient to pick the best answer on the PCAT Reading Comprehension test. In using the question analysis strategy, however, you read the question first so you know what to look for; then you search the passage for the passage sentence (usually only one) that gives the answer. Note that this step follows only after you have carefully highlighted the passage and drawn your mind map.

You will know when you have found the right passage sentence because of the number of important words (primarily *significant* nouns) that it has in common with the question. For example, if a question asks, "In what historical period was U.S. population growth the lowest," you can scan the passage given for "population growth" and "lowest." The passage sentence that provides the answer in this case reads: "This was the lowest rate of population growth recorded until the 'Great Depression' when the net growth rate fell to 7 per 1,000 population during the 1930–1935 period." Once you have found the passage sentence, which you can learn to do quickly with practice, choosing the right answer depends on precise understanding. Once again, this may require you to SLOW DOWN.

At first, you may find the question analysis strategy awkward and time-consuming. It is unlikely you have ever read this way before. However, practice will perfect this skill, which in turn will both increase your accuracy and ensure that you have enough time to complete this section of the test.

Question analysis is a bit like going to a grocery store with a shopping list. You can zip through the aisles checking items off on the list instead of wandering around and backtracking as you try to recall where you have seen the items you need.

With the question analysis strategy, follow these six steps:

1. Read the question first, working with one question at a time.

2. Underline the significant words in the question, primarily the nouns and active verbs.

3. Scan the passage looking for the passage sentence that contains the same words that you have underlined. Note that these words may appear in the passage sentence in a different order than the way they appear in the question, but you know you have found the right passage sentence by the number of words it shares with the question.

4. Put the number of the question in the margin of your test booklet.

5. You can learn to do steps 1–4 quickly, but now SLOW DOWN because you are looking for what the test maker thought was difficult, that is, you need to look for the right answer and the "almost-right" answer.

6. Answer the question carefully, working back and forth between passage and question. Pay special attention to the remaining words in the sentence, especially to the precise meaning of conjunctions, qualifiers such as adverbs and adjectives, and restrictive phrases.

Since part of your strategy is to read the questions first, analyze each question for the following:

- Can you pick out the significant nouns and verbs?
- Can you begin to anticipate where the difficulty in choosing the right answer might lie?

Look to the marked passage (fig. 3.1) for examples of what to look for in the passage. In addition, leave ample space for your own notes when you read passages.

At this time, do not worry about speed; you need to get the correct answer consistently before you attempt to get it quickly!

3.2.5 Remembering

Memorization and recall are linked to the reasoning skills and diagramming methods you worked on earlier. Developing your reasoning skills (chapter 1) will help to improve your short-term memory. Visual mapping skills are an aid to remembering details.

To remember important concepts, building your vocabulary and learn to extract information from the texts you read. Aids for locating and extracting information are given below.

Integrated with your reasoning ability, these skills and techniques will help you to become a highly skilled critical reader.

AIDS TO RECALLING FACTS AND DETAIL

To remember important concepts, follow these information locating aids:

1. Read with interest. This will help you recall facts. Associate facts and details with your needs regarding the outcome of the PCAT. These may include achieving a good PCAT score or being accepted into pharmacy school. This level of interest will keep facts at the surface of your memory for instant recall and use.

2. Observe and concentrate to develop good recall. We remember best those things that we find interesting, that require careful examination, and that invoke serious thought.

3. Read with the intention of recalling facts. As you read, decide which facts are important; not all printed facts are worth recalling. It is impractical to try to recall everything you read.

4. Develop optimal speed. This is tied to your rate of reading. Your rate of reading should never be so high as to interfere with understanding. Comprehension should never be sacrificed in favor of speed. Excessive speed will only compound problems for a student who has difficulty comprehending ideas and recalling facts. Your reading rate will increase over time as techniques improve. Taking a speed reading course will hurt and not help you to improve reading comprehension.

3.3 COMPREHENSION OF "CURRENT" INFORMATION

3.3.1 Definition

Current information includes but is not limited to lecture notes, laboratory notes, the information you gather from friends and learn through the news media, your textbooks, and study guides. To master any information, you must first comprehend it and decipher the various forms of reasoning embedded within the information. Good comprehension aims at developing reasoning skills, perceiving interrelationships between the various kinds of information, understanding given and implied assumptions, and, finally, deriving direct and indirect (or implied) conclusions.

The material below includes sections on logic, interpretation, a discussion of reading comprehension questions, and error analysis.

3.3.2 Applying Logic to Comprehension

In our culture generally, and on national standardized tests in particular, form and syntax in written text are governed by the language and rules of logic. Thus, we use logical reasoning both to understand what we read and to determine the way we organize our thoughts when we write. Logical reasoning should also govern our understanding of test questions, of what is being asked and how to choose an answer.

In logic, there are premises, at least three by convention. "Premise" is a logician's term. Although each academic discipline is governed by the use of logic, each has developed its own specialized language. In law, for example, the word for premise is "evidence"; in medicine, "symptoms"; in biology, "data." No matter what the discipline, logic supplies the rules; that is, although the "labels" might change from discipline to discipline, the "rules" of academic thinking stay the same. Thus, if you recognize a pattern in the data, the evidence, or the symptoms, you might draw a conclusion. In logic, recognizing a pattern to draw a conclusion is called "making an inference." Just as each discipline has its own word for premise, so each has its own word for conclusion. In law, this would be "verdict"; in medicine, "diagnosis"; in biology "results" or "conclusions"; and in an essay, it would be "thesis."

Conclusions come in three degrees of certainty. First, a hypothesis is a conclusion drawn that has not yet been tested. Second, a conclusion suggested is one that has been tested somewhat, but not enough to make it a conclusion confirmed. The third and most certain is a conclusion confirmed.

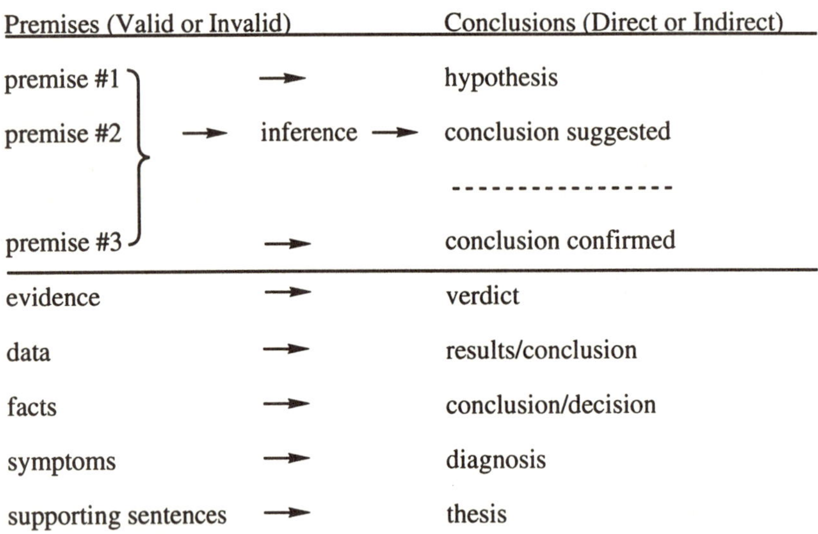

Fig. 3.3 — Model of a Logical Argument

The broken line between "conclusion suggested" and "conclusion confirmed" represents a standard we often set for ourselves. This helps determine when a conclusion moves from one that is suggested to one that is confirmed. For example, the Food and Drug Administration sets the standard that governs when a medicine is declared effective and can be put on the market. That is, if a certain percentage of patients taking the drug are made to feel better, and the side effects are acceptable, and when a certain amount of time has passed to make sure that there are no undesirable long-term side-effects, etc., the medicine is declared effective, or, in the language of the model, the conclusion suggested becomes a conclusion confirmed.

In a text, you can tell by the syntax whether a sentence is a conclusion suggested or a conclusion confirmed. That is, if the sentence is a conclusion suggested, it will contain the conditional verbs: may, seem, can (as in "it *can* be inferred"), etc.; or adverbs such as *probably, primarily, most likely, most nearly,* etc. In logic, these conditional verbs and/or adverbs signify to you, the reader, that you are to read the sentence according to the rules of inductive logic, that is, the conclusion is to be judged according to probability. This is different from a deductively phrased statement that you are to judge according to logical validity. Logical validity states that if the premises are true, then the conclusion must also be true.

Perhaps an example will help: you ask me to dinner at your house and I say "I may come." This is a very different from "I will come." The first statement is to be read as "I may, or I may not" and you must judge whether to expect me or not on the basis of probability. On the other hand, if I say "I will come," I mean "all other things being equal, I will be there." Clever students have an additional difficulty. They tend to look for the obscure but possible answer rather than choose the probable answer that seems too easy. Do not base your answer on either possibility or certainty. Remember: the directions on the PCAT tell you to pick the "one best answer."

3.3.3 Interpretation of Scientific Information

This section will help you understand the patterns you apply to the comprehension of scientific reading material and show you how to overcome any shortcomings you may have.

The interpretation of scientific reading material is linked to the following statements of reading comprehension skills. Examine your understanding of scientific reading material by applying the questions given here.

1. Extracting the central idea:
   - How is the central idea extracted from a passage?

2. Cause and effect statements:
   - Which statements in the passage are related as cause (C) and effect (E)? Mark them with the symbol C/E for use in answering test items.

3. Developing interrelationships including chronological mapping:
   - Is there a set of time-related events in the passage? Draw a time-line as a chronological map to understand the variations with time.

4. Developing comparison/contrast abilities:
   - Are there compare/contrast items or issues? Mark them with the symbol C/C. Look through the practice passage on connective tissues (Exercise 1) and review the skills taught there.

5. Understanding assumptions:
   - Are there any direct or stated assumptions? Indirect or unstated assumptions?

6. Conclusions:
   - Are there any direct or obvious conclusions?
     Indirect or implied conclusions?

Some students find that they frequently score less than 80 percent correct even though they are working for accuracy rather than for speed. If this is true for you, take time to work on your basic reading skills. A speed reading course will not help. Instead, we recommend *Active Reading in the Arts and Sciences* by Shirley Quinn and Susan Irvings which may be purchased from Betz Publishing and is an excellent reading development book.

One key component in learning to read better is to try reading new and difficult material. Work out a program for active reading by selecting new material from school texts. In addition, read at least one of the national science magazines such as *Scientific American,* or the weeklies *Science* and *Science News.* These magazines and the *Encyclopaedia Britannica*, for example, are especially good reading resources for PCAT preparation for the following reasons:

- they are approximately the same difficulty as PCAT passages;
- they are similar to the information given in your textbook; and
- they are written for a generally well-educated but not necessarily scientifically educated audience. This means that each article helps you to review the basic scientific knowledge that is tested in the PCAT. Reading a scientific magazine each week has the added bonus of keeping you abreast of current issues in science.

3.3.4 Reading Comprehension Questions

The reading comprehension questions on the PCAT measure your ability to read and understand a passage. The test generally will have one passage taken from each of the following categories:

Biological Sciences:	medicine, botany, zoology, human biology, pharmacology
Physical Sciences:	chemistry, astronomy, technology, ecology, geology
Argument:	the presentation of a definite point of view on a current subject (physical or biological sciences)

The purpose of the reading comprehension questions is to measure the ability to read with understanding, insight, and discrimination. Reading comprehension questions explore the examinee's ability to analyze a written passage from several perspectives. These perspectives are the ability to recognize both explicitly stated elements in the passage and assumptions underlying statements or arguments in the passage, as well as the implications of those statements or arguments. Because the written passage upon which reading comprehension questions are based presents discussion of a particular topic, there is ample context for analyzing a variety of relationships; for example, the function of a word in relation to a later segment of the passage, the relationships and connections among the various ideas in the passage, or the relation of the author to his or her topic or to the audience.

There are six types of reading comprehension questions. These types focus on:

(1) the main idea or primary purpose of the passage
(2) information explicitly stated in the passage
(3) information or ideas implied or suggested by the author
(4) possible application of the author's ideas to other situations
(5) the author's logic, reasoning, or persuasive techniques
(6) the tone of the passage or the author's attitude as it is revealed in the language used

In the PCAT, usually there are at least two relatively long reading comprehension passages, each providing the basis for answering seven to twelve questions, and two relatively short passages, each providing the basis for answering three or four questions. Each of the four passages are usually drawn from different subject matter areas (either biological sciences or physical sciences).

Possible Reading Comprehension Approaches:

1. Since reading passages are drawn from many different disciplines and sources, <u>you should not expect to be familiar with the material in all the passages</u>. However, you should not be discouraged by encountering material with which you are not familiar. Questions are to be

answered on the basis of the information provided in the passage, and you are not expected to rely on outside knowledge, which you may or may not have, of a particular topic.

2. There are different strategies for approaching reading comprehension questions; you must decide which one works most effectively for you. Try using the different strategies as you work with the reading comprehension questions. The choice of strategies includes: reading the passage very closely and then proceeding to the questions; or scanning the passage closely; and reading the questions first, then reading the passage closely. You may find that different strategies work better for different kinds of passages; for example, it might be helpful with a difficult or unfamiliar passage to read through the questions first.

3. You should analyze the passage carefully before answering the questions. As with any kind of close and thoughtful reading, you should be sensitive to clues that will help you understand less explicit aspects of the passage.

4. Try to separate main ideas from supporting ideas or evidence; try also to separate the author's own ideas or attitudes from information he or she is merely presenting.

5. It is important to note transitions from one idea to the next and to examine the relationships among the different ideas or parts of the passage: Are they contrasting? Are they complementary?

6. Consider both the points the author makes and the conclusions he or she draws and also how and why those points are made or conclusions drawn.

7. You may find it helpful to underline or mark key parts of the passage. For example, you might underline main ideas or important arguments or circle transitional words that will help you map the logical structure of the passage (*although, nevertheless, correspondingly,* and the like) or descriptive words that will help you identify the author's attitude toward a particular idea or person.

8. You may want to mark an important fact or idea, but don't waste too much time underlining or making notes in the margin of the test book. Try to get a sense of the principal ideas, facts, and organization of the passage.

9. Read each question carefully and be certain that you understand exactly what is being asked.

10. *Always* read all the answer choices before selecting the best answer.

11. The best answer is the one that most accurately and most completely answers the question being posed. Be careful not to pick an answer choice simply because it is a true statement; be careful also not to be misled by answer choices that are only partially true or only partially satisfy the problem posed in the question.

12. Answer the questions on the basis of the information (stated or implied) as provided in the passage and do not rely on outside knowledge. Your own views or opinions may sometimes conflict with the views expressed or the information provided in the passage; be sure that you work within the context provided by the passage. You should not expect to agree with everything you encounter in reading passages.

13. Read each passage carefully. Follow the author's reasoning. Notice attitude, tone, and general style.

14. In answering main idea questions, don't be distracted by statements that are true according to the passage but that are secondary to the central point.

3.3.5 Errors in Reading and How to Avoid Them

1. Continued Analytical Reading Problems

Analytical reading requires a precise, problem-solving approach. If you have trouble reading the questions precisely enough to reason out the correct answer, you need to obtain a copy of *Problem Solving and Comprehension* by Arthur Whimbey and Jack Lochhead. Almost any college student can benefit from doing the exercises they prescribe.

2. Careless Reading of the Questions

Do you read each question analytically? Do you circle important qualifiers such as "some"? In compare/contrast questions, do you pay attention to which set the question refers to? Do you recognize when a question has more than one proposition? If your errors result from reading the question too quickly, SLOW DOWN until you are getting all or nearly all of the answers correct; then slowly build for speed.

3. Careless or Hasty Reading of the Passage

Are you finding the correct sentence in the passage but still failing to get the correct answer? Finding the correct passage sentence is only the first step. Learn to do this quickly. After that, SLOW DOWN to make sure that you thoroughly understand what is said, carefully working back and forth between the question and the passage sentence until you are certain of the meaning. The passage should be read as evidence and you, as the reader, are the detective looking for very precise clues.

4. Variations in Degree of Concentration

Do you find some passages more interesting and some less interesting than others? This is natural. Nonetheless, finding the passage *too* interesting can cause you to waste precious time, while finding the passage uninteresting can cause you to lose concentration. Instead, approach each passage and its attendant set of questions as though it were an enclosed puzzle.

For the PCAT, as a first step to improve your concentration, eliminate unconscious breaks by taking a deliberate break as soon as you need it. Work with a clock in front of you. Make your break deliberate by standing, stretching, or moving around for 2 to 5 minutes. Then, when you get back to studying, try to concentrate for just a little longer before your next break. Just as you need to build your speed slowly, you should also increase your concentration little by little. To prepare for the PCAT in its entirety, you need to work on building your concentration.

When you analyze practice tests (or class tests), do you notice that your correct answers and wrong answers tend to come in groups? That is, you will be doing well and then suddenly get three or more answers wrong in a cluster? This pattern indicates that you slip in and out of focus.

To correct for this, you need to develop your concentration. In this situation, do not blame question difficulty if you get the wrong answers.

5. Slow Start, Slow Finish

Do you perform better on the second reading passage than on the first? It is a good idea to bring a practice reading passage (newspaper or journal article) with you on the test day itself. Working on a practice reading set in the last minutes of your break will enable you to get a running start for the reading test.

Does your performance slack off as you progress toward the end of the test? If so, you need to build for stamina. After all, 45 minutes is a long time for sustained concentration when you are not reading for entertainment or pleasure. As with speed, build for stamina slowly.

6. Early Panic, Late Anxiety

Do you look at the first question and sense your mind go blank? If so, don't answer it. Move on until you find a question you can answer with confidence. Then come back to the first one. You may find your anxiety rising as the time passes and you become increasingly aware that you are never going to finish unless you speed up. Try to get your pacing under control *before* you take the PCAT. Speeding up under pressure tends to increase the number of careless errors. You do not get extra points for answering every question on the reading test. Your score will depend on how many questions you answer *correctly*. In the real PCAT, save the last minute on each subtest to fill in a preselected guess answer for any unanswered question (choose any number, but use it consistently). Unlike the SATs, there is no penalty for wrong answers.

7. Question Type Preference

Do you find you do better on one type of question than another? If so, increase your practice on the type that gives you more difficulty. Each of us tends to work hardest on what we do best, so you must practice to reverse that habit. The best learning strategy for improvement dictates that you work to overcome your weaknesses.

8. Problems with Multiple-Choice Questions

Multiple-choice questions take more analyzing time than conventional questions (open-ended or true/false). When working multiple-choice questions, you should eliminate three answer choices after careful scrutiny. You should slow down to consider the remaining two out of the four possibilities. When choosing the right answer proves difficult, put slash marks through clearly wrong answers or you will waste time by rereading them. It is a good idea to practice multiple-choice reading questions until you are consistent in both accuracy and speed because multiple-choice questions tend to dominate the reading comprehension portion of the PCAT.

9. Trouble with Negative Stems

The presence of negative words in a question or answer makes the item more difficult. We are not accustomed to reading for what is not, for what is false, or for the exception. The test maker knows this. You will find more negative-stemmed questions in the biology subtest than in chemistry, since biology does not offer as many options for definition questions. A test maker creates a problem by posing a negative-stemmed question.

When you see a negative-stemmed item, circle the negative word and SLOW DOWN. You need a separate strategy for these items. Consider each answer and decide whether it is true or false, writing a "T" or "F" next to each. If you aren't sure, mark "?T" or "?F". Force yourself to choose. When you do this, the answer should be apparent; but pay attention when you choose your answer—true answers are easier to approve than false answers.

Especially time consuming are the questions that start, "All of the following are true **EXCEPT**...." As the exam date approaches, if you find you are still working too slowly in the reading section, consider answering all **EXCEPT** questions last. Remember, answering the single hardest or most time-consuming PCAT question is not rewarded with extra points. It is a better strategy to spend the same amount of time answering two or three easy questions correctly.

10. Practicing Keyed-Choice (I, II, III, IV) Questions

Many students continue to have problems with inductively phrased questions. If this is true for you, reread section 1.2 (Reasoning Skills for PCAT Preparation) in Chapter 1. Compare inductively phrased questions with deductively phrased questions. Do you see why they are written inductively? Do you see how inductive phrasing allows for more than one possible answer? Do you remind yourself that inductive phrasing is a clue to remind you that you should choose the *best* or most likely answer?

If most of your reading has been in textbooks, you may be unfamiliar with inductive reasoning in text. Regular reading of research reports and *Scientific American* will help familiarize you with this type of reasoning.

These are advanced level, logical reading questions and have appeared in some versions of the PCAT. Each question or test item consists of a given logical statement. Your job is to classify the given statement using one of the keyed-choices (I, II, II or IV).

I = explicitly supported
II = implicitly supported
III = contradicted
IV = neither supported nor contradicted

Two scientific passages (I and II) each with four questions are being provided here to illustrate the format of such questions and how to answer them.

Passage I:

From the earliest medical records to the present, physicians and laymen have postulated an association between diet and the development of cancer. This has proved a fertile area for a wide range of speculation extending from food faddists to epidemiologists. An objective approach views diet composition and practices in food preparation as possible environmental factors which may influence tumor development.

There are large demographic differences in the prevalence of gastric cancer. Japan, Chile, Austria, Finland, and Iceland have rates (predominantly in males) four or more times those of U.S. Caucasians. In the U.S. and Europe, higher rates are noted for gastric as well as esophageal cancer among low income groups.

Certain ethnic groups in the U.S. appear to have increased risk. Studies of dietary practices in patients with gastric cancer have yielded few or no significant differences from control groups. An association with alcohol intake has been suggested and denied. The increased use of laxatives or mineral oil in affected individuals has been noted. It has been suggested, but remains unproved, that the high incidence of this tumor in Iceland is related to the large intake of smoked food in association with a low intake of vitamin C. It has been pointed out that Japanese prefer talc-dusted rice and that the talc may contain asbestos. The latter is implicated in the development of gastrointestinal cancer, especially gastric cancer. It is postulated that the asbestos-contaminated talc on rice is the carcinogen or cocarcinogen responsible for the high incidence of stomach cancer in Japan.

Death rates for carcinoma of the large bowel (colonic cancer) have a strong negative correlation with those of gastric cancer, the one being common where the other is rare. In the U.S. and England, colonic cancer is second only to lung cancer in numbers of deaths. It has been suggested that cancer of the colon in New Yorkers is associated with a high fat intake. In Japan where colonic cancer is uncommon, fat intake is about 12% of calories and mostly of the unsaturated type compared to the 40 to 44$ figure in the United States.

Japanese immigrants, and especially their children born in the U.S., have a much higher incidence of this disease than those in Japan. The same has been noted for Puerto Ricans living in Puerto Rico and on the mainland of the United States.

Japanese with colonic cancer have a higher socioeconomic status than those with rectal cancer and tend to eat diets with more calories in the form of fats and fresh fruit. Czechs have approximately twice the U.S. rate for intestinal cancer. Their dietary intake is appreciably lower in animal-derived protein and fat and in vitamins. While their caloric intake is the same, it is derived more from vegetable sources than is the American diet. Contrary to the observations with carcinoma of the esophagus and stomach, the incidence of colonic cancer in the U.S. does not vary appreciably with color or socioeconomic status.

Read the items numbered (1 through 4) and classify them as (I, II, III or IV). Only one keyed-choice is possible per item. Pick the best response after reading the above passage.

Possible Keyed-Choices:

I. explicitly supported
II. implicitly supported
III. contradicted
IV. neither supported nor contradicted

1. Environmental factors, like cooking methods such as frying (high fat) or steaming (low fat) may mitigate the effects of cocarcinogens like the talc used on Japanese rice.

2. The incidence of colon cancer is likely to be related to the amount of unsaturated fat present in the diet regardless of ethnic origin.

3. Scientists have not yet determined which factors in socioeconomic status, diet, and other environmental conditions are most pertinent in determining the risk of cancer, but certain patterns in isolated ethnic groups are at least partially useful as predictors of risk of specific cancers.

4. A diet high in vegetables, but low in fat, is a reliable prophylaxis for intestinal carcinomas.

Passage II:

Proton magnetic resonance testing enables researchers to distinguish magnetically different protons present in a molecule by counting the signal emitted. Each magnetically different proton sends a separate signal.

There are two means by which protons can be considered "identical"—by symmetry or by being geminal (twins on the same carbon atom). The four protons of methane are all geminal and so only one signal is observed. Similarly, all six protons of ethane are identical by symmetry. But the two methyl groups of methyl ethanoate (methyl acetate) are not identical. One methyl group is attached to a carbonyl carbon while the other is attached to an oxygen. Each methyl group is then in a different magnetic environment. Propane is symmetrical about carbon-2 and so has two magnetically different types of protons. Propane offers the chance to make a careless error in selecting the number of magnetically different protons present. There are four.

Protons (c) and (d) are not identical. Proton (c) is cis to a methyl group while proton (d) is trans to the methyl group. Again, this gives a different magnetic environment to these protons. In an analogous fashion, protons (c) and (d) of 1,2-dimethyl-cyclopropane are not identical. Here (d) is cis to two methyl group while (c) is cis to two protons. Different magnetic environments. (S)-2-bromobutane is a more difficult case. Protons (c) and (d) here are again superficially the same, but in fact they are not. They are "diastereotopic" protons. Replacing each of these protons with some other group will give diastereomers—easily distinguished by chemical and physical properties. Proton (d) will "feel" the effects of the bromine atom of carbon-2 more than will proton (c) in the configuration shown. Each is in a magnetically different environment. If replacement of each of two suspected identical protons with another group yields enantiomers, the protons are called "enantiotopic" and are magnetically indistinguishable.

Read the items numbered (5 through 8) and classify them as (I, II, III or IV). See directions given after Passage I.

5. The author advocates the use of diastereomers to distinguish geminally identical proton nuclei in methane.

6. Diastereotopic protons are either geminal or symmetrical.

7. If apparently identical protons yield enantiomers when another group is substituted for each member of the original pair, then the original proton pair may be considered identical.

8. Propane offers a good example of diastereotopic protons.

Answers to Passage I:

1. IV neither supported nor contradicted (cooking is only mentioned as food preparation in paragraph 1; no relationship between cooking and talc or cooking and cancer is made; no mention of ameliorating any environmental factors is introduced as a remedy or preventative).

2. II supported in paragraphs 4 and 5.

3. II this sentence should be a fair statement of the key idea of the passage, and is therefore implicitly supported.

4. III contradicted in paragraph 6—see Czech diet (despite current thinking on the advisability of vegetarian, low fat diets!!

Answers to Passage II:

5. IV neither supported nor contradicted, this statement is primarily nonsense, and depends on a misreading of the entire passage. The tip-off is that the author advocates absolutely nothing.

6. III definition in lines 8-10.

7. I supported in lines 35-39.

8. II information in lines 19 and 31 combined.

If you need more practice with questions that primarily test your logical and analytical reasoning, you can find extra practice materials either in an LSAT or GRE guide (GRE test books are available from Betz Publishing Company). Whenever an actual test is used it obviously provides the most accurate material from which to study. An excellent first book in learning how to improve reasoning ability is *With Good Reason: An Introduction to Informal Fallacies* by S. Morris Engel.

11. Verbal Ability

Synonyms may cause problems. If you encounter words or phrases that appear to be synonymous and you know synonyms cause you trouble, SLOW DOWN and DOUBLE CHECK. Do the words *really* mean the same thing?

To be synonymous, words must be on the same level of classification. As an example, "dog" and "German shepherd" are not synonyms because "German shepherd" is only one kind of canine. A discussion of synonyms is actually a discussion about the relationship between the two terms under consideration. There are three ways to illustrate this relationship: with outlines, Venn diagrams, and analogical reasoning.

- An outline would look like this:
  I. Canine
     A. Dog
        1. German shepherd
        2. poodle
     B. Wolf
        1. red
        2. grey
- A Venn diagram illustrating the same relationship would look as follows:

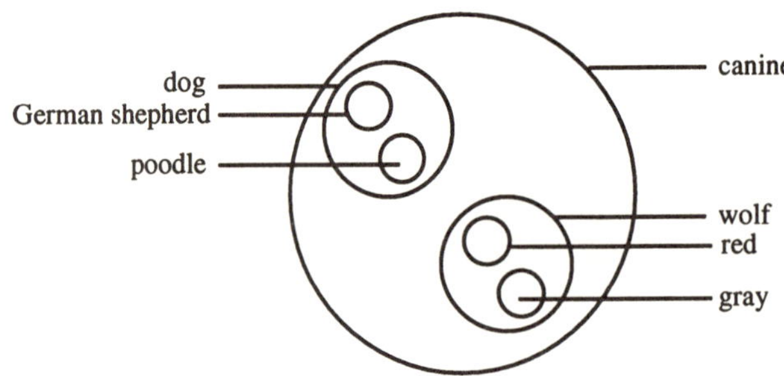

  Learn how to draw Venn diagrams if they are unfamiliar to you. Venn diagrams can clarify the concept "not." Practice exercises using Venn diagrams can be found in both the LSAT and GRE practice guides.

- See item 3 (section 1.2 in chapter 1) to review analogical reasoning.

12. Double Propositions

Questions with more than one proposition, or answers with more than one variable, can also cause trouble. Once again, SLOW DOWN. Remember the correct answer must satisfy all the conditions given.

13. Proportional Reasoning

Students often have trouble with questions that include the words "increase" and "decrease," especially when they require proportional reasoning. This is true in PCAT Biology, Chemistry, and Quantitative Ability as well. Draw a sketch in the margin of the test booklet and use arrows to help you visualize what is being asked and to facilitate choosing the right answer.

14. Speed, Accuracy, and Concentration

The most common PCAT error pattern is misunderstanding the outcomes of speed, accuracy, and concentration. Managing time during the exam is a complex matter. Figuring out how many minutes per question on average you have for each section of the test does not help, simply because the test maker does not expect you to spend the same amount of time on each question. Rather, the test maker carefully balances relatively quick-to-answer questions with those that take longer. As a sophisticated test taker, you need to develop sense of timing for working on the questions.

Moreover, keep in mind that speed is always a trade-off for accuracy. This is as true on the PCAT as it is on the highway. Too many students confuse the two; that is, they believe their primary problem on tests is speed, whereas they really have an accuracy problem that must be dealt with first. If you work on speed first, you will only get the wrong answer faster. Once your accuracy is high, then (and *only* then) build for speed SLOWLY.

Negative-stem test questions (i.e., questions that contain **false** or **not** or **except**) usually take longer to answer because you must be careful in checking your answer against what is being asked. Negative-stem questions cause added difficulties simply because students neither slow down nor change strategy when answering them. When you see a negative-stem question, SLOW DOWN first, then ask yourself whether each answer choice is TRUE or FALSE and put a "T" or "F" next to the letter. If you are not sure, guess with a "?T" or an "?F"; when you are finished, check your answer choice against the question stem one more time.

Do not let your unconscious mind determine when you take your breaks. Rather, go into the examination knowing that after every thirty questions or so you are going to sit back and stretch and roll your head around to ease the strain in your neck and shoulders. If you do this, you will be taking the test rather than letting the test take you!

15. Learning Error Patterns

Finally, remember to analyze your errors! As you continue to work reading passages, add your errors to the error journal you started in chapter 1 (section 1.1.3) and analyze the data for repeated error patterns. An important part of improving your performance is developing your skills as a self-conscious test taker. Refer also to section 3.3.4 in this chapter.

When you study, you should spend about two-thirds of your time working to correct your errors, that is, working from your error journal, and only one-third of your time reviewing what you already know or do well. Unless you do this deliberately, you will tend to work longest on what you already know and can do well. After all, success feels better than concentrating on errors. Correcting error patterns is not easy because we all tend to revert carelessly to old habits. Breaking error patterns requires long-term dedicated and conscious effort, but it can be done!

3.4 Practice Passages and Items
Passage #1:

Growth and Formation of Bones

The "cartilage" skeleton is completely formed at the end of three months of pregnancy. During subsequent months of gestation, ossification and growth occur.

Longitudinal growth of bones continues in a definite sequence until approximately fifteen years of age in the female and sixteen in the male. Longitudinal growth should not be confused with bone maturation and remodeling, which are processes continuing until the age of twenty-one in both the male and female. This pattern of maturation is so regular that an individual's age can be determined with amazing accuracy from radiologic examination of his or her bones.

It is sometimes stated that bone is preformed in the cartilage, since the majority of embryonic bones do resemble the future skeleton in shape and composition; however, it is incorrect to state that cartilage actually turns into bone. Cartilage merely represents the environment in which the bone develops.

Formation

Chemical Composition
The strong protein matrix of bone is responsible for its resilience when tension is applied, whereas the salts deposited in this matrix prevent crushing when pressure is applied. A substance known as hydroxyapatite $[Ca_3 (PO_4)_2]_3 \cdot Ca(OH)_2$ makes up the major portion of salts present in bone. Small amounts of calcium carbonate ($CaCO_3$) are also present.

Deposition of Bone
Bone develops from spindle-shaped cells called **osteoblasts**, which are found beneath the periosteum (the fibrovascular membrane covering the bone) and in the endosteum, which lines the marrow cavity. The first function of the osteoblasts is that of secreting a protein substance that polymerizes to form the tough, leather-like matrix. Calcium salts are then precipitated within the matrix, giving the bone its characteristic quality of hardness. For these salts to be deposited it is necessary that calcium first combine with phosphate, producing calciumphosphate ($CaH PO_4$); this substance is slowly converted over a period of several weeks into hydroxyapatite.

Regulation of Deposition
Deposition of bone is regulated partially by the amount of strain on the bone—the more strain the greater the deposition. Bones in casts, therefore, will waste away, whereas continued and excessive strain will cause the bone to grow thick and strong. In addition, a break in the bone will stimulate injured osteocytes to proliferate, secreting large quantities of matrix for the deposition of new bone.

Reabsorption of Bone
Large cells called **osteoclasts** are present in almost all cavities of bone, and function to cause reabsorption of bone. It is thought that this is brought about by the secretion of enzymes that digest the protein portion of bone and split the salts. These phosphate and calcium salts are then absorbed into the surrounding extracellular fluid.

The strength and, in some instances, the size of the skeletal bone will depend on the comparative activity of the bone. For example, it is obvious that during the growth period deposition is more active than reabsorption. The role of the osteoclast has not been definitely established, but it is known to be associated with the removal of dead bone from the inner side during remodeling. As a result, the medullary cavity enlarges, and the bone itself is prevented from becoming overly thick and heavy. Osteoblastic deposition continues to counteract the never ending process of reabsorption, even when the bones are no longer capable of growth.

It is possible for crooked bones to become straight due to this continual process. A broken bone that has healed crooked in a child will straighten in a matter of a few years.

During the four-day flight of Gemini IV in 1965, one of the astronauts lost between 1 and 12 percent of his bone mass, as measured by x-ray of his hands and feet. The flight of Gemini V, which lasted eight days, caused losses of more than 20 percent. As a result of these findings, exercises in flight were prescribed that were found to reduce this loss.

Intramembranous Ossification

There are two types of ossification. The first of these is intramembranous ossification, a process in which dense connective membranes are replaced by deposits of inorganic calcium salts, thus forming bone. The membrane itself becomes the **periosteum** (around bone), while immediately within the periosteum can be found compact bone with an inner core of **spongy** or **cancellous bone.**

Endochondral Ossification

Most bones form by the process of **endochondral ossification,** the replacement of cartilaginous structures with bone. Growth in length of a bone occurs at the growth plate, which consists of a number of layers of cartilage cells lying between the epiphysis (knoblike extremity of a bone) and the diaphysis (the shaft or central portion of a bone). The basal layer of cells is abundantly supplied with blood, and this layer proliferates, producing more cartilage cells and adding to the length of the bone. The upper layers of cells are thus lifted away from the source of blood and nutrients and are subsequently ossified.

As a long bone increases in length, there is a proportional increase in its diameter, owing to periosteal deposition of layers of compact tissue. These layers are thickest in the middle of the shaft and taper toward the epiphysis, which remains essentially cancellous. Simultaneously, the cancellous interior of the diaphysis is destroyed, leading to the formation of the marrow canal. The spongy bone of the epiphysis is left intact.

Ossification of the epiphysis follows a generally predictable pattern. The age of the skeleton can be determined by the presence and size of various mesossification centers. For instance, the physician can determine if a baby is at term by ascertaining whether or not the distal femoral epiphysis is ossified.

Longitudinal growth is dependent, then, on the growth plate at the junction of the diaphysis and epiphysis. Growth in the diameter of bone occurs primarily by the deposit of bony tissue beneath the periosteum. In a short time, only two thin strips of tissue, the growth plates, remain between the epiphysis and the diaphysis. When these two final sites have filled with osseous tissue, longitudinal growth is complete and growth is no longer possible. The initial shape assumed by a bone during its formation is genetically determined. Extrinsic factors such as muscle strength, mechanical stress, and biochemical environment assume a function in determining the shape of a bone. Wolff's law reflects the role of mechanical forces acting on bone and, briefly stated, suggests that the structure of a bone is dependent on its function.

1. Which of the following is NOT a function of the skeletal system?
   A. Support tissues
   B. Protect vital organs and other tissues
   C. Hematopoiesis
   D. Filtration of blood

2. The skeletal system is composed of ________ bones?
   A. 1,206
   B. 601
   C. 2,010
   D. 206

3. Which of the following is NOT a part of the appendicular skeletal system?
   A. Shoulders
   B. Vertebrae
   C. Pelvic girdle
   D. Arms

4. Ossification of the skeletal system begin
   A. in utero.
   B. during puberty.
   C. during first three months of pregnancy.
   D. after the first three months of pregnancy.

5. The major portion of salts found in bone is represented by
   A. hydroxyapatite.
   B. calcium carbonate.
   C. calcium chloride.
   D. sodium chloride.

6. Bone develops from cells responsible for secreting a protein matrix, in which salts are precipitated. These cells are called
   A. fibroblast.
   B. ameloblast.
   C. osteocytes.
   D. osteoblast.

7. Bone deposition is regulated *primarily* by
   A. genetic coding.
   B. stress.
   C. age.
   D. cartilage.

8. Before hydroxyapatite can be formed, calcium must first combine with
   A. phosphate.
   B. protein.
   C. oxygen.
   D. carbon.

9. Phosphate and calcium salts freed as a result of bone reabsorption are absorbed into the
   A. small intestine.
   B. lymphatic system.
   C. extracellular fluids.
   D. bone matrix.

10. Bones of the face and skull are formed by the process of
    A. endochondral ossification.
    B. osteoclastic activity.
    C. intramembranous ossification.
    D. Wolff's Law.

11. Longitudinal growth of bones continue until age
    A. 25 in males and 24 in females.
    B. 16 in males and 15 in females.
    C. 19 in males and 18 in females.
    D. puberty in males and females.

12. The bone found immediately beneath the periosteum is called
    A. spongy bone.
    B. compact bone.
    C. cancellous bone.
    D. long bone.

13. Growth in bone length occurs
    A. in the shaft.
    B. at the sutures.
    C. at the epiphysis.
    D. in the growth plate.

14. Which statement is incorrect?
   - **A.** Longitudinal growth of bone is complete when the growth plates are completely ossified.
   - **B.** Cartilage skeletal will turn to bony skeletal.
   - **C.** Strain and injury will cause bone to grow thick and strong.
   - **D.** Osteoclast is known to be associated with bone reabsorption.

15. The fibrovascular membrane covering bone is called the
   - **A.** peritoneum.
   - **B.** osseous membrane.
   - **C.** endosteum.
   - **D.** periosteum.

16. All of the following statements are correct EXCEPT:
   - **A.** Reabsorption is less active than deposition in the growth period of the bone.
   - **B.** Some bones form by the process of mitrochondrial ossification.
   - **C.** In a long bone, the periosteal deposition of layers makes the bone taper toward the cancellous epiphysis.
   - **D.** The age of the skeleton can be determined by the location and size of mesossification centers.

Passage #2:

Mitosis and Meiosis

All organisms that reproduce sexually develop from a single cell, the **zygote**, produced by the union of two cells, the **germ cells** or **gametes** (a **spermatozoon** from the male and an **ovum** from the female). The union of an egg and a spermatozoon is called **fertilization**. The zygote produced by fertilization develops into a new individual of the same species as the parents. Every cell of the individual, with the exception of gametes, contains the same number of chromosomes. In the somatic cells of a plant or an animal, chromosomes are paired, one member of each pair originally derived from one parent, the other member from the other parent. A member of a pair of chromosomes is called a **homologue**, and commonly we speak of pairs of chromosomes (or homologues) when we refer to the chromosome number of a species. Man has forty-six chromosomes or twenty-three pairs, an onion has eight pairs, a toad has eleven pairs, a mosquito has three pairs, and so on. Homologues of each pair are alike, but the pairs are generally different. The original chromosome number of each cell (diploid number) is preserved during successive nuclear divisions involved in the growth and development of a multicellular organism.

Mitosis

The continuity of the chromosomal set is maintained by **cell division**, which is called **mitosis.** At the time of cell division the nucleus becomes completely reorganized. Mitosis takes place in a series of consecutive stages known as prophase, anaphase, and telophase. In a somatic cell the nucleus divides by mitosis in such a fashion that each of the two daughter cells receives exactly the same number and kind of chromosomes as the parent cell.

Each chromosome duplicates some time during **interphase,** before the visible mitotic process begins. At this stage and at early **prophase** chromosomes appear as extended and slender threads. At late prophase chromosomes become short, compact rods by a process of spiral packing. A spindle arises between the two centrioles and the chromosomes line up across the equatorial plane of the spindle at the **metaphase** plate. At **anaphase** each chromosome separates, forming two daughter chromosomes, which go to opposite poles of the cell. Finally, at **telophase** the daughter chromosomes at each pole resolve themselves into a reticulum and two daughter nuclei are formed.

In mitosis the original chromosome number is preserved during the successive nuclear division. Since the somatic cells are derived from the zygote by mitosis, they all contain the normal double set, or diploid number (2^n), of chromosomes.

Meiosis

If the gametes (ovum and spermatozoon) were diploid, the resulting zygote would have twice the diploid chromosomes number. To avoid this, each gamete undergoes a special type of cell division called **meiosis**, which reduces the normal diploid set of chromosomes to a single (**haploid**) set (**n**). Thus, when the ovum and spermatozoon unite in fertilization, the resulting **zygote** is diploid. The meiotic process is characteristic of all plants and animals that reproduce sexually and it takes place in the course of gametogenesis.

Meiosis is the reduction of the chromosome number by means of two nuclear divisions, the **first** and **second meiotic divisions**, that involve only a single division of the chromosomes.

The essentials of the process are simple. The homologous chromosomes, distinguished by their identical morphologic characteristics, pair longitudinally; they lie in close contact, forming a bivalent. Each chromosome is composed of two spiral filaments called the **chromatids**. The bivalent thus contains four chromatids and is also called a **tetrad**. In the tetrad each chromatid of the homologue has a single pairing partner. Portions of these paired chromatids may be exchanged from one homologue to the other, giving rise to cross-shaped figures, which are called **chiasmata**. Chiasma is a cytologic manifestation of an underlying genetic phenomenon called **crossing over**.

At metaphase I the bivalents arrange themselves on the spindle, and at anaphase I the homologous chromosomes and their two associated chromatids migrate to opposite poles. Thus, in the first meiotic division the monologous pairs of chromosomes are segregated. After a short interphase, the two chromatids of each homologue separate in the second meiotic division, so that the original four chromatids are distributed into each of the four gametes. The result is four nuclei with only a single set of chromosomes.

In the male, all four cells develop into spermatozoa. In the female, one cell develops into an ovum, and the other three become small **polar bodies**. The formation of germ cells in plants is complicated because before fertilization the haploid products of meiosis undergo two or more mitotic divisions. However, the essential features of the meiotic process are similar in all sexually reproducing plants and animals.

17. All organisms that reproduce sexually develop from the
   A. gamete.
   B. zygote.
   C. ovum.
   D. homologue.

18. The chromosomes duplicate during
   A. anaphase.
   B. telophase.
   C. interphase.
   D. prophase.

19. The zygote contains the _____ number of chromosomes
   A. haploid
   B. tetraploid
   C. quadroploid
   D. diploid

20. Which statement is NOT true of mitosis?
   A. It is a process of cell division.
   B. In mitosis the original chromosome number is preserved.
   C. The daughter cells will have the haploid number of chromosomes.
   D. The nucleus is completely reorganized.

21. The process of gametogenesis occurs during
   A. mitosis.
   B. fertilization.
   C. implantation.
   D. meiosis.

22. Meiosis is the process by which
   A. the zygote is formed.
   B. The diploid number of chromosomes is preserved.
   C. continuity of chromosomal set is maintained.
   D. nuclear division occurs with a reduction in the chromosomes to the haploid number.

23. The bivalent contains four chromatids. It is also called
   A. tetrad.
   B. polar bodies.
   C. homologues.
   D. gametes.

24. During meiosis the homologous chromosomes and their chromatids migrate to opposite poles during
   A. second meiotic division.
   B. metaphase I.
   C. first meiotic division.
   D. anaphase II.

25. In mitosis the chromosomes line up across the equatorial plate during
   A. anaphase.
   B. metaphase.
   C. prophase.
   D. interphase.

26. During the first meiotic division the major accomplishment is when
   A. tetrads are formed.
   B. gametes are formed.
   C. chromosomes come together to form the bivalent.
   D. the homologous chromosomes are segregated.

27. A member of a pair of chromosomes is called a
   A. polar body.
   B. ovum.
   C. sperm cell.
   D. homologue.

28. The chromosomes become coiled and visible and the nuclear membrane disintegrates. This is what phase of mitosis?
   A. Interphase
   B. Prophase
   C. Metaphase
   D. Telophase

29. The correct sequence of steps in mitosis is
  A. Prophase, metaphase, interphase, anaphase, telophase.
  B. Interphase, anaphase, metaphase, prophase, telophase.
  C. Interphase, prophase, metaphase, anaphase, telophase.
  D. Anaphase, prophase, interphase, metaphase, telophase.

30. The number of mature gametes resulting from meiosis in the male is
  A. 1.
  B. 2.
  C. 3.
  D. 4.

31. The key difference between anaphase I of meiosis and anaphase of mitosis is
  A. crossing over occurs in anaphase I of meiosis.
  B. centromeres divide in anaphase I of meiosis.
  C. homologous chromosomes move to opposite poles in anaphase I of meiosis.
  D. anaphase in mitosis creates polar bodies.

32. A key difference in the mechanism of mitosis and meiosis is
  A. mitosis has crossing over of homologous chromosomes during prophase.
  B. meiosis has a second duplication of DNA during interphase I.
  C. meiosis has alignment of homologous chromosomes in metaphase I and separation of homologous chromosomes in anaphase I.
  D. mitosis has a reductional division.

33. The main difference in the outcome of mitosis versus meiosis is
  A. meiosis produces identical daughter cells and mitosis produces different daughter cells.
  B. mitosis occurs only in vertebrates.
  C. meiosis produces somatic cells.
  D. meiosis results in haploid cells and mitosis results in diploid cells when the parent cells are diploid.

Passage #3
Viruses and Bacteria (Procaryotes)

Procaryotes (bacteria and blue-green algae) differ from eucaryotes by the latter having (1) genetic material in a nucleus and DNA conjugated with proteins, (2) organelles bound within membranes, (3) subcellular structural units to carry out specific functions (e.g., ATP production, photosynthesis), and (4) presence of cell walls made of cellulose or chitin versus murein (amino sugars and amino acids) as in procaryotes. The DNA of procaryotes is found in a nonmembrane region called the nucleoid; enzymes for metabolism and energy production are either free in the cytoplasm or bound to the cell membrane, and the ribosomes are smaller than in eucaryotes. Viruses are not procaryotes or eucaryotes but constitute their own group.

Viruses

Viruses are usually called "nonliving" and differ from bacteria and other "living" organisms because they (1) don't contain both DNA and RNA, (2) have no metabolic machinery for energy production or protein synthesis, (3) do not arise directly from other viruses but depend on the host's metabolic machinery to synthesize them, and (4) have no membranes to regulate exit and entry. Structurally, most viruses consist of a protein coat surrounding a core (center) of either DNA or RNA.

The many variations of the basic life cycle of a virus are given below. A cell may have a special receptor or region that is recognized by the virus. The virus attaches and may enter via a process similar to phagocytosis. In the cell, the central core of DNA or RNA and occasionally special enzymes or proteins take over the host's metabolic machinery to produce new coat proteins and new viral DNA or RNA. This may occur in the nucleus or the cytoplasm or both. The viral coat and viral core (DNA or RNA) then combine to form complete viral particles. At a certain point, the host cell lyses (bursts) and releases the new viral particles as well as uncombined viral coats and viral cores. Sometimes the viral particles exit by a process similar to reverse phagocytosis and incorporates part of the host's cell membrane onto their protein coat in doing so. The above is typical of a virus that attacks an animal or plant cell.

Viruses that attack bacteria are called bacteriophages. Bacteriophages in general consist of a head made of a protein coat and a core as before, and they also contain a tail made of protein that is specialized for attaching to bacteria. A bacteriophage attaches to the surface of a bacteria and the core of RNA or DNA is injected into the bacteria and the protein coat/remains on the surface. Then the cycle may proceed as described above for viruses and is called lytic or virulent. However, the bacteriophage nucleic acid may become combined with the bacterial nucleic acid and remain as such for long periods before new bacteriophages are produced and cell rupture occurs. In this case, the bacteriophage is called lysogenic or temperate. The nucleic acid from the bacteriophage is called a prophage. Newly-released bacteriophages may contain some of the bacterias' nucleic acid that may be passed onto other bacteria when they are attacked by these bacteriophages. This is the mechanism of transduction.

Bacteria

The general characteristics of bacterial structure are discussed above under procaryotes. More specifically, from inside out, a bacteria may have a capsule that is usually made of a polysaccharide mucoid-like material and protects the bacteria from phagocytosis. Inside the capsule is the cell wall, and this prevents the hyperosmotic bacteria from bursting. Inside the cell wall is the cell membrane that may contain invaginations called mesosomes where localization of enzymes concerned with similar functions may be found. The cytoplasm and nucleoid are as described above. The DNA is circular and is haploid. Some bacterias contain flagella or cilia for locomotion—these are structurally different than their eucaryotic counterparts.

Bacteria have three common shapes: cocci (spherical or ovoid), bacilli (cylindrical or rod-like), and spirillia (helically coiled). The cocci are often found in clusters: diplococci (two bacteria together), streptococci (linear chains of cocci), or staphylococci (grape-like clusters of cocci). All of these are made up of individual bacteria with distinct cell walls.

Metabolically, bacteria may be aerobic or anaerobic. Anaerobic bacteria may use fermentation (where an organic molecule such as pyruvate lactate is the final electron acceptor) or inorganic substances as final electron receptors (such as S — H_2S). An obligate anaerobe is one that is killed if exposed to oxygen. This is usually because they cannot handle the peroxides (very toxic) produced in oxidative metabolism. A facultative anaerobe can metabolize in the presence or absence of oxygen. Bacteria may use a great variety of molecules as nutrients. Some are photosynthetic, others heterotrophic (using organic molecules made by other organisms) and others are chemosynthetic (making organic molecules and energy from inorganic precursors). The last group are important in fixation of nitrogen for use by all organisms. The variety of metabolic nutrients required and products produced are extremely important in studying basic questions of genetics as well as biochemistry, and also in differentiating between the different types of bacteria.

Most bacteria reproduce asexually by the process of binary fission that produces two identical haploid daughter cells by the simple process of mitosis. Genetic recombination (e.g., transfer and rearrangement of genetic information) may occur by three distinct means: transformation, transduction, and conjugation. Transformation involves a bacterium picking up free DNA from a medium, the free DNA being from a different bacterium. Transduction is the transfer of parts of DNA between bacteria by bacteriophages. In conjugation there is pairing of "male" and "female" forms. DNA is passed sequentially between them via structures called pili. All or a fraction of the DNA may be passed in this way. The above three genetic mechanisms allow extraordinary adaptability and variability of bacterium. Since bacteria can reproduce in a span as short as twenty minutes, a new trait such as drug resistance can spread rapidly in a given population.

34. Bacteriophages
   A. cause disease in humans.
   B. are viruses.
   C. are bacteria.
   D. can reproduce by binary fission.

35. Select the substance(s) not ordinarily found in viruses.
   A. Carbohydrates
   B. Proteins
   C. RNA
   D. DNA

36. Viruses
   A. are considered to be living organisms.
   B. consist of protein, lipids, and carbohydrates only.
   C. do not arise from other viruses directly.
   D. have an incomplete metabolic machinery for energy production.

37. Eucaryotes are characterized by all except
   A. genetic material in a nucleus.
   B. organelles bound within membranes.
   C. presence of cell walls made of murein.
   D. subcellular structural units to carry out specific functions.

38. "Contains DNA or RNA, no means of energy production, cannot reproduce self directly" would be a description of a/an
   A. animal cell.
   B. plant cell.
   C. bacteria.
   D. virus.

39. In the replication of a virus in a host cell
   A. the virus directs the metabolic machinery of the host.
   B. the host directs synthesis of new viral particles.
   C. viral particles are made as a single unite (i.e., coat and core).
   D. coat and core structures are released from the host and then combined.

40. Structurally, bacteriophages differ from the usual virus by
   A. having a protein coat.
   B. having a core of DNA or RNA.
   C. being able to replicate independent of a host cell.
   D. having a tail region made of protein for attaching to cells.

41. The part of the cycle of a bacteriophage that may be different from that of a typical virus is
   A. taking over of host cells metabolic machinery.
   B. incorporation of its nucleic acid into the host cell's.
   C. lysis of host cell.
   D. synthesis by host cell of coat and core separately and then combining to form complete particle.

42. Which structure may protect a bacteria from phagocytosis by white blood cells?
   A. Mesosome
   B. Capsule
   C. Nucleoid
   D. Cell wall

43. Select the incorrect association.
   A. Cocci–spherical
   B. Bacilli–rod-like
   C. Diplococci–two cocci
   D. Staphylococci–linear combinations of cocci

44. The process whereby a bacterium picks up DNA from a medium and incorporates it into its own DNA is called
   A. binary fission.
   B. conjugation.
   C. transformation.
   D. transduction.

45. Bacteria transfer (exchange) genetic information between themselves by all except
   A. transformation.
   B. transduction.
   C. budding.
   D. conjugation.

46. Methods used to distinguish between bacteria may include all of the following except
   A. shape.
   B. nutrient requirements.
   C. products of metabolism.
   D. all are possible methods.

47. A form of hepatitis (inflammation of the liver) is caused by a virus. The serum of patients with hepatitis may contain antigens from the virus, HB_SAg (hepatitis B surface antigen) and HB_CAg (hepatitis B core antigen). (An antigen is a substance foreign to the body capable of eliciting an immune response.) Select the correct statement.
   A. This information is inconsistent with what is known about modes of viral replication.
   B. The HB_CAg is probably a lipid.
   C. The HB_SAg is probably a protein.
   D. Enzymes found in liver cells probably do not increase in the serum during the acute disease.

48. Which of the following would interfere most with the replication of a virus? Assume all agents can only affect the host cell and its contents.
   A. An agent that blocks synthesis of lipids.
   B. An agent that blocks synthesis of carbohydrates.
   C. An agent that blocks synthesis of proteins.
   D. An agent that blocks synthesis of lysogenic enzymes.

49. In the treatment of viral infections, a drug is discovered that directly blocks the synthesis of the viral protein coat. This drug
   A. probably adversely affects protein synthesis by the host cell and hence may cause side affects in the host.
   B. probably does not affect host protein synthesis.
   C. probably destroys final electron receptors.
   D. probably makes the viral protein coat thicker to penetrate.

50. Given a bacterial population without resistance to a certain drug, all of the following may cause introduction of bacterial resistance except
   A. transformation.
   B. binary fission.
   C. transduction.
   D. conjugation.

3.5 ANSWERS TO PRACTICE PASSAGES

1. D	**10.** C	**19.** D	**28.** B	**37.** C	**46.** D
2. D	**11.** B	**20.** C	**29.** C	**38.** D	**47.** C
3. B	**12.** B	**21.** D	**30.** D	**39.** A	**48.** C
4. D	**13.** D	**22.** D	**31.** C	**40.** D	**49.** A
5. A	**14.** B	**23.** A	**32.** C	**41.** B	**50.** B
6. D	**15.** D	**24.** C	**33.** D	**42.** B	
7. B	**16.** B	**25.** B	**34.** B	**43.** D	
8. A	**17.** B	**26.** D	**35.** A	**44.** C	
9. C	**18.** C	**27.** D	**36.** C	**45.** C	

3.6 REFERENCES

Atkinson, R. H., and Debbie G. Longman. *Reading Enhancement and Development,* 4th ed. (St. Paul, Minn.: West Publishing, 1992). (Available from Betz Publishing Co.)

Finegold and Baron. *Diagnostic Microbiology*, 7th ed. (St. Louis: Mosby Yearbook, 1986).

Flesch, R. F. *The Art of Clear Thinking* (San Francisco: Harper & Row, 1973).

Giroux, James A., and Glenn R. Williston. *Comprehension Skills, Isolating Details to Recalling Specific Facts*, Advanced Level (Providence, R.I.: Jamestown Publishers, 1974).

Quinn, Shirley, and Susan Irvings. *Active Reading in the Arts and Sciences*, 2nd ed. (Boston: Allyn and Bacon, 1991). (Available from Betz Publishing Co.)

PART II

SCIENCE AND MATHEMATICS REVIEW FOR THE PCAT

Chapter 4

Preparing for PCAT Biology

4.0 INTRODUCTION TO THE PCAT BIOLOGY SECTION

The PCAT biology section measures a student's knowledge of the principles and concepts of basic biology with an emphasis on human biology (introduction to human anatomy and physiology). Topics include cell biology, heredity, human structure and function, bacteria, viruses, evolution and plants. There are usually 50 questions. In this chapter, are illustrated the types of questions and level of subject matter tested on the PCAT. There is <u>no</u> formal review provided in this manual. Biology should be reviewed from college textbooks using the detailed subject outline provided below. As mentioned earlier, do <u>not</u> forget to blend the various reading comprehension skills, quantitative reasoning skills, and problem-solving skills in your review of biology.

In various parts of this chapter, certain salient features of a specific topic are explained briefly to show what subject matter is relatively more important. Do *not* assume that this brief exposure to certain concepts is enough for the PCAT review.

4.1 BIOLOGY

This section outlines the subject of biology. The material is divided into content groups with a short listing of the topics that should be mastered. A biology review test is included to illustrate the level of difficulty of PCAT biology and to identify specific topics requiring more independent study and biology review. To measure your competency, use the book *A Complete Preparation for the MCAT* for review and the Graduate Record Examination (GRE) subject books (biology, general, and organic chemistry) to test your aptitude. The GRE general and subject test books are printed by Educational Testing Service and may be purchased from Betz Publishing Company, the publishers of this book. We also encourage you to use biology review software available from Betz Publishing Company if you have a PC or Macintosh computer.

4.1.1 Biology Outline

A. Origin of Life
- **1.** Introduction
- **2.** Review of Various Theories

B. Cell Metabolism
- **1.** Definition, example
  - **a.** Cellular Respiration
    - **(i)** Aerobic Respiration
    - **(ii)** Anaerobic Respiration
  - **b.** Photosynthesis

(i) Autotrophs
(ii) Heterotrophs
(iii) Definition, equation

c. Respiration vs. photosynthesis

C. Enzymology

1. Review of enzymes
   a. Definition, function, and example
   b. Coenzymes
   c. Specificity of an enzyme
   d. Enzyme and Substrate (Lock and Key) model
   e. Feedback inhibition
      (i) Definition
      (ii) Graphic Enzyme Reaction
      (iii) Chart of Digestive Enzymes

D. Thermodynamics and Cellular Bioenergetics

1. Definitions
   a. Heat and Internal Energy
   b. Thermal Equilibrium and Temperature
2. Scales for temperature measurement
   a. Thermometer
      (i) Freezing Point
      (ii) Boiling Point
   b. Four Temperature Scales
      (i) Celsius
      (ii) Fahrenheit
      (iii) Rankine
      (iv) Absolute
3. Heat Capacity
   a. Specific Heat Capacity
      (i) Equation
      (ii) Calorie and Joule
4. Thermodynamics
   a. 1st Law of Thermodynamics
      (i) Entropy
      (ii) Enthalpy
   b. 2nd Law of Thermodynamics
5. Bioenergetics
   a. Basic Definitions
   b. Energy production
      (i) Glycolysis
      (ii) Citric Acid Cycle
      (iii) Electron Transport System
      (iv) Oxidative Phosphorylation

E. Organelle Structure and Function

1. Definition of a Cell, Organelle
   a. Eukaryotic Cell
   b. Prokaryotic Cell
2. Parts of Eukaryotic Cell
   a. Cell Membrane and Transport

- (i) Phospholipids
- (ii) Unit Membrane Model
- (iii) Fluid Mosaic Model
- (iv) Diffusion
- (v) Osmosis
- (vi) Tonicity
- (vii) Facilitated Diffusion
- (viii) Active Transport
- (ix) Phagocytosis
- (x) Pinocytosis

b. Cytoplasm and Cytoplasm Organelles
- (i) Location of various organelles
- (ii) Function of various organelles

c. The Nucleus and Cell Mitosis
- (i) Chromatin
- (ii) Chromosomes
- (iii) Cell Division
- (iv) Cell Cycle
  - (a) Interphase
  - (b) Prophase
  - (c) Metaphase
  - (d) Telophase
- (v) Centrioles

3. Example of Eukaryotic Cell

a. Fungus
- (i) Characteristics
- (ii) Life Cycle and Reproduction

F. Biological Organization and Relationship of major Taxa

1. Linnaeus's Classification Chart

a. Five Kingdom Classification Chart
- (i) Characteristics of Kingdoms
- (ii) Examples of Kingdoms

b. Kingdom Animalia — Phylum chordata
- (i) Invertebrates (subphylum)
- (ii) Vertebrates (subphylum)
  - (a) Class Amphibian
  - (b) Class Reptilia
  - (c) Class Birds (Avis)
  - (d) Class Mammalia
  - (e) Class Fish (Osteichthyes)

c. Plant Kingdom
- (i) Prokaryota
- (ii) Eukaryota

G. Integumentary System

1. Review of the Skin and Thermodynamics

a. The Skin Layers

b. Functions of the Skin

c. Thermoregulation
- (i) Mechanisms of heat conservation
- (ii) Mechanisms of heat loss

H. Skeletal System
- **1.** Structure of Bones
  - **a.** Spongy Bone
  - **b.** Compact Bone
  - **c.** Human Bone
    - **(i)** Flat
    - **(ii)** Long
- **2.** Human Skeleton

I. Muscular System
- **1.** Types of Muscles
  - **a.** Smooth
  - **b.** Striated
  - **c.** Cardiac
- **2.** Structure of a Muscle
  - **a.** Antagonistic muscle
  - **b.** Synergistic muscle
  - **c.** Muscle Groups
    - **(i)** Flexor and Extensor
    - **(ii)** Abductor and Adductor
  - **d.** Functional Units of Muscle
    - (i) Myofibril
      - **(a)** Sarcomeres
      - **(b)** Myosin
      - **(c)** Actin Complex
    - **(ii)** Sarcoplasmic Reticulum
- **3.** Oxygen Debt and Voluntary Muscle Control
  - **a.** Oxidative Metabolism
  - **b.** Endurance and Cramps

J. Circulatory System
- **1.** The Heat
  - **a.** Structural Features of Heart
  - **b.** Heart Beats
    - **(i)** Systole
    - **(ii)** Diastole
- **2.** Circulatory Blood Vessels
  - **a.** Arteries
  - **b.** Veins
  - **c.** Arterioles
  - **d.** Capillaries
- **3.** The Blood
  - **a.** RBCs
  - **b.** WBCs
  - **c.** Platelets
  - **d.** Lymphocytes
- **4.** Fundamental Principles of Blood Circulation
  - **a.** Resistance
  - **b.** Ejection Fraction
  - **c.** Critical Velocity
  - **d.** Cardiac Output

K. Immunological System

1. Review of Bacteria and Viruses
    a. Structure, Shape, Metabolism, and Life Cycle
    b. HIV Virus Life History and AIDS
2. Characteristics of Bacteriophages and Rickettsiae
3. Types of Bacterial Classes
    a. Schizomycetes Class
        (i) Order Eubacteriales
            (a) Suborder Eubacteriineae
            (b) Suborder Caulobacteriineae
            (c) Suborder Rhodobacteriineae
        (ii) Order Actinomycetales
        (iii) Order Chlamydobacteriales
        (iv) Order Myxobacteriales
        (v) Order Spirochaetales
        (vi) Order Beggiatoales
4. Nutritional Grouping of Bacteria
    a. Autotrophic Bacteria
    b. Saphrophytic Bacteria
    c. Parasitic Bacteria
5. Bacteria and Enzyme Relationship
    a. Hydrolytic Enzymes
        (i) Amylolytic Enzymes
            (a) Diastase
            (b) Cellulase
            (c) Disaccharidases
        (ii) Lipolytic Enzymes
        (iii) Proteolytic Enzymes
    b. Oxidizing Enzymes
        (i) Alcoholnidase
        (ii) Zymase
6. Bacterial Respiration
7. The Mechanism of Infection
    a. Virulence of Pathogenic Bacteria
        (i) Virulence of Organism
        (ii) Specificity
    b. Sources of Infection
        (i) Outside the Host
        (ii) Within the Host
        (iii) Transmission of Disease-producing Organisms
8. Kinds of Immunity
    a. Natural
        (i) Racial
        (ii) Individual
    b. Acquired
        (i) Active
        (ii) Passive
9. The Mechanism of Immunity
    a. Opsonins
    b. Bacteriolysins
    c. Agglutinins

- **d.** Precipitins
- **e.** Antitoxins
- **f.** Hypersensitivity
  - **(i)** Anaphylaxis
  - **(ii)** Allergy

10. Viral and Rickettsial Diseases

L. Digestive System

1. Structure and Functional Relationships
2. Digestive Functions of Key Nutrients
3. Origins and Functional Chart for Digestive Enzymes

M. Respiratory System

1. Structure and Functional Characteristics
2. Effects of Smoking

N. Renal Fluid Composition

1. Body Fluid Composition
   - **a.** Extracellular
   - **b.** Intracellular
   - **c.** Acidity of Plasma
2. The Renal System
   - **a.** Structure
   - **b.** Functional Characteristics
3. Homeostasis of Body Fluids
4. Buffers in the Renal System

O. Nervous System

1. Central and Peripheral Systems
   - **a.** Neurons
     - **(i)** Sensory Neurons
     - **(ii)** Motor Neurons
     - **(iii)** Associate Neurons
   - **b.** Neurotransmitters and Impulse Transmission
2. Autonomic System
   - **a.** Sympathetic System
   - **b.** Parasympathetic System
3. Hindbrain
   - **a.** Structure
   - **b.** Functions
4. Spinal Cord
5. Types of Nerves
   - **a.** Cranial Nerves
   - **b.** Spinal Nerves

P. Endocrine System

1. Endocrine Glands (Anatomy and Functions)
2. Major Hormones of Endocrine Glands

Q. Reproductive System

1. Female and Male Anatomy
2. Gametogenesis
   - **a.** Females
   - **b.** Males
3. Meiosis
4. The Menstrual Period

- **R.** Fertilization, Descriptive Embryology, and Developmental Mechanics
  - **1.** Fertilization
  - **2.** Developmental Mechanics of Embryo
  - **3.** Descriptive Embryology
    - **a.** Differentiation
    - **b.** Determination
    - **c.** Induction
- **S.** Mendelian Inheritance, Chromosomal Genetics, Molecular and Human Genetics
  - **1.** Nucleic Acids
    - **a.** Nucleotides
    - **b.** Nucleosides
    - **c.** Nucleic Acids
  - **2.** RNA Structure
    - **a.** Types of RNA
    - **b.** Differences between DNA and RNA
  - **3.** Biosynthesis and Molecular Genetics
    - **a.** Genetic Code
    - **b.** DNA Duplication, Transcription
    - **c.** RNA Translation
    - **d.** Activation of Amino Acid by Activating Enzyme
    - **e.** Protein Synthesis
      - **(i)** Base-Pairing Rule
      - **(ii)** Amino Acids and DNA Codons Chart
  - **4.** Chromosomes and Mendelian Genetics
    - **a.** Alleles
      - **(i)** Homozygous
      - **(ii)** Heterozygous
    - **b.** Mendelian Inheritance
      - **(i)** First Law of Segregation
      - **(ii)** Second Law of Independent Assortment
    - **c.** Chromosomal Mutations
    - **d.** Pedigree Charts/Punnett Squares
    - **e.** Hardy-Weinberg Principle and Application
- **T.** Evolution and Adaptation
  - **1.** Mechanism of Evolution
    - **a.** Mutations and Hardy-Weinberg Law
  - **2.** Consequences of Evolution
    - **a.** Speciation
      - **(i)** Reproductive Isolation
      - **(ii)** Geographic Isolation
    - **b.** Patterns of Evolution
      - **(i)** Convergent
      - **(ii)** Divergent
      - **(iii)** Parallel
  - **3.** Population Growth
    - **a.** Growth Curves
    - **b.** Parallel
- **U.** Animal Behavior with Social Behavior
  - **1.** Basic Behavioral Responses (Terms and Graphs)
  - **2.** Effect of Evolution of Neurological Structures on Behavior

3. Behavioral Modes in Populations
    a. Social Factors
    b. Interspecific Interactions
4. Communication Between Individuals

V. Plant Biology
1. Cellular Anatomy and Physiology
    a. ATP and energy-producing pathways
        (i) Respiration
        (ii) Fermentation
        (iii) Photosynthesis
        (iv) Experimental Biosynthesis
        (v) Guttation
    b. Extracellular Matrix
        (i) Plant Cell Walls
        (ii) Collagen
2. Plant Structure and Function (Morphology)
    a. Roots, Stems, Leaves and Their Tissues
    b. Meristems
        (i) Growth
    c. Water Relations
        (i) Absorption
        (ii) Transport
        (iii) Transpiration
    d. Mineral Nutrition
    e. Translocation and Storage
    f. Control Mechanisms
        (i) Hormones
        (ii) Photoperiods
        (iii) Tropisms
3. Plant Reproduction and Development
    a. Sex and Alternation of Generations
    b. Flowers, Fruits, and Seeds
    c. Mendelian Genetics in Plants
4. Miscellaneous Topics in Plant Biology
    a. Histology (lab techniques)
    b. Mycology
    c. Phycology
    d. Paleobotany
    e. Taxonomy
    f. Pathology

4.1.2 BIOLOGY SAMPLE TEST

Select the one best answer for each question. Eliminate all responses that you know are incorrect before selecting an answer from the remaining responses.

1. All autotrophic organisms
- **A.** must obtain all organic molecules from their environment.
- **B.** are capable of nitrogen fixation.
- **C.** belong to the Kingdom Plantae.
- **D.** can synthesize organic molecules from inorganic raw materials.

2. Select the substance that is not an electron carrier in cellular energy production.
- **A.** ATP
- **B.** NAD+
- **C.** FAD
- **D.** Ubiquinone

3. The conversion of the code sequence in DNA to a code sequence in mRNA is
- **A.** secretion.
- **B.** transcription.
- **C.** translation.
- **D.** condensation.

4. The substance(s) below *not* ordinarily found in cell membranes is (are)
- **A.** globular proteins.
- **B.** phospholipids.
- **C.** DNA.
- **D.** all of the above.

5. The main difference in the outcome of mitosis versus meiosis is
- **A.** meiosis produces identical daughter cells and mitosis produces different daughter cells.
- **B.** mitosis occurs only in vertebrates.
- **C.** meiosis produces somatic cells.
- **D.** meiosis results in haploid cells and mitosis results in diploid-cells when the parents are diploid.

6. Which of the following substances probably would not cross a membrane by simple diffusion?
- **A.** Ethanol
- **B.** Chloride ion
- **C.** Glucose
- **D.** Water

7. The function of molecular oxygen in cellular respiration is to
- **A.** oxidize the fuel molecule.
- **B.** combine with carbon to form carbon dioxide.
- **C.** generate ATP.
- **D.** serve as a final hydrogen acceptor.

8. All of the following hormones are secreted by the anterior pituitary gland *except*
   A. oxytocin.
   B. prolactin.
   C. luteinizing hormone.
   D. thyroid stimulating hormone.

9. Factors important in the differentiation of cells include
   A. cytoplasmic composition and distribution of constituents.
   B. characteristics of neighboring cells.
   C. physical environmental agents.
   D. all of the above.

10. The control center of respiration is in the
   A. cerebrum.
   B. cerebellum.
   C. diaphragm.
   D. medulla.

11. The secretion of pepsinogen is stimulated by
   A. enterogastrone.
   B. secretin.
   C. gastrin.
   D. enterokinase.

12. The doctrine that living things arise form other living things is
   A. biogenesis.
   B. cellularity.
   C. development.
   D. heredity.

13. The tropic level with the largest biomass in a natural ecosystem is formed by
   A. decomposers.
   B. primary consumers.
   C. producers.
   D. secondary consumers.

14. Below are structures of a typical fatty acid and a hexose.

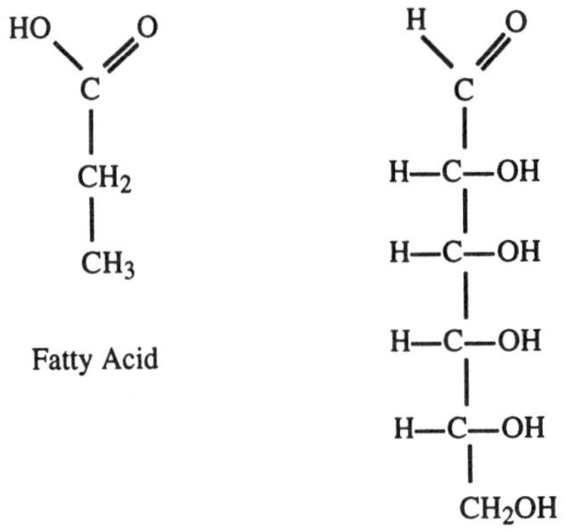

HO–C(=O)–CH_2–CH_3

Fatty Acid

H–C(=O)–(H–C–OH)$_4$–CH_2OH

Hexose

If both were degraded bioenergetically to CO_2 and H_2O, equal weights of fatty acid would yield

A. more energy because it is more reduced than hexose.
B. less energy because it is more reduced than hexose.
C. less energy because it is more oxidized than hexose.
D. more energy because it is more oxidized than hexose.

15. Sex-linked traits

A. are found more in females than males.
B. are found on the X and Y chromosomes.
C. allow recessive alleles to be expressed when one such allele is present in the male.
D. occur in males who have a 50 percent chance of receiving sex-linked alleles from the father.

16. Since enzymes are proteins, they are affected by the same factors that affect proteins. An enzyme is "designed" to function under a certain set of conditions. Which of the following conditions would be most conducive to the normal function of a human cellular enzyme?

A. Temperature = 25°C
B. Temperature = 37°C
C. pH = 1.0
D. pH = 7.0

17. Fungi

A. are prokaryotes.
B. may be unicellular.
C. contain hyphae in unicellular stages.
D. are not saphrophytic.

18. What probably limits the size a cell may attain?

A. Surface area
B. Volume of a cell
C. Balance of surface area and volume
D. Osmotic pressure

19. Which type of muscle is a syncytium?
- **A.** Skeletal
- **B.** Cardiac
- **C.** Smooth
- **D.** All

20. Lymph nodes
- **A.** are found in veins.
- **B.** contain lymphocytes only.
- **C.** may contain lymphocytes and macrophages.
- **D.** are not directly important in protecting the body against disease.

21. Select the *incorrect* statement concerning bile salts.
- **A.** Break down (digest) lipids
- **B.** Emulsify and solubilize lipids
- **C.** Synthesize in the liver
- **D.** Are stored in the gall bladder

22. During inspiration of air into the lungs
- **A.** the chest cavity has a positive pressure.
- **B.** the diaphragm moves upward.
- **C.** the diaphragm contracts.
- **D.** all of the above.

23. All are part of the human kidney except
- **A.** glomerulus.
- **B.** loop of Henle.
- **C.** Malpighian tubules.
- **D.** collecting ducts.

24. All are specifically associated with a neuron except
- **A.** lack of a nucleus.
- **B.** Nissl bodies.
- **C.** dendrite.
- **D.** axon.

25. Select the *incorrectly* paired hormone and disease or deranged process associated with an excess/deficiency of it
- **A.** growth hormone — acromegaly
- **B.** insulin — diabetes mellitus
- **C.** cortisol — abnormal calcium/phosphate metabolism
- **D.** thyroxin — altered metabolic rate

26. One of the scientists who helped the disapproval of spontaneous generation was
- **A.** van Leeuwenhoek.
- **B.** Redi.
- **C.** Einstein.
- **D.** Miller.

27. The five major categories to which most living things belong according to Linnaeus are the animalia, plantae, protista, fungi, and monera
  A. kingdoms.
  B. species.
  C. classes.
  D. grouped phyla.

28. Diseases such as blights, wilts, and galls are caused by
  A. fungi.
  B. viroids.
  C. bacteria.
  D. virions.

29. NAD^+ is a noncovalently bound coenzyme for the enzyme a-glycerol-phosphate dehydrogenase. NAD^+ picks up an H^{-1} (hydride) and becomes NADH; the enzyme is not affected by the reaction. The activation energy is lowered by the system.
  A. This is not true catalysis because the NAD^+ is changed in the reaction.
  B. This is true catalysis because the NAD^+ is not covalently bonded to the enzyme.
  C. This is true catalysis because the activation energy of the reaction is lowered by the enzyme which is unchanged in the reaction.
  D. This is true catalysis because the activation energy of the reaction is raised by the enzyme which is unchanged in the reaction.

30. What entity of neurons allows for one-way conduction of impulses in the nervous system?
  A. Axons
  B. Dendrites
  C. Synapses
  D. Somas

31. Melatonin is produced by the
  A. pineal gland.
  B. skin.
  C. liver.
  D. pituitary gland.

32. Lymph moves toward the veins due to
  A. tissue pressure.
  B. muscle action.
  C. pumping action of heart.
  D. gravity.

33. Iron is absorbed in the
  A. stomach.
  B. jejunum.
  C. ileum.
  D. duodenum.

34. The autonomic nervous system includes
- **A.** sympathetic system.
- **B.** parasympathetic system.
- **C.** somatic nervous system.
- **D.** both A and B.

35. Which of the following tissues secrete hormones?
- **A.** Pancreas
- **B.** Ovaries
- **C.** Gastrointestinal tract
- **D.** All of the above

36. Filtration of blood occurs at which structure in the kidney?
- **A.** Loop of Henle
- **B.** Collecting ducts
- **C.** Tubules
- **D.** Glomerulus

37. Heterotrophs are organisms that
- **A.** feed on inorganic compounds.
- **B.** feed on organic molecules.
- **C.** use anaerobic fermentation of nitric acid.
- **D.** use aerobic fermentation of nitric acid.

38. Mollusks are most closely related to
- **A.** roundworms.
- **B.** coelenterates.
- **C.** annelids.
- **D.** flatworms.

39. Which of the following is a viral disease?
- **A.** anthrax.
- **B.** syphilis.
- **C.** polio.
- **D.** tuberculosis.

40. All of the following are associated with reproductive functions in fungi except
- **A.** conidia.
- **B.** sporangium.
- **C.** basidium.
- **D.** mesenchymal.

41. The A-band of striated muscle represents
- **A.** myosin only.
- **B.** actin only.
- **C.** both A and B.
- **D.** calcium channels.

42. An enlarged lymph node may mean
   A. infection.
   B. inflammation.
   C. metastasis.
   D. all of the above.

43. The enzyme responsible for the activation of trypsinogen in the intestine is
   A. pepsin.
   B. enterokinase.
   C. chymotrypsin.
   D. carboxypeptidase.

44. What structure(s) is(are) used to prevent the bronchi from collapsing?
   A. Cartilage rings
   B. Bony rings
   C. Fibrous tissue
   D. All of the above

45. Select the correct statement concerning the antidiuretic hormone (ADH).
   A. Synthesized in the posterior pituitary gland
   B. Acts on the collecting duct of the kidney
   C. Also called aldosterone
   D. All of the above are correct

46. Reabsorption of most of the water, glucose, amino acids, sodium and other nutrients occurs at
   A. loop of Henle.
   B. collecting duct.
   C. proximal convoluted tubule.
   D. distal convoluted tubule.

47. Myelin sheaths are found
   A. surrounding tendons.
   B. covering the brain.
   C. covering muscles.
   D. around axons of neurons.

48. All of the following hormones are correctly paired with one of its major functions except
   A. thyroxin-increases metabolic rate.
   B. glucocorticoids-increases blood sugar levels.
   C. aldosterone-role in "fight or flight" sympathetic response.
   D. parathyroid hormone-regulation of calcium/phosphorous metabolism.

49. Ethyl alcohol is converted into lactic acid during the process of
   A. aerobic respiration.
   B. excretion.
   C. coenzyme production.
   D. anaerobic respiration.

50. All of the following are vertebrates except
   A. sponge.
   B. cow.
   C. shark.
   D. eagle.

51. Which of the following is (are) fungal disease(s)?
   A. influenza.
   B. pneumonia.
   C. both A and B.
   D. ringworm.

52. Select the correct sequence of filtered blood through the kidney.
   A. Bowman's capsule, glomerulus, tubules, collecting duct
   B. Glomerulus, Bowman's capsule, collecting ducts, tubules
   C. Bowman's capsule, collecting ducts, glomerulus, tubules
   D. Glomerulus, Bowman's capsule, tubules, collecting ducts

53. Which of the following substances probably would not cross a membrane by simple diffusion?
   A. Ethanol
   B. Chloride ion
   C. Glucose
   D. Water

54. In the fungus
   A. the haploid phase tends to dominate.
   B. the diploid phase tends to dominate.
   C. there is only asexual reproduction.
   D. spores are sexual structures only.

55. Which structure does not play a part in motion of cells?
   A. Microvilli
   B. Cilia
   C. Flagella
   D. Pseudopods

56. The products of triglyceride hydrolysis by lipases in the intestine may include
   A. fatty acids.
   B. monoglycerides.
   C. diglycerides.
   D. all of the above.

57. All of the following may cause an increase in respiratory rate except
   A. increased hydrogen ion concentration.
   B. increased carbon dioxide tension.
   C. increased oxygen tension.
   D. decreased oxygen tension.

58. The acidity of the plasma is caused by
   - **A.** oxidation of glucose and fat.
   - **B.** metabolism of sulfur containing amino acids.
   - **C.** production of CO_2 by the tissues.
   - **D.** all of the above.

59. What ion(s) determine(s) the resting potential of a nerve cell?
   - **A.** Sodium
   - **B.** Potassium
   - **C.** Calcium
   - **D.** Both A and B

60. All of the following are arthropods except
   - **A.** jumping spiders.
   - **B.** dragonflies.
   - **C.** snails.
   - **D.** soft shell crabs.

61. Infectious diseases
   - **A.** are inherited.
   - **B.** are caused by pathogens.
   - **C.** are caused by rickettsias.
   - **D.** are caused by bacterial respiration.

62. All of the following substances are filtered at the glomerulus except
   - **A.** platelets.
   - **B.** proteins.
   - **C.** glucose.
   - **D.** sodium.

63. Secretion of bicarbonate and fluid from the pancreas is stimulated by
   - **A.** secretin.
   - **B.** cholecystokinin.
   - **C.** enterokinase.
   - **D.** gastrin.

64. All are functions of the medulla except
   - **A.** voluntary movements.
   - **B.** respiratory regulation.
   - **C.** circulatory regulation.
   - **D.** cough reflex.

65. In the hypothalamic-pituitary-adrenal axis, if the long feedback loop holds then
   - **A.** ACTH inhibits the production of ACTH-RF by the hypothalamus.
   - **B.** cortisol inhibits the production of ACTH by the pituitary.
   - **C.** cortisol inhibits the ACTH-RF produced by the hypothalamus.
   - **D.** all of the above.

66. Urea
A. is a product of protein metabolism.
B. contains only carbon, hydrogen, and oxygen.
C. is excreted by the lungs.
D. all of the above.

67. During the early phase of the action potential
A. only Na^+ moves.
B. only K^+ moves.
C. only Ca^{++} moves.
D. Na^+ moves into the cell and K^+ moves out.

68. All of the following are types of bacteria except
A. metatrophic.
B. parasitic.
C. autotrophic.
D. tsutsugamuchi.

69. Select the correct sequence of the meninges from outside inward: (A = arachnoid, D = dura, P = pia).
A. A, D, P
B. D, P, A
C. P, A, D
D. D, A, P

70. A vaccine mostly results in
A. passive immunity.
B. active immunity.
C. production of antibodies.
D. both B and C.

71. An organism makes and gives off useful chemical compounds. It is carrying on the life process of
A. secretion.
B. photosynthesis.
C. catalysis.
D. cellular respiration.

72. Calcitonin
A. decreases serum calcium.
B. has no effect on serum calcium.
C. is made in the parathyroid gland.
D. is a steroid.

73. All of the following are families in Suborder Eubacteriineae, except
A. rhizobiaceae.
B. chlamydobacteriales.
C. achromobacteriaceae.
D. parvobacteriaceae.

74. Select the *incorrect* statement concerning the parasympathetic system.
   A. Ganglia are located near the end-organ
   B. Increases the heart rate
   C. Maintains homeostasis
   D. Increases digestive actions

75. All of the following are *infections* except
   A. typhoid.
   B. botulism.
   C. common flu.
   D. strep throat.

4.1.3 EXPLANATORY SOLUTIONS FOR BIOLOGY SAMPLE TEST

Question 1: [D] Topic: diversity of life. Choice **A** refers to heterotrophic organisms, and the other choices to some, not all, autotrophs.

Question 2: [A] Topic: cell and molecular biology. ATP is the main short term energy storage molecule and is not an electron carrier.

Question 3: [B] Topic: cell and molecular biology. Translation is the conversion of a nucleotide sequence to an amino acid sequence. Responses **A**, **C**, and **D** have no connection at all to the question.

Question 4: [C] Topic: cell and molecular biology. The cell membrane is composed of phospholipids and proteins.

Question 5: [D] Topic: cell and molecular biology. Mitosis is a nucleocytoplasmic division. There is only one division of the cell into two identical diploid (2n) daughter cells. Meiosis has two phases, (i) is a reduction division in which daughter cells contain the haploid number of chromosomes and (ii) is similar to mitosis except that the cell has the haploid number of chromosomes.

Question 6: [C] Topic: cell and molecular biology. Some ions, lipid soluble substances, and very small molecules (such as ethanol, glycerol, and urea) can diffuse through membranes. Polar molecules, ions (especially cations), and larger molecules such as sugars and amino acids must cross the membrane by other means.

Question 7: [D] Topic: cell and molecular biology. Oxidation is the removal of hydrogen, or more generally a loss of electrons. Water is formed as a by-product of oxidation; it is not the primary function of oxidation.

Question 8: [A] Topic: vertebrate anatomy and physiology. This question specifically requires knowledge of the hormones secreted by the posterior pituitary gland. All of the other hormones are secreted by the anterior pituitary gland.

Question 9: [D] Topic: developmental biology. This question tests your knowledge of embryology, specifically those factors that cause cells to differentiate.

Question 10: [D] Topic: vertebrate anatomy and physiology. This question tests your knowledge of the brain and its role in respiration. The key in selecting the correct answer is to know the function of the parts of the brain as well as the diaphragm.

Question 11: [C] Topic: vertebrate anatomy and physiology. None of the other hormones are associated with the stomach.

Question 12: [A] Topic: cellular and molecular biology, origin of life. This question tests your general knowledge of the theories relating to the origin of living things.

Question 13: [C] Topic: evolution, ecology, and behavior. This question tests your understanding of the ecosystem and its composition at various levels.

Question 14: [A] Topic: cellular and molecular biology. A reduced compound has all (or mostly) hydrogens and not oxygens. The fatty acid has many more hydrogens and fewer oxygens so it is more reduced. The more reduced a compound, the higher the energy that can be released when it is oxidized to CO_2 and H_2O.

Question 15: [C] Topic: genetics. This question tests your understanding of alleles carried on the X or Y chromosomes and the probability of this trait being expressed based on which chromosome it is attached to.

Question 16: [B] Topic: enzymology. This question discusses conditions under which enzymes function. The function of a cellular enzyme should be maximal at those conditions found in the internal milieu of a cell or a particular compartment of a cell. This would generally be conditions similar to the whole organism. The temperature of 37°C is the normal human body temperature and the normal pH of blood is 7.40. The other conditions are extreme, but there are enzymes that can function at or near most of these—some in the human, some not.

Question 17: [B] Topic: organelle structure and function. This question tests your understanding of characteristics of fungi.

Question 18: [C] Topic: organelle structure and function. This question discusses cell geometry. The reasoning is a follows: the nutritional and energy requirements and waste production are proportional to the volume of the cell. The volume of a cell is proportional to a linear dimension (l = length) cubed, i.e., l^3. The flux (i.e., the exchange rates) of materials in (nutrients) and out (wastes) is proportional to the surface area of a cell. The surface area is proportional to a linear dimension squared, i.e., l^2. As the cell increases in size (as volume increases), the requirements, given by l^3, increase much more rapidly than supply and waste removal, give by l^2. Hence, a balance between surface area and volume is required such that supply (and waste removal) can keep in balance with cell requirements.

Question 19: [D] Topic: structure and function of muscular system. This question tests your understanding of various types of muscle.

Question 20: [C] Topic: structure and function of the immunological system. The structure and functions of lymph nodes are tested in this question.

Question 21: [A] Topic: structure and function of the digestive system. This question tests your understanding of bile composition and production.

Question 22: [C] Topic: structure and function of the respiratory system. This question tests your understanding of physiology of the respiratory system.

Question 23: [C] Topic: structure and function of the urinary system. This question tests your understanding of anatomy of the kidney.

Question 24: [A] Topic: structure and function of the nervous system. This question tests your understanding of anatomy of a neuron.

Question 25: [C] Topic: structure and function of the endocrine system. This question is designed to check if you remember the major glands and hormones secreted by them.

Question 26: [B] Topic: origin of life. This question checks your understanding of work done on spontaneous generation.

Question 27: [A] Topic: biological organization and relationship of major taxa. This question checks your fundamental knowledge of major taxonomic groups.

Question 28: [C] Topic: structure and function of the immunological system. This question relates causes of various diseases to the type of microorganism.

Question 29: [C] Topic: cell metabolism. True catalysis occurs when the activation energy is lowered and this lowering is accomplished by the enzyme's active site environment. Coenzymes serve the accessory function of transferring chemical groups.

Question 30: [C] Topic: structure and function of the nervous system. Impulse transmission in neurons is tested in this question. Draw a clear sketch showing one-way impulse conduction to understand neuronal pathways for impulses.

Question 31: [A] Topic: structure and function of the endocrine system. This question checks to see if you remember hormonal secretion glands and hormones secreted by each gland.

Question 32: [B] Topic: structure and function of the immunological system. This question tests your understanding of the lymphatic system, in particular the flow pattern of lymphatic fluid.

Question 33: [D] Topic: structure and function of the digestive system. The absorption of chemical elements or compounds occurs in various parts of the digestive system. You should memorize with reasons what chemicals are absorbed in which specific parts of the digestive system.

Question 34: [D] Topic: structure and function of the nervous system. This question tests your understanding of anatomy of the autonomic nervous system.

Question 35: [D] Topic: structure and function of the endocrine system. This question tests your understanding of the endocrine glands.

Question 36: [D] Topic: structure and function of the urinary system. Understanding the functions of different parts of the kidney, e.g., nephron, glomerulus, calyx, etc. is being tested in this question.

Question 37: [B] Topic: structure and function of the immunological system. This question tests your understanding of heterotrophs and autotrophs.

Question 38: [C] Topic: relationship of major taxonomic groups. This question tests your understanding of classification characteristics of taxonomic groups.

Question 39: [C] Topic: structure and function of immunological systems. This question tests your understanding of viral diseases, infections, and microbiological characteristics.

Question 40: [D] Topic: major differences between eukaryotic and prokaryotic cells. This question tests your understanding of reproductive characteristics of fungi.

Question 41: [C] Topic: structure and function of muscular system. This question tests your understanding of striated muscle anatomy. Technically, the band is visible as such because of the myosin, but within the limits of the band, actin is also present.

Question 42: [D] Topic: structure and function of immunological system. This question tests your understanding of characteristics of lymph nodes and factors which cause swelling of the node.

Question 43: [B] Topic: structure and function of the digestive system. This question tests your understanding of digestive enzymes.

Question 44: [A] Topic: structure and function of respiratory system. This question tests your understanding of the anatomic structures in the respiratory system.

Question 45: [B] Topic: structure and function of the endocrine system. This question tests your understanding of secretion of ADH and its functions.

Question 46: [C] Topic: structure and function of the urinary system. This question tests your understanding of reabsorption sites in the renal system.

Question 47: [D] Topic: structure and function of the nervous system. This question tests your understanding of myelin sheaths encasing the neuron.

Question 48: [C] Topic: structure and function of the endocrine system. This question tests your understanding of endocrine glands, hormones, and their effects and functions.

Question 49: [D] Topic: cell metabolism (including photosynthesis). This question tests your understanding of biochemical reactions and conversions.

Question 50: [A] Topic: biological organization of chordates. This question is designed to see if you remember characteristics of vertebrates.

Question 51: [D] Topic: immunology and basic pathology. This question tests your knowledge about fungal diseases.

Question 52: [D] Topic: structure and function of the renal system. The question discusses the flow of filtered blood through the kidney. A flow diagram of the renal system would be helpful to develop visual skills.

Question 53: [C] Topic: characteristics of prokaryotes and eukaryotes. Some ions, lipid soluble substances, and very small molecules (such as ethanol, glycerol, urea) can diffuse through membranes. Polar molecules, ions (especially cations) and larger molecules must enter by other processes.

Question 54: [A] Topic: reproduction in eukaryotic cells. This question tests your understanding of sexual and asexual reproduction.

Question 55: [A] Topic: characteristics of prokaryotic and eukaryotic cells. Pseudopods are cytoplasmic extensions that aid in motion as found in amoeba. Microvilli are evaginations (out pouches) of the cell membrane which increase its surface area. Microvilli provide more area for flux of materials in and out of cells, as in the gut.

Question 56: [D] Topic: structure and function of the digestive system. This question tests your understanding of enzymology of the digestive system.

Question 57: [C] Topic: structure and function of the respiratory system. This question tests your understanding of respiratory rate and how it is changed by ionic tension.

Question 58: [D] Topic: structure and function of the circulatory system. This question tests your understanding of components of blood and their chemical characteristics.

Question 59: [D] Topic: structure and function of the nervous system. This question tests your understanding of nerve cells and chemistry of ionic transmission.

Question 60: [C] Topic: biological classification. This question tests your knowledge of arthropods.

Question 61: [B] Topic: infectious diseases. This question tests your understanding of microorganisms and diseases caused by these organisms.

Question 62: [A] Topic: structure and function of the renal system. Your knowledge of the function of glomerulus is tested in this question.

Question 63: [A] Topic: structure and function of endocrine glands. This question tests your understanding of pancreatic enzymes.

Question 64: [A] Topic: structure and function of the nervous system. Your understanding of neurophysiology is tested through this question.

Question 65: [C] Topic: structure and function of the nervous and endocrine system. In the long feedback loop, the specific hormone (cortisol) of the gland (adrenal) feeds back past the pituitary to the hypothalamus.

Question 66: [A] Topic: structure and function of the urinary system. This question tests your understanding of chemical structure of urea.

Question 67: [A] Topic: modes of cellular transport. This question tests your understanding of ionic equilibrium between extracellular and intracellular fluids.

Question 68: [D] Topic: bacteria types and their origins. This question tests your memory on various types of bacteria.

Question 69: [D] Topic: structure and function of the nervous system. This question is best answered if you have a sequential diagram of the meninges from outside inward.

Question 70: [D] Topic: structure and function of the immune system. This question tests your understanding of the immune system (antibodies and antigens).

Question 71: [A] Topic: cellular metabolism. This question tests your understanding of the biochemical reactions of various organisms.

Question 72: [A] Topic: structure and function of the endocrine system. This question tests your understanding of hormonal effects.

Question 73: [B] Topic: bacterial classification. This question tests your understanding of bacterial classes and subclasses.

Question 74: [B] Topic: structure and function of the parasympathetic system. This question tests your understanding of neuroanatomy related to the parasympathetic system.

Question 75: [B] Topic: infectious diseases. This question tests your understanding of infectious diseases.

4.2 INTRODUCTION TO BIOLOGY TOPICS

4.2.1 Origin of Life

The earth is about 4.5 billion years old. Life on the planet earth started some three billion years ago. It is believed by most scientists that probabilistic chemical events occurred over hundreds of millions of years, resulting in the formation of bioorganic cells. For thousands of years people believed in "spontaneous generation," the routine appearance of living organisms from nonliving matter. Francesco Redi, an Italian scientist, disproved spontaneous generation in 1668 by laboratory experiments on maggots. The theory of spontaneous generation met its death in 1850 at the hands of Louis Pasteur in France.

The origin of life is rooted in four basic requirements:

- (a) presence of certain chemicals
- (b) absence of oxygen gas
- (c) energy source of some kind
- (d) millions of years in time

The four requirements mentioned above were tested in a laboratory apparatus based on ideas by a Russian, Alexander Oparin, in 1924 and later by an American, Stanley Miller, in 1953. The laboratory equipment was rich in hydrogen, ammonia, and methane and used to produce proteinoids (chains of amino acids). Adding water to proteinoids formed microspheres—similar to living cells. Review various theories explaining origin of life and note assumptions (express or implied), hypotheses and conclusions.

4.2.2 Bioorganic Molecules

Review the chemical composition of structures present in eukaryotic cells and constituents of body fluids. Proteins, amino acids, phospholipids and carbohydrates have complex classification techniques and experimental analysis techniques. Keep a biological focus to understand types and configurations of biologically significant molecules. Memorize the twenty-two a-Amino acids and their structures along with the RNA genetic code showing base sequence. Note all *possible* distinction between anomers and epimers versus phospholipids and sphingolipids. Understand the basic classification and experimentation techniques for bioorganic molecules e.g., how are steroids classified? how are steroids tested in the laboratory to determine pK_{a1}, pK_{a2} and isoelectric points?

4.2.3 Enzymology

Focus on the molecular structure and functions of enzymes for the human body. Understand that enzymes are chiral molecules and behave as stereospecific or geometry specific biochemicals. Remember classification of enzymes as isomerases, ligases, oxidoreductases, transferases, hydrolases and lysases. Review special functions of elastase, plasmin, trypsin, urease, a-amylase, enterokinase and bovine pancreatic ribonuclease. Recognize allosteric effectors and the role they play in enzymology. Identify important coenzymes such as biotin, nicotinamide and lipoic acid. Learn how to graph enzyme reactions and feedback inhibition characteristics of enzymes.

4.2.4 Understanding DNA and RNA Structure

Review the structure and function of DNA and RNA as complex biomolecules. The Watson-Crick model (traditionally proposed as right-handed double helix) for DNA was challenged and a new Z-DNA model (considered as left-handed double helix) was suggested. Compare the old and new DNA models with special focus on assumptions (given and implied), molecular biology applications and current research trends. Understand terms such as target and vehicle DNA, plasmids, genomes, modern DNA cloning techniques, and genetic repair. The specific roles of mRNA, tRNA and rRNA should be linked to translation and transcription mechanisms.

4.2.5 Introduction to Protein Synthesis

Protein synthesis (also called biosynthesis) is made up of two subprocesses: translation and transcription. Link biological molecules (structure and chemistry) to the mechanics of translation and transcription. Each process (translation and transcription) consists of three major steps: initiation, elongation, and termination or release of the biochain. The emphasis is to comprehend Crick's law of molecular biology. The law states "DNA information is passed onto the RNA which in turn transfers it to the proteins." Focus on how information is passed from DNA to RNA. How is information passed from RNA to proteins? How is experimental research done to prove the law?

4.2.6 Introduction to Cellular Metabolism

Cellular metabolism consists of a series of complex biochemical reactions. There are four types of reactions: (1) carbon bond reactions (making and breaking of C bonds), (2) isomerization, substitution and reorganizing reactions, (3) oxidation and reduction reactions, and (4) electrophilic group-transfer reactions (nucleophile to nucleophile). Learn to apply and integrate these four reactions with the four major bioechemical processes of glycolysis, citric acid cycle, electron transport chain and oxidative phosphorylation. Understand various mechanisms, which determine and control biochemical synthesis of lipids, fatty acids, lipoproteins, amino acids and urea. Relate biochemical synthesis to basal metabolic rate. Carefully review Gibbs free energy linked to cellular metabolism. In doing so, compare and contrast exergonic, isogonic and endergonic reactions related to $\Delta G = \Delta G° + RT\ (\ln[P_1][P_2]/[R_1][R_2])$. P_1, P_2 are the biochemical products and R_1, R_2 are the biochemical reactants. Understand Lipmann's law as it applies to eukaryotes and prokaryotes. Lipmann's law states that "The ADP-ATP coupling is the receptor and distributor of biochemical energy in *all* living organisms (or more complex systems)."

4.2.7 Cell Metabolism

All the chemical metabolic reactions that occur in a living cell consist of: cellular respiration, release of energy; use of energy to build other substances for use, storage, or excretion. Examine a rather complex biochemical pathway of metabolism (metabolic pathway)—cellular respiration. ATP (Adenosine triphosphate) is produced as a result of cellular respiration. ATP is the source of energy for most endothermic reactions in cells. Cellular respiration may be divided into two types:

(a) Aerobic Cellular Respiration (with oxygen):

$$C_6H_{12}O_6 + 6O_2 \xrightarrow[2ATP]{} 6CO_2 + 6H_2O + 38ATP$$
(Glucose)

Net ATP gained = 36 ATP

(b) Anaerobic Cellular Respiration (without oxygen):

$$C_6H_{12}O_6 \xrightarrow[2ATP]{} 2C_2H_5OH + 2CO_2 + 4ATP$$

Net ATP gained = 2 ATP

Autotrophs are organisms that make food from inorganic molecules. Heterotrophs, on the other hand, feed on organic molecules. Autotrophs and Heterotrophs are further classified as:

(A) Chemoautotrophs or Photoautotrophs
(B) Chemoheterotrophs or Photoheterotrophs

Photosynthesis is a complex set of reactions in the metabolic cycle. It is a process by which autotrophic organisms make food.

Photosynthesis can be represented by

$$6CO_2 + 6H_2O \xrightarrow[\text{Sunlight}]{\text{Chlorophyll}} C_6H_{12}O_6 + 6O_2$$

Chlorophyll is the green pigment in plants and leaves. Photosynthesis made up of chemical reactions is exactly opposite to aerobic cellular respiration. Respiration is endothermic whereas photosynthesis is exothermic. The sunlight is converted into ATP during respiration. Glucose is the most important molecule for life to exist in any form.

4.2.8 Introduction to Prokaryotic and Eukaryotic Cells

Learn the microbiology of a prokaryotic cell and fungus as compared to the microbiology of a eukaryotic cell. Learn the structures, life history and sources of disease for bacteria, bacteriophage, virus and fungus. Learn the detailed structure and functions of eukaryotic cells. Connect the study of generalized eukaryotic cells to specialized eukaryotic cells such as neural cells (neurons), contractile cells (sarcomeres), epithelial cells and connective cells. Evaluate the physical and chemical aspects of cell membrane transport models, ion channels, chromosome movement mechanics, cellular adhesion and membrane receptors. A basic review of fundamentals of microbiology and microbial diseases appears in section 4.3.

4.2.9 Introduction to Evolution and Genetics

Molecular genetics, mutations and comparative chordate anatomy should be studied as parts of the large scale evolution process. The history and mechanisms controlling evolution (for various organisms) should be directly applied to problem solving in gene flow, genetic drift and genetic (chromosomal) mapping. Recognize and appraise this section as a series of hypotheses, theories and conclusions. Determine how given information is used to solve special mathematical problems in genetics. Review chapter 5 (sections on problem solving and probability mathematics) before working with genetics problems.

4.2.10 The Mechanism of Evolution

Evolution is the study of the changes that occur in organisms, how the changes occur, and the results of the changes. These changes may be minor and lead to better adaptation to an environment, or they may be major and lead to a totally different species. Changes come about when organisms are *"selected"* on the basis of *phenotypic differences* to survive. These phenotypic differences must be based upon underlying *genetic differences,* as found in the germ cells that lead to evolutionary change. (The survival of selected organisms leads to *changes in the gene frequencies and gene combinations* in the population, which in turn leads to *changes in phenotypic characteristics* and, hence, evolution.)

4.2.11 Evolution of Species

The consequences of evolution are seen in the changes that may occur in a given species. These changes can be minor and reflected as clines. *Clines* are gradual variations in a species due to geographic (environmental) variations such as altitude or latitude. *Subspecies (races)* result when an abrupt environmental change is associated with an abrupt change in characteristics. Finally, the evolutionary changes may be so great as to result in a totally new species—a process called speciation.

A *species* is viewed as a set of genetically distinct organisms that share a common gene pool (i.e., gene flow is possible between them) and are reproductively isolated from all other such groups. The first step in *speciation* is usually *geographic isolation* of two populations of the same species. A *barrier* (e.g., rivers, oceans, canyons, mountains, etc.) prevent the populations from coming together to mate. The two separate populations will tend to differ because: (1) gene frequencies usually differ, (2) each population experiences different mutations, (3) the different environments will exert different selection pressures, and (4) if small, genetic drift can cause differences. The second factor in speciation then comes into play; it is *reproductive isolation.* The two populations will begin to differ such that gene flow between them is no longer possible even if they are brought together. This is brought about by *intrinsic reproductive isolating mechanisms* which act at all the steps of reproduction discussed earlier. These are: (1) *ecogeographic isolation* (organisms can no longer survive in each other's environment), (2) *habitat isolation* (organisms may occupy only certain, but different, habitats within the same range), (3) *seasonal isolation* (the breeding periods may be at different times of the year), (4) *behavioral isolation* (mating rituals differ), (5) *mechanical isolation* (nonfitting of genitals), (6) *gametic isolation* (fertilization cannot occur), (7) *hybrid unviability* (the offspring cannot reproduce), and (8) *developmental isolation* (fertilization can occur, but the embryo dies). So, by geographic isolation followed by reproductive isolation, the mechanisms of evolution lead to new species.

General *patterns* of evolution are *divergent* (moving from one species to different species, the usual pattern), *convergent* (moving from separate to common species), or *parallel* (two species resulting from one but evolving in a parallel fashion). *Adaptive radiation* is the gradual divergent differentiation of a species, usually as a response to environmental variations. *Homologous* structures are those that arose from a common structure even though functions may be different. *Analogous* structures have common functions but arose from different structures.

4.2.12 Comparative Anatomy for Chordates (Optional for the PCAT)

The major adaptive evolutionary changes are discussed for chordates. *Chordates* are distinguished by (1) a dorsal, hollow nerve cord, (2) gill slits in the throat region, and (3) a notochord. Chordates are divided into invertebrate chordates (tunicates, acorn worms, cephalochordates or amphioxus) and vertebrates. *Vertebrates* have a vertebral column, closed circulatory system (enabling large growth), a better developed nervous system and improved sensory apparatus. *Fish* include the Agnatha (jawless, e.g., lampreys), Chondrichthyes (e.g., sharks, all cartilage except inner ears) and Osteichthyes (bony fish). The pectoral fins, pelvic fins and lateral line system are important for balance. Lobe fin fish (or crossopterygians, e.g., latimeria) invaded land, had lungs, had stubby fins (bones into fins—was a crucial step for land invasion) and gave rise to the amphibians. *Amphibians* (frogs, toads, salamanders) are still tied to water because their eggs are easily dessicated. *Reptiles* (snakes, turtles, lizards, crocodiles and alligators) arose from amphibians. Total land life was possible because of the amniotic egg which wouldn't dessicate and which had a sufficient food supply. Reptiles are also advanced beyond amphibians by (1) internal fertilization by copulation, (2) ventricle of heart is partly divided to separate oxygenated and unoxygenated blood, (3) ribs aid in respiration, and (4) the brain has small cerebral hemispheres. The pterosaurs (extinct) gave rise to the birds. *Aves* (birds) can fly because of special feathers (modified reptile scales, large quills for flying surface, fanlike tail feathers for stabilization, contour and down feathers for insulation), light skeleton and a special breastbone for flight muscles, warm-blooded, efficient respiration with the four-chambered heart, advanced sight and muscular coordination by the brain. *Mammals* arose from a different type of reptile than did the birds. Key distinguishing features of mammals are: (1) internal development of young and nutrition by mammary glands, (2) jaw is strengthened and teeth are differentiated, (3) a diaphragm is present to separate thorax and abdomen and is used in breathing, (4) legs are swung underneath the body, and (5) the brain is greatly enlarged.

TABLE 3: Evolutionary Timetable

Geologic Era	**Period**	**Time***	**Features**
Precambrian	--------	2,700	Marine invertebrates; protozoans
Paleozoic	Cambrian	600	Trilobites; brachiopods
	Ordovician	500	First fish
	Silurian	430	First air-breathing animals; first insects
	Devonian	410	First amphibians; sharks; sea lilies
	Carboniferous	350	First reptiles; insects
	Permian	275	Mammal-like reptiles; emergence of modern insects
Mesozoic	Triassic	225	First dinosaurs
	Jurassic	175	First birds, flying reptiles; dinosaurs; first mammals
	Cretaceous	130	Primitive mammals; first modern birds; dinosaurs become extinct
Cenozoic	Tertiary	60	Rapid development of higher mammals and birds
	Quaternary	2	Appearance of modern humans; extinction of giant mammals

* Time in millions of years

4.2.13 TAXONOMY: Biological Organization of Major Taxa

A hierarchical classification that exists for organisms was due primarily to *Linnaeus*. Organisms are grouped at each level on the basis of similarities. As the hierarchy is ascended (shown below), the similarities become more general. A well-known mnemonic is given with the hierarchy:

Kings	Kingdom
Play	Phyllum
Chess	Class
On	Order
Fine	Family
Grain	Genus
Sand	Species

All organisms are given a two-component Latin name. The first is the genus (capitalized), and the second is the species (not capitalized), e.g., *Homo sapiens.*

For a long time all living organisms were placed in the animal kingdom or plant kingdom. To classify certain microorganisms the five-kingdom system is strongly supported by biologists.

TABLE 4: Five-Kingdom Classification Chart

Name of Kingdom	**Kingdom Characteristics**	**Examples**
Animalia	Mobile, multicellular organisms. Heterotrophic. They eat other organisms.	lobsters, snakes, insects, mammals, eagles, fish
Plantae	Multicellular, autotrophic organisms. They make their food with chlorophyll and sunlight.	pine tree, oak tree, ferns, seed plants
Protista	Mostly unicellular. Some are heterotrophic and others are autotrophic organism. They do have nuclei.	algae, paramecium, amoeba, euglena, diatoms
Fungi	Multicellular organisms. Heterotrophic and absorb food molecules from living/dead organisms	mushrooms, puffballs, molds, yeasts
Monera	Prokaryotic, single cell organisms. They do *not* have nuclei.	bacteria, blue-green algae

4.2.14 Classification/Characteristics of Various Kingdoms

Students should learn examples of each class shown in this section:

Animal Kingdom
They are subclassified as vertebrates and invertebrates.
Platyhelminthes = blood flukes, tapeworms
Porifera = sponges
Coelenterata = jelly fish, anemones, corals
Nematoda = roundworms, Trichinella
Annelida = earthworms, leeches
Mollusca = clams, octopus, squid
Echinodermata = sand dollars, sea urchins
Arthropoda = crabs, spiders, lobsters, insects
Chordata = fish, snakes, birds, frogs, mammals

Kingdom Plantae
This kingdom is composed of five phyla, three of which are algae—green, brown, and red.

Green algae = volvox, spirogyra
Brown algae = seaweeds, kelp
Red algae = Irish moss, agar

The two major phyla in the plant kingdom are nonvascular and vascular plants. Examples of nonvascular plants are mosses and liverworts.

Vascular plants belong to phylum Tracheophyta. These include ferns and seed plants. Seed plants are grouped as Angiosperms and Gymnosperms. Angiosperms produce fruit to cover their seeds. Gymnosperms have uncovered seeds, e.g., pines, spruces, cedars.

Kingdom Protista
They can be algae or protozoans. Protozoans are classified into four phyla based on the way that they move—Paramecium, Flagellate, Amoeba, and Malaria Plasmodium.

Kingdom Fungi
Fungi do not contain chlorophyll. Common examples are molds, mildews, yeasts, and mushrooms. They are subclassified as thread-like fungi, sac fungi, club fungi, and imperfect fungi.

Kingdom Monera
Bacteria and blue-green bacteria are members of this kingdom. The classification is based on shape, type of nutrition, requirements for oxygen, and other characteristics.

4.2.15 The Classification of Plants

Plant Kingdom (EUKARYOTA)

Subkingdom THALLOPHYTA/Subkingdom CHLORONTA

THE ALGAE

Phylum Cyanophyta
- Class Cyanophyceae

Phylum Chlorophyta
- Class Chlorophyceae
  - Order Volvocales
  - Order Ulotrichales
  - Order Ulvales
  - Order Oedogoniales
  - Order Conjugales
  - Order Chlorococcales
  - Order Dasycladales
- Class Charophyceae

Phylum Euglenophyta
- Class Euglenophyceae

Phylum Pyrrophyta
- Class Dinophyceae

Phylum Chrysophyta
- Class Xanthophyceae
- Class Chrysophyceae
- Class Bacillariophyceae

Phylum Phaeophyta
- Class Phaeophyceae
  - Order Ectocarpales
  - Order Laminariales
  - Order Fucales

Subkingdom BILONTA

Phylum Rhodophyta
Phylum Glaucophyta
Phylum Cryptophyta

Subkingdom MYCONTA

THE FUNGI (Myconta)

Phylum Schizomycophyta
- Class Schizomycetae
- Class Actinomycetae

Phylum Myxomycophyta
- Class Myxomycetae
- Class Acrasieae
- Class Plasmodiophoreae

Phylum Eumycophyta
- Class Phycomycetae
- Class Ascomycetae
- Class Basidiomycetae

Class Deuteromycetae
Class Chytridiomycetae
Class Oomycetae
Class Zygomycetae

Subkingdom EMBRYOPHYTA

Phylum Bryophyta
- Class Hepaticae
  - Order Marchantiales
  - Order Jungermanniales
- Class Anthocerotae
- Class Musci
  - Order Sphagnales
  - Order Bryales

Phylum Tracheophyta
- Subphylum Psilopsida
  - Class Psilophytineae
    - Order Psilotales
    - Order Psilophytales
- Subphylum Lycopsida
  - Class Lycopodineae
    - Order Lycopodiales
    - Order Selaginellales
    - Order Lepidodendrales
    - Order Isoetales
    - Order Pleuromeiales
- Subphylum Rhyniopsida
- Subphylum Zosterophyllopsida
- Subphylum Trimerophytopsida
- Subphylum Progymnospermopsida
- Subphylum Filicopsida
- Subphylum Sphenopsida
  - Class Equisetineae
    - Order Hyeniales
    - Order Sphenophyllales
    - Order Calamitales
    - Order Equisetales
- Subphylum Peteropsida
  - Class Filicineae
    - Order Coenopteridales
    - Order Ophioglossales
    - Order Marattiales
    - Order Filicales
  - Class Gymnospermae
    - Subclass Cycadophytae
    - Subclass Coniferophytae
    - Subclass Gnetophytae
  - Class Angiosperm

Subclass Dicotyledonae
Subclass Monocotyledonae
- Order Anthocerotales

Plant Kingdom (PROKARYOTA)

Subkingdom SCHIZONTA
Phylum Archaebacteria
Phylum Eubacteria
Phylum Actinobacteria
Phylum Mollicutes

Subkingdom CYANOCHLORONTA

Subkingdom PROCHLORONTA

As an example, yucca is commonly called soaptree, palmilla, and Spanish bayonet.

In scientific terminology it is classified as follows:

Subkingdom	—	Embryophyta
Phylum	—	Tracheophyta
Subphylum	—	Pteropsida
Class	—	Angiospermae
Subclass	—	Monocotyledonae
Order	—	Liliales
Family	—	Liliaceae
Genus	—	Yucca
species	—	elata

4.2.16 Reproductive System Concepts

Review reproductive system essentials as they link to the endocrine system, Mendelian genetics (sex-linked characteristics) and major differences and similarities between embryogenesis and gametogenesis. Familiarize yourself with current issues and problems related to the reproductive systems of females and males, e.g., in-vitro fertilization and embryo transfer technology. Review both plant and animal reproduction.

4.2.17 Concepts Related to Respiratory, Integumentary, and Skeletal Systems

The respiratory and integumentary systems are both subjected to external environmental factors. Pollution and ozone layer depletion lead to various breathing and skin problems. The health sections of newspapers and magazines are good sources to discover new techniques and current problems. Students should review racing, running and aerobic actions which affect ventilation of lungs and sweating. The mechanisms controlling inspiration, expiration and protective actions of the skin are closely linked. Review these for small and large animals and plants. Review the design construction and working of a spirometer and a bronchoscope as used in a clinical setting. Review the skeletal system with focus on the axial skeleton, appendicular skeleton and articulations (arthrology is a medical specialty). Understand the six types of synovial joints (ball-and-socket, ellipsoidal, gliding, hinged, pivot and saddle).

4.2.18 Muscle System Concepts

The student should learn nervous control of muscles. Compare and contrast characteristics of motor and sensory control. Distinguish between the control mechanisms for voluntary and involuntary muscles. Develop a detailed understanding of the sliding filament theory and mechanisms of muscular contractions (emphasize myosin binding mechanism in contractile process). Review differences between isotonic and isometric contractions. Do not memorize but realize that there are 700 skeletal muscles (focus on the location, shape and size of important muscles)

4.2.19 Circulatory System Concepts

Identify the complex structure and working of contractile cells and tissues with emphasis on the cardiac muscle. Identify the thermoregulatory function of the cardiovascular system and its components: heart, blood and arterial/venous systems. Visit a hospital or clinic if permitted, to understand heart transplants, artificial heart machine and blood bank operations. Learn the following laws and their limitations (do *not* forget both stated and unstated assumptions behind these laws) as applied to the circulatory system:

(i) *Marey's Law:* If blood pressure *falls* the heart beats *faster* (an inversely proportional relationship)

(ii) *Starling's Law:* relates length of stretched cardiac muscle fibers to strength of contraction (a directly proportional relationship, the longer the stretched fiber, the stronger the contraction)

(iii) *Frank-Starling Law:* The heart automatically adjusts its pumping capability depending on blood volume to be pumped by it (a directly proportional relationship, the more the blood volume to be pumped, the higher the pumping capability)

Do *not* forget to understand why these laws are true and under what conditions are they valid. In understanding these laws remember, cardiac muscle is not plastic, the tone of the heart makes it contract continuously. Also, review the circulatory system in various animals.

4.2.20 Concepts Related to Lymphatic and Immune Systems

Review the basic structures and functions of these systems. Understand the mechanisms which work these systems to regulate various processes in the human body. Examine the composition of blood on both a physical and chemical basis and the mechanisms which control flow of lymph at various lymph nodes. Review the physical structure, physical properties, chemical properties and stereochemistry of helper T-cells, killer T-cells, suppressor T-cells and T-cell receptors. Review auto immunity, active immunity and passive immunity in studying immunological publications and current medical literature. Examine and recognize current research involving bone marrow transplants, spleen and thymus surgical procedures. Connect your knowledge to microbiology (especially virus and bacteria life history).

4.2.21 Digestive System Concepts

Understand the histology and mechanisms associated with the digestive system, e.g., the GI tract has the peritoneum and other muscular control layers such as tunica serosa, tunica muscularis, tunica submucosa and tunic mucosa. Review the microscopic structure of muscularis mucosae, lamina propria, circular and longitudinal muscle to understand the role and mechanisms of the digestive process. Review histology of the digestive system integrated with the biochemical and muscular actions within the system.

4.2.22 Excretory System Concepts

Focus on the functional unit of a kidney—the nephron. Remember there are 1 million nephrons per kidney, each nephron is made up of glomerulus and the tubule (made up of renal corpuscles, podocytes, distal and proximal tubules). Familiarize yourself with the histology of podocytes. Draw a sketch showing tubular reabsorption (both active and passive), definition and use of milliosmol as a concentration unit and various hydrostatic forces involved in effective filtration.

4.2.23 Nervous System Concepts

The complexity of this system is partly due to current and ongoing research efforts linking it to the enormous details associated with sensory reception and processing. Review the four major parts of the nervous system, i.e., Central Nervous System, Peripheral nervous system, autonomic nervous system (sympathetic and parasympathetic) and the sense organs (eyes, nose, ears, tongue and skin). The central nervous system is the command center (messages or impulses arrive there and are sent to various glands, organs and muscles). Understand the similarities and differences between the motor (efferent) and the sensory (afferent) systems. The efferent system is then divided into the autonomic and somatic nervous systems. The most efficient way to review the nervous system is to understand the biological (structural or anatomical) aspects (functions of each part, physiological role of each part including dimensions and equations) of the four major parts. Understand the concepts behind the labeled-line law which states, "Each type of sensory nerve fiber transmits only one modality of sensation."

4.2.24 Endocrine System Concepts

Learn the cellular mechanisms of hormone action to understand specificity and target tissues connected to each hormone. Review the organic structure, physical and some chemical properties (mol. weight, density, melting/boiling point, interaction with other body hormones or chemicals) of various hormones.

4.3 REVIEW OF BACTERIA AND VIRUSES

This is a quick overview for all students and details should not be memorized for the PCAT.

4.3.1 Types of Bacteria

Bacteria are now considered as one *class* of the lowest *division* of the plant *kingdom.* This class has five *orders;* some of the orders are subdivided into suborders and all into *families*, the families into tribes, the tribes into *genera,* and the genera into *species*. Following the binomial system of Linnaeus, long ago adopted by botanists and zoologists, a generic and a specific name are assigned to each species. For example, *Streptococcus lactis* is the organism chiefly responsible for the souring of milk. The generic name should begin with an upper case letter, and the specific name with a lower case letter.

4.3.2 Classification of Bacteria

The chaotic condition of bacterial classification caused the Society of American Bacteriologists to set up as a major project the construction of a more satisfactory system. At its annual meeting in Urbana, Illinois, in 1915, the Society of American Bacteriologists assigned to the Committee on Classification, of which A. Winslow was chairman, the task of formulating a new system of classification.

4.3.3 Characteristics of Class Schizomycetes

These are mostly unicellular plants. Individual cells may be spherical, curved, or spiral rods. Some species produce pigments. The sulfur purple and green bacteria possess pigments much like or related to the true chlorophylls of higher plants. These pigments have photosynthetic properties. The phycocyanin found in the blue-green algae does not occur in the *Schizomycetes.* Multiplication is typically by cell division. Endospores are formed by some species included in *Eubacteriales.* Sporocysts are found in *Myxobacteriales.* Ultramicroscopic reproductive bodies are found in *Borrelomycetaceae.* The latter types cause diseases of either plants or animals. Five orders are recognized.

4.3.4 Key to the Orders and Suborders of the Class Schizomycetes

A. Cells rigid, not flexuous. Motility by means of flagella or by a gliding movement.
  1. Cells single, in chains or masses. Not branching and mycelial in character. Not arranged in filaments. Not acid-fast (bacteria do not retain the primary stain, carbol fuchsin and decolorize with acid alcohol). Motility, when present, by means of flagella.
     Order I: Eubacteriales
     (a) Do not possess photosynthetic pigments. Cells do not contain free sulfur.
     (b) Not attached by a stalk. Do not deposit oxide.
     Suborder I: Eubacteriineae
     (i) Attached to substrate, usually by a stalk. Some deposit iron oxide.
     Suborder II: Caulobacteriineae
     (ii) Possesses photosynthetic purple or green pigments. Some cells contain free sulfur.
     Suborder III: Rhodobacteriineae
  2. Organisms forming elongated, usually branching, mycelial cells. Multiply by special oidiospores and conidia. Sometimes acid-fast. Nonmotile.
     Order II: Actinomycetales
  3. Cells in filaments frequently enclosed in tubular sheath with or without a deposit of iron oxide. Sometimes attached. Motile flagellate and nonmotile conidia. Filaments sometimes motile with a gliding movement. Cells sometimes contain free sulfur.
     Order III: Chlamydobacteriales

B. Cells flexuous, not rigid
  1. Cells elongated. Motility by creeping on substrate.
     Order IV: Myxobacteriales

2. Cells spiral. Motility, free swimming by flexion of cells.
Order V: Spirochaetales

C. *Supplement:* Groups whose relationships are uncertain.
1. Obligate intracellular parasites or dependent directly on living cells.
(a) Not ultramicroscopic. More than 0.1 micron in diameter.
(b) Ultramicroscopic. Less than 0.1 micron in diameter.
Group II: Order Virales
2. Grown in cell-free culture media with the development of polymorphic structures including rings, globules, filaments, and minute reproductive bodies (less than 0.3 micron in diameter).
Group III: Family Borrelomycetaceae

4.3.5 The Order Eubacteriales

This order consists of simple and undifferentiated rigid cells that are either spherical or rod shaped. The rods may be short or long, straight or curved, or spiral. Some groups or species are nonmotile, others show locomotion by means of flagella. Elongated cells divide by transverse fission and may remain attached to each other in chains. Spherical organisms divide either by parallel fission producing chains, or by fission alternating in two or three planes producing either tetrads or cubes of 8 and multiples of 8 cells. Many spherical cells form irregular masses in which the plane of division cannot be ascertained. Endospores occur in some species. Some species are chromogenic, but only in a few is the pigment photosynthetic (bacteriopurpurin and chlorophyll).

4.3.6 The Suborder Eubacteriineae

These are, as the name *Eubacteriineae* implies, the true bacteria in the narrower sense of the word. The cells are rigid and free. Branching occurs only under abnormal conditions of life. They are not attached by holdfasts or stalks. They form no sheaths. One-third of the species form pigments, but these have no photosynthetic properties. Endospores occur in one family (Bacillaceae), rarely in others.

This suborder includes most of the common bacteria studied in the laboratory, both saprophytes and parasites, and some of the autotrophic species. Its importance is indicated by the fact that it contains many more species than all the other orders combined.

4.3.7 Families in Eubacteriineae

There are *thirteen* families in this suborder, and a brief description of each follows.

Nitrobacteriaceae. Mostly gram negative rods, nonspore-forming, and autotrophic, obtaining energy by the oxidation of hydrogen, methane, carbon dioxide, ammonia, nitrites, sulfur, or thiosulfates. They are nonparasitic and mostly inhabitants of soil and water.

While this is a relatively small family, with only 9 genera and about 22 species, it is of tremendous economic importance to humans. It contains the nitrifying organisms that, living in enormous numbers in nearly all well aerated soils, change the ammonia of decaying organic matter to the nitrates so essential to soil fertility. The benefits thus obtained from the action of these bacteria more than offset the harm done by all disease-producing species combined.

Pseudomonadaceae. Gram negative, nonspore-forming rods, usually motile by polar flagella that are single or in small or large tufts. Some are straight and others spirally curved but rigid and dividing transversely. Many are saprophytes in soil or water, and others are parasitic on plants or animals. This is a large and important family of 12 genera and about 250 species. Here are to be found *Vibrio comma,* and cause of Asiatic cholera, and other species of the same genus that cause diseases of lesser importance. Three other genera are worthy of mention. *Pseudomonas* from soil, water, and diseased plants sometimes produce pigments of a greenish hue, flourescent, and water soluble, which diffuse into the surrounding medium, making colored halos around the colonies. *Xanthomonas* is a large genus of plant pathogens that cause many important diseases, including blights of bean, walnut, and cotton. *Acetobacter* is a genus having pleomorphic organisms that are important in completing the carbon cycle and for producing vinegar and commercial acetic acid by the oxidation of alcohol.

Azotobacteriaceae. Pleomorphic with motile or nonmotile forms and large cocci. Strongly aerobic, oxidizing carbohydrates for energy, and fixing atmospheric nitrogen when growing in media or soils deficient in nitrogen compounds.

There is but one genus and the typespecies is *Azotobacter chroococcum.* They are widely distributed in the soil, where they carry on nonsymbiotic nitrogen fixation. These species, with those of *Rhizobium,* are the chief agencies in the recovery of nitrogen from the atmosphere.

Rhizobiaceae. Straight, nonspore-forming rods, mostly gram negative.

Micrococcaeceae. A moderate sized family of coccus forms by dividing in two or three planes and forming sheets, tetrads, packets, or irregular masses. Nearly all are gram positive and nonmotile. Many species are pigmented, usually yellow, orange, pink, or red. There are 3 genera. The most important, *Micrococcus,* has cells arranged in plates or irregular masses as a result of the successive planes of division being oblique to each other and perhaps because of some reorientation after division. Some species cause boils, abscesses, infection of wounds, etc. *Sarcina* contains species of saprophytes and faculative parasites. They are mostly gram positive and pigmented orange or yellow. By division in three planes they form definite packets. Common in air, water, soil, and milk.

Neisseriaceae. Gram negative cocci forming pairs or masses. They grow best at 37°C, but most of them require special media, preferably one containing blood, serum, or ascitic fluid. There are 2 genera and 13 species.

Neisseria is a genus made up of species that are nearly strict mammalian parasites, growing best on blood media and some of them poorly even on such media. By division in two planes they form pairs or small irregular masses. This genus is of great importance, for one species, N. *gonorrhoeae* causes a serious widespread venereal disease, and another, N. *meningitis,* causes one of the most common forms of meningitis.

Lactobacteriaceae. Includes two tribes: streptococceae, composed of spheres or short rods in chains, and Lactacilleae, composed of longer rods. This family is mostly nonmotile and gram positive. It ferments carbohydrates with the formation of lactic acid and other products.

This is a medium sized family of 7 genera and 62 species. It contains some very important species, both saprophytic and pathogenic. *Streptococcus lactis* and the different species of

Lactobacillus are responsible for the souring of milk. Several species of *Streptococcus* are pathogenic, causing wound infections, septicemia, puerperal fever, erysipelas, scarlet fever, etc. *Diplococcus pheumoniae* is responsible for the most common types of pneumonia in humans and animals. Members of this family are used extensively in the microbiological assay of vitamins and amino acids.

Corynebacteriaceae. This is a new family made up of 3 genera and 29 species. Generally gram positive, slender, straight to slightly curved rods with irregularly stained segments or granules. Its members are usually nonmotile, and may or may not show positive reactions in various physiological tests. One species, *Corynebacterium diphtheriae,* produces a powerful exotoxin that causes diphtheria in humans.

Achromobacteriaceae. This is also a new family composed of 3 genera and 45 species. Gram negative to gram variable, small to medium sized rods, usually uniform in shape. If motile, cells have peritrichic flagella. Growth on agar slants nonchromogenic to grayish-yellow in milk. Many organisms of this family occur in water and soil. None are active in the fermentation of sugars, especially lactose.

Enterobacteriaceae. Nonspore-forming rods. Gram negative. Mostly with peritrichic flagella. Carbohydrates are fermented, and nitrates reduced to nitrites.

This is a large family of 8 genera and 198 species. While many species are harmless saprophytes, widely distributed in nature, others inhabit the alimentary tract of humans and other mammals, either as part of the normal flora or as causative organisms of specific diseases. Thus *Shigella dysenteriae* causes bacillary dysentery, *Salmonella typhosa* causes typhoid fever, and *Salmonella pullorum* causes white diarrhea of chicks. In the genus *Salmonella,* serological relationships are the chief means of identifying new strains of which there are at present about 150, called serotypes rather than species.

One genus, *Erwinia*, contains species of plant pathogens, including *E. amylovora,* the cause of the destructive fire blight of apples and pears.

Parvobacteriaceae. Gram negative rods, mostly parasitic, growing poorly on artificial media except those that contain body fluids. Do not form gas in fermentation of carbohydrates.

This family of 10 genera and 56 species is very important in medical bacteriology. In the genus *Pasteurella, P. multocida* is the type species and includes the hemorrhagic septicemic bacteria. *Pasteurellae* are encountered in fowl, swine plague, and bubonic plague of humans and rodents. *P. tularensis* causes tularemia in humans and animals. *Malleomyces mallei* is causes glanders in horses and other animals, including humans; and *Brucella melintensis, B. abortus,* and *B. suis* produce brucellosis in humans and domestic animals. *Hemophillus pertussis* is the probable cause of whooping cough and *Noguchia granulosis* of trachoma in humans.

Bacteriaceae. Nonspore-forming rods forming a heterogeneous collection of species whose relationship to one another and to other groups of bacteria are not determined. This is a large collection of bacteria that require further study. There is one genus and 56 species. Most of them are harmless saprophytes but a few cause diseases of minor importance. One species, *Bacterium bibula,* is important in the soil, where it digests the cellulose of plant refuse.

Bacillaceae. This family is distinguished from all others by the production of endospores, more resistant than vegetative cells to unfavorable environmental conditions. All members are rod shaped, and most are gram positive. There are but two genera; *Bacillus,* containing 33 species of aerobes, and *Clostridium,* consisting of 61 species that are anaerobes or microaerophiles.

The family is an important one. The ability to decompose proteins makes its members valuable scavengers. Most species of *Bacillus* are saprophytic, but the dread disease, anthrax, is caused by B. *anthroacis.* Although the majority of species of *Clostridium* are nonpathogenic, some are pathogenic. C. *perfringens* and related species cause the fatal gas gangrene or wounds and C. *botulinim,* growing saprophytically in the absence of air, produces the deadly toxin of botulinus poisoning.

4.3.8 The Suborder Caulobacteriineae (Stalked Bacteria)

This suborder contains 4 families of organisms that constitute another group of "iron bacteria" in that they store ferric hydroxide, not in a sheath (which is absent), as do the organisms in the order Chlamydobacteriales, but in a stalk by which the cells are attached to a solid support.

The cells are single and kidney shaped or spherical. the stalk is secreted from the concave surface of the cell. Cell division is transverse in most genera but longitudinal in the family Pasteuriaceae. As the cell divides, the tip of the stalk at the point of attachment divides also, resulting in branched colonies. In most genera reproduction is by fission only, but in the Pasteuriaceae budding also takes place.

A characteristic of the suborder is the stalked condition. The stalks vary from quite slender, thread-like structures many times the length of the cell at its tip to short, broad disk-like holdfasts.

Most species of the Caulocateriineae are harmless saprophytes or autophytes of minor importance. One species, *Pasteuria ramosa,* is parasitic in the body cavities of the crustaceans, *Daphnia pulex* and D. *magna.*

4.3.9 The Suborder Rhodobacteriineae (Purple and Green Bacteria)

This suborder has 3 families, 21 genera, and 48 species of organisms that possess photosynthetic purple or green pigments. Some purple cells contain free sulfur. In certain genera the cells are spherical or ellipsoidal and divide in two or three planes within a gelatinous matrix that holds them together for a time in groups or a mass. Later they escape and in some species develop motility.

It is believed that two types of chemical reaction are carried on in the photosynthetic process of different members of the Rhodobacteriineae:

1. $CO_2 + 2H_2S \rightarrow HCHO + H_2O + 2S$
2. $3CO_2 + 2S + 8H_2O \rightarrow 3HCHO + 3H_2O + 2H_2SO_4$

It will be noted that in the first reaction hydrogen sulfide replaces the water used in photosynthesis by the typical green plant, and that in the second both water and sulfur are used. Both reactions are carried out anaerobically, and oxygen is not an end product.

Thiorhodaceae. Members of this family make up 13 genera and 34 species of organisms, the cells of which contain bacteriopurpurin with or without sulfur granules. Most of these organisms are found in soil and water.

Athiorhodaceae. The members of this family contain bacteriopurpurin, which gives them a red, purple, or violet color when seen in masses, and are sometimes striking and beautiful in appearance. The two genera are rod shaped or spiral and generally motile with polar flagella.

The family is especially interesting because of the ability of its members to carry on photosynthesis. The bacteriopurpurin, which gives the organisms their red or purple color, has been shown to be complex of two or more pigments. One of these, the bacteriochlorophyll, is green in color and appears to play an active part in using the energy of light for photosynthesis. The function of the red pigment is, as yet, uncertain. In this process carbon from carbon dioxide is used in the formation of organic compounds, perhaps carbohydrates, which are at once used in the growth of the bacteria. Red and infrared light rays are more effective in supplying energy for this process than are those with shorter wavelengths.

Unlike most bacteria, Athiorhodoaceae thrive better in light than in darkness. They lose their red color in the absence of light and regain it when light is supplied. In an unevenly lighted field or one in which the rays of light have been separated by passage through a prism, motile forms will swim about until a region of the right intensity or color of light is found, then they come to rest.

Chlorobacteriodaceae. This is a new family that includes the green bacteria that do not contain sulfur. There are 6 genera and 8 species.

4.3.10 The Order Actinomycetales (Fungus Bacteria)

Compared with the great order Eubacteriales, the order Actinomycetales is very small. It has only 3 families, 5 genera, and about 125 species.

The cells are cylindrical, and in certain genera, notable *Actinomyces,* they are firmly united to form filaments resembling the mycelium of a true fungus but much more slender. True branching is fairly common in this order. True endospores are not produced. The members of this order are, in general, less aquatic than those of the Eubacteriales, as shown by their lack of motility and their usual absence from natural waters. Most of them are aerobic and gram positive.

Mycobacteriaceae. This family has much in common with the Eubacteriineae in that the cells occur singly or in short chains, and there is no differentiation into vegetative and reproductive parts. Branching is rare.

There is but one genus, *Mycobacterium*, which is highly significant in medical bacteriology. This genus includes 12 species, about half of which are pathogenic, causing different forms of tuberculosis in humans and other vertebrates and leprosy in humans. The rods are slender, nonmotile, and acid-fast. Most species grow poorly or not at all on the common laboratory culture media.

Actinomycetaceae. In this family the tendency to form filaments is very pronounced. In several genera there is no differentiation into vegetative and reproductive portions. One such genus, *Nocardia*, is quite remarkable in that some of its species can use paraffin, phenol, and m-cresol for energy.

The morphology of *Actinomyces* is so radically different from that of other bacteria that some regard it as a true fungus of the *Fungi Imperfecti.* It is very definitely filamentous and has been called the "ray fungus." The filaments are very slender, only about a micron in diameter, and without cross walls. This much-branched, mycelium-like structure forms a definite vegetative body that may fragment into elements of various sizes but does not produce conidia.

A number of species are pathogenic to animals. *Actinomyces bovis* causes actinomycosis or "lumpy jaw" in cattle, *A. isreali* causes actinomycosis in humans, and *Norcardia madurae* causes madura foot in humans.

Crenothrichaceae. Crenothrix polyspora is a species the filaments of which are not branched by are attached at the base to a rock or other submerged object. The sheath of young filaments is composed of organic material that, with age, becomes incrusted with ferric hydroxide, especially the basal portion. As the filament matures, its terminal portion expands and opens, giving it a trumpet shape.

Reproduction takes place by the formation of nonmotile conidia. These are ovoid in shape and formed by three-plane division of the cells at the tip of the filament. Escaping through the open end of the sheath, they become attached and form new filaments by growth and transverse division.

This species often develops luxuriantly in water supplies where it would do no harm but for the fact that masses of it die and decay, thus giving a disagreeable odor and flavor to the water.

Beggiatoaceae. The members of this family form filaments, the tips of which usually have an oscillating motion similar to that of the blue-green algae *Oscillatoria.* Some move by a gliding motion also. No conidia are formed. The cells reproduce by constriction and the filaments by fragmentation. Sulfur granules but no bacteriopurpurin are formed. There are 4 genera and 18 species.

The best known representative of the family is *Beggiatoa alba,* which forms gray, slimy masses on the vegetation of swamps, sulfur springs, and sewage-polluted streams. This species is reported to be highly pleomorphic, the cells of the thick filament within a delicate sheath breaking up into free-swimming cells grow into few filaments.

Many species oxidize hydrogen sulfide as a source of energy and are called "sulfur bacteria."

4.3.11 The Order Chlamydobacteriales (Sheathed Bacteria)

This is a small order, having 3 families, 8 genera, and 27 species. Their normal habitat is water, and partly for this reason and partly because of their structure they are spoken of as alga-like bacteria. They form long slender filaments, mostly 1 to 2 microns in diameter. In some genera these are attached at the base to some object, while in others they are free floating.

4.3.12 The Order Myxobacteriales (Slime Bacteria)

This order is characterized by the production of a mass of slime that enables these bacteria to carry on a communal life that is quite remarkable and not found elsewhere in the bacterial world.

Vegetative or Swarm Stage. The bacterial cells live and multiply within a slimy matrix that forms a flat, irregularly shaped pseudoplasmodium. This is called the "swarm stage." The cells are at this time slender flexible rods. They have no flagella but show slow motility both individually and in mass. As the cells grow and multiply they secrete more slime, with two results. The pseudoplasmodium enlarges and moves slowly along, carrying the bacteria in its terminal portion. The movement is supposedly due to asymmetrical slime production that, increasing in the back portion of the mass, crowds the colony along. Probably the individual movement of the cells aids in the process. The entire mechanics of the process is perplexing and not well understood. The gliding motion of the individual cells is suggestive of that of *Ossillatoria* and certain diatoms.

Encystment or Fruiting Stage. When the pseudoplasmodium has reached a certain degree of maturity a striking change takes place. The cells collect in a compact on a gelatinous base. Thus a "fruiting body" or cyst is formed that may be simple and round or variously lobed. The size, shape, and color are characteristic of the species. In most species the cysts have stalks composed of slime devoid of bacteria, these having collected in the sellings at the top. The fruiting bodies are rarely more than 1 millimeter high, generally yellow, orange, or red in color. In some species, e.g., *Chondromyces crocatus*, they are exquisite in appearance, though so tiny as to require a hand lens for detailed observation.

As the cysts mature, the cells become shorter and thicker (in some species nearly spherical), and their activity ceases for a time, the slime drying below and about the cells.

After a short resting period the cells, singly or in tiny masses bound together by the dried slime, escape from the cysts, largely through the action of wind and air. Under favorable conditions they then start new swarms and excrete slime as before.

In this order there are 5 families, 13 genera, and 71 species. For the most part they are saprophytes, absorbing food from their substratum, which at best is decaying wood, fleshy fungi, or the dung of animals. One species, *Polyangium parasiticum*, is parasitic on the green alga *Cladophora.* Another, *Podangium lichenicolum*, is parasitic on lichens.

These bacteria are interesting because of the communal life of their cells by which, through mutual and coordinated production of slime, there has evolved a method of locomotion and dissemination.

4.3.13 The Order Spirochaetales (Flexuous Spiral Bacteria)

The organisms in this small order are flexuous spiral rods. The pointed ends of some species taper into a slender thread that is probably *not a true* flagellum. In some species an axial filament has been observed. This consists of a relatively straight, cylindrical, protoplasmic core about which the spiral ridges of the cell are wound. Movement in the Spirochaetales is brought about by the contraction of the protoplasm, which gives the flexible cell an undulating movement, propelling it through the water. In some cases this is a wriggling motion; in others the cell is made to revolve screwlike on its major axis.

Most members of the order are not readily stained by methods generally successful with other kinds of bacteria. Special stains have been devised for some, and dark-field illumination has been extensively used to supplement stained preparations.

The flexible body, the character of movement, and the axial filament are strongly suggestive of certain kinds of protozoa, and it is possible that, as a result of further study, some members of the Spirochaetales will be transferred to that group. However, their apparent lack of nuclei, lack of sexuality, and transverse division justify placing them with the bacteria.

There are two families in this order. Spirochaetaceae, with 3 genera and 11 species, contains some harmless saprophytes found in water, especially water polluted with sewage, and some parasites found in the intestinal tract of bivalve mollusks. The family Treponemataceae consists of 3 genera and 26 species, many of which are parasitic on vertebrates and some of which are pathogenic. Species of *Borrelia* cause different forms of relapsing fever, often transmitted by insects, and *Treponema pallidum* is the cause of syphilis, one of the worst scourges of the human race.

4.3.14 Class Schizomycetes (Bacteria) Chart

- Order I: Eubacteriales
  - Suborder I: Eubacteriineae (true bacteria)
    - Family I: Nitrobacteriaceae
      - 3 tribes, 9 genera, 22 species
        - Example: *Nitrobacter winogradskyi*
    - Family II: Pseudomonadaceae
      - 2 tribes, 12 genera, 250 species
        - Example: *Pseudomonas aeruginosa*
    - Family III: Azotobacteriaceae
      - 1 genus, 3 species
        - Example: *Azotobacter chroococcum*
    - Family IV: Rhizobiaceae
      - 3 genera, 13 species
        - Example: *Rhizobium leguminosarum*
    - Family V: Micrococcaceae
      - 3 genera, 33 species
        - Example: *Micrococcus luteus*
    - Family VI: Neisseriaceae
      - 2 genera, 13 species
        - Example: *Neisseeria gonorrhoeae*
    - Family VII: Lactobacteriaceae
      - 2 tribes, 7 genera, 62 species
        - Example: *Lactobacillus acidophillus*
    - Family VIII: Corynebacteriaceae
      - 3 genera, 29 species
        - Example: *Corynebacterium diphtheriae*
    - Family IX: Achromobacteriaceae
      - 3 genera, 45 species
        - Example: *Alcaligenes faecalis*
    - Family X: Enterobacteriaceae
      - 5 tribes, 8 genera, 198 species
        - Example: *Escherichia coli*
    - Family XI: Parvobacteriaceae
      - 4 tribes, 10 genera, 56 species
        - Example: *Brucella abortus*

Family XII: Bacteriaceae
1 genus, 56 species
Example: *Bacterium triloculare*
Family XIII: Bacillaceae
2 genera, 94 species
Example: *Bacillus subtilis*
Suborder II: Caulobacteriineae (Stalked bacteria)
Family: Nevskiaceae
1 genus, 2 species
Example: *Nevskia ramosa*
Family II: Gallionellaceae
1 genus, 4 species
Example: *Gallionella ferruginea*
Family III: Caulobacteriaceae
1 genus, 1 species
Example: *Caulobacter vibrioides*
Family IV: Siderocapsaceae
2 genera, 3 species
Example: *Siderocapsa trubii*
Suborder III: Rhodobacteriineae (Purple and green bacteria)
Family I: Thiorhodaceae
13 genera, 31 species
Example: *Thiosarcina rosea*
Family II: Athiorhodaceae
2 genera, 6 species
Example: *Rhodopseudomonas palustris*
Family III: Chlorobacteriaceae
6 genera, 8 species
Example: *Chlorobium limicola*
Order II: Actinomycetales (Fungus-like bacteria)
Family I: Mycobacteriaceae
1 genus, 12 species
Example: *Mycobacterium tuberculosis*
Family II: Actinomycetaceae
2 genera, 35 species
Example: *Actinomyces bovis*
Family III: Strepmycetaceae
2 genera, 78 species
Example: *Streptomyces albus*
Order III: Chlamydobacteriales (alga-like bacteria)
Family I: Chlamydobacteriaceae
3 genera, 12 species
Example: *Leptothrix ochracea*
Family II: Crenothrichaceae
1 genus, 1 species
Example: *Crenothrix polyspora*
Family III: Beggiatoaceae
4 genera, 18 species
Example: *Beggiatoa alba*
Order IV: Myxobacteriales (Slime bacteria)

Family I: Cytophagaceae
1 genus, 9 species
Example: *Cytophaga hutchisonii*
Family II: Archangiaceae
2 genera, 6 species
Example: Archanium gephyra
Family III: Sorangiaceae
1 genus, 8 species
Example: *Sorangium schroeter*
Family IV: Polyangiaceae
5 genera, 30 species
Example: *Chondromyces aurantiacus*
Family V: Myxococcaceae
4 genera, 18 species
Example: *Myxococcus fulvus*
Order V: Spirochaetales (Flexuous spiral bacteria)
Family I: Spirochaetaceae
3 genera, 11 species
Example: *Spirochaeta plicatilis*
Family II: Treponemataceae
3 genera, 26 species
Example: *Treponema pallidum*
Supplement I: Order Rickettsiales
10 genera, 35 species
Example: *Rickettsia prowazekii*
Supplement II: Order Virales
242 species described
Supplement III: Family Borrelomycetaceae
1 genus, 7 species
Example: *Asterococcus mycoides*

SUMMARY

Eubacteriales	90 genera	929 species
Actinomycetales	5 genera	125 species
Chlamydobacteriales	8 genera	31 species
Myxobacteriales	13 genera	71 species
Spirochaetales	6 genera	37 species
TOTAL:	122 genera	1,193 species

4.3.15 Nutritional Grouping of Bacteria

The kinds of bacteria that now live on the earth differ greatly from one another in their food requirements, particularly as to the sources of carbon and nitrogen and the substances that can be oxidized for the release of energy. One convenient way of grouping bacteria is into *autotrophic, saprophytic,* and *parasitic* species.

Autotrophic Bacteria. It seems probable that millions of years ago, when the first primitive bacteria appeared on the earth, few or no other forms of life were present, and consequently little or no organic matter was available for food. It is obvious that this first living substance had to subsist on inorganic food and obtain energy from it. Forms of life that can do this are called autotrophic. The inorganic substances that various kinds of bacteria are known to oxidize include ammonia, nitrites, hydrogen, sulfide, sulfur, and ferrous compounds. Also, a few species can oxidize hydrogen and a few others carbon monoxide. Most of these substances appear to have been dissolved in the sea water where primitive bacteria came into being. Carbon dioxide and perhaps carbon monoxide were probably the source of carbon.

Based on the source of the energy used for the synthesis of simple compounds or elements into more complex ones, we recognize *photosynthetic* and *chemosynthetic* plants.

Photosynthetic plants include most of the seed plants and the ferns, mosses, and algae. In the process of photosynthesis these plants, with the aid of their chlorophyll, use the energy of light to combine the carbon dioxide and water into some form of carbohydrate. A few of the Rhodobacteriineae do this with the aid of a green pigment, bacteriochlorophyll, which is one of the constituents of bacteriopurpurin and performs a function similar to that of chlorophyll. It is doubtful if the most primitive bacteria could carry on photosynthesis, as both chlorophyll and bacteriochlorophyll seem to have been products of evolution. It is conceivable that a simple form of photosynthesis not requiring these pigments may have been used in the earliest forms of life.

Chemosynthetic plants, most of which are bacteria, appear to be the most primitive of any now in existence. By the oxidation of such simple inorganic compounds as those mentioned above, they obtain the energy by which carbon dioxide is broken up and combined with other simple inorganic compounds to produce the various constituents of protoplasm.

The majority of autotrophic bacterial species obtain most of their food from nonliving organic material—plant and animal bodies and their secretions and excretions. In addition, most of them make use of some inorganic compounds such as ammonia, nitrates, chlorides, phosphates, and sulfates.

The organic compounds, carbohydrates, fats, and proteins, supplemented by a few inorganic salts, are easily used by saprophytes to supply materials for growth and for the energy required in synthesis of substances in the cell. Some of this material, such as glucose, is ready for use without preliminary treatment. Other kinds, such as starches and fats, have to be digested. Practically all culture media consists of combinations of organic and inorganic foods for saprophytes and *facultative parasites*, e.g., organisms that can grow either saprophytically or parasitically.

Parasitic Bacteria. Some bacteria have evolved the parasitic habit—that is, they have developed the ability to live intimately associated with the living cells of an organism or a different species, usually a higher animal or plant, and to take nourishment from it. These kinds of bacteria commonly cause disease, and if so they are also called *pathogenic.*

Strict parasites are those that cannot multiply except within the cells or fluids of a living host. They will not grow in a culture medium unless it contains living tissue. Strict parasites are very few among the true bacteria, exclusive of the Rickettsias and viruses. One of the few bacterial species that appear to be strictly parasitic is that which causes leprosy.

Facultative parasites are those that can multiply either within the cells or fluids of a suitable host or in nonliving substance such as those found in culture media.

Bacterial parasitism was once supposed to be restricted to humans and the higher animals but now more than one hundred species are known that are parasitic on plants, some of them causing destructive diseases such as fire blight of apple and pear trees.

Prototrophic, Metatrophic, and Paratrophic Bacteria. Some authorities use the term *prototrophic* for those bacteria that can live without organic food, e.g., the autotrophic species. Indeed, some of these find the presence of organic matter such as sugars and gelatin unfavorable for their development. In the same grouping the saprophytic bacteria are called *metatrophic,* and the parasitic bacteria are called *paratrophic.* While there is considerable overlapping among these three groups in that most bacteria can obtain their food in more than one way, the terms are convenient and widely used where sharp distinctions are not required.

Nutritional grouping vs. Relationship. For convenience it is often desirable to group living things in ways that have little to do with actual relationship. Thus, "carnivorous" animals may be mammals, birds, fishes, or insects; "parasitic" plants may be flowering plants, fungi, or bacteria; and "aquatic" plants include representatives of all four plant divisions. Assuming that the system of classification of bacteria used in this book is, for the most part, phylogenetic, it should be noted that the grouping given above does not correspond with phylogenetic relationships. Probably some of the autotrophic bacteria are actually primitive in that they have changed relatively little from the ancestral condition, while others have come from ancestors that were saprophytic. Some are included in the Eubacteriales, and some in the Chlamydobacteriales.

Origin of Saprophytism. It seems probable that, as there was little or no organic food on the earth when the first bacteria came into existence, these bacteria must all have been autotrophic. With the passage of time other kinds of plants and animals came into being, lived their lives, and died leaving a supply of organic matter. Some of the autophytes could not adapt themselves by evolutionary changes to the use of this organic food and remained autophytes as we have them today. Others, however, did undergo such evolutionary changes. They acquired the ability to produce digestive enzymes, underwent other less obvious changes, and became saprophytes while still making use of some inorganic salts.

Origin of Parasitism. Probably there was a time when both autophytes and saprophytes existed, but there were no parasites. Parasitism undoubtedly came about through evolutionary changes from saprophytism. Such changes probably took place repeatedly, separated by long intervals of time. The steps in this evolution are not known, but very likely they included the following events.

In the parasitism of plants certain saprophytic bacteria, having been introduced into wounds, stomata, water pores, nectaries, etc., were able to survive there and pass through evolutionary changes that enabled them to live and multiply in their new environment and penetrate deeper into their hosts. Thus they became plant pathogens.

Most bacteria that cause disease of plants are placed in two genera: *Xanthomonas,* rods usually with monotichic flagella, related to *Pseudomonas;* and *Erwinia,* rods with peritrichic flagella, some species of which are probably related to *Aerobacter* or *Escherichia.*

In animals, it is logical to assume there are at least three methods by which parasitism originated: (1) saprophytes, accidentally introduced into wounds, evolved into wound parasites; (2) saprophytes of the intestinal contents evolved into parasites such as those that cause typhoid fever, dysentery, and Asiatic cholera; and (3) saprophytes drawn into the respiratory tract evolved into parasites such as those that cause pneumonia and perhaps tuberculosis.

In the most highly developed form of parasitism, such as that of the protozoan *Gregarena melanopli* in the grasshopper or of *Trypanosoma lewisi* in the rat, the parasite obtains the full benefit of a parasitic life without doing serious damage to the host, leaving it alive to support the parasite.

4.3.16 Bacteria and Enzymes Relationship

It seems rather remarkable that organisms such as bacteria have evolved the power to produce enzymes corresponding closely to most of those produced by other kinds of plants and animals, including humans. These enzymes must be thought of as absolutely necessary products to the life of organisms.

Formation and properties of Enzymes. Enzymes are secretion products formed within the cells by the living protoplasm. Some of them remain within the cell during its lifetime and are called *intracellular* enzymes or endoenzymes. Others diffuse through the cell membranes into the surrounding medium and are called *extracellular* enzymes or exoenzymes. In some cases the secretion from the cell is not the true enzymes but a *proenzyme* or *zymogen,* which is changed into the true enzymes after it leaves the cell.

Probably some kinds of enzymes, such as oxidases, are produced by living things and aid in their respiration. Others are produced only by certain species.

The best known of the enzymatic changes are analytic, resulting in products chemically simpler than the substance destroyed. Others, however, are *synthetic* and thus aid in building up more complex substances, even protoplasm itself. In the naming of enzymes no system was followed for the first few that were discovered, but the ending -ase is not quite generally applied as a suffix to the name of the material affected, as maltase, gelatinase, urease, inulase, etc. This method of naming is complicated by the fact that different kinds of enzymes may act on the same substance with the formation of different product. From glucose, alcohol may be formed, or glycerol, or lactic acid, or oxalic acid. Enzymes cannot be classified by their appearance, for we do not know what most of them look like in a pure state; neither can they be classified by their chemical composition until we learn it more definitely for each one. There are two methods of classifying enzymes that are in common use. One is based on the kind of substance acted upon—carbohydrates, fats, proteins, etc. The other is based on the way in which chemical change is brought about—hydrolysis, oxidation, reduction, etc.

On the basis of the nature of chemical change brought about by the enzyme, two main classes may be distinguished: (1) hyrolases, which promote hydrolysis, and (2) oxidases (including reductases), which promote oxidation and reduction.

4.3.17 Enzyme Classification

The following partial classification of enzymes will, perhaps, serve better here than a more complete and elaborate one. The hydrolytic group includes enzymes that cause one or more molecules of water to combine with each molecule of substance, such as starch, with the formation of new substances. Most of the amylolytic and proteolytic enzymes bring about their changes by hydrolysis, making this a very large group.

A. The amylolytic group (carbohydrases) consists of enzymes that hydrolyze complex carbohydrates into simpler ones.

1. The amylolytic group (carbohydrases) consists of enzymes that hydrolyze complex carbohydrates into simpler ones.
   (a) Diastase (amylase, ptyalin). This enzyme, which varies slightly, depending on the source, hydrolyzes starch to maltose.
   (b) Cellulase is an enzyme that converts cellulose into the sugar cellobiose by a reaction similar to that given above for the destruction of starch, as cellulose has the same empirical formulas as starch. Cellulase is produced by many fungi but by only a few kinds of bacteria, chiefly certain species in the genus *Bacterium,* and also by some species of *Clostridium.* Both diastase and cellulase are exoenzymes.
   (c) Disaccharidases. These related enzymes change disaccharides into monosaccharides. The action of maltase, for example, is given below:

$$\underset{\text{Maltose}}{C_{12}H_{22}O_{11}} + H_2O \rightarrow \underset{\text{Glucose}}{2C_6H_{12}O_6}$$

   Invertase likewise converts sucrose into glucose and fructose, and lactase converts lactose into glucose and galactose. Disaccharidasses are produced by many species of fungi, yeasts, and bacteria. They are exoenzymes.

2. The lipolytic group (streatolytic group) includes the exoenzymes that hydrolyze fats, esters, etc. There are about a dozen members in the group. Lipases hydrolyze fats into fatty acids and glycerol. Comparatively few kinds of bacteria produce lipase, but when sufficient water occurs in fats and oils to support bacterial life, fats are hydrolyzed by certain species of bacteria. The keeping quality of fats is largely due to their dryness.

3. The proteolytic group includes extracellular enzymes that hydrolyze proteins and related substances. Best known of these are pepsin and trypsin, so important in animal digestion. No bacteria are known to produce pepsin. The proteases produced by many kinds of bacteria and fungi are similar in action to trypsin. Gelatinase, which hydrolyzes and liquefies gelatin if the latter is mixed with water to form a gel, is produced by many bacteria and fungi. Rennin hydrolyzes the casein of milk, forming paracasein, which combines with calcium to form a precipitate. The enzymes is produced abundantly by the stomachs of young mammals such as pigs, sheep, and calves. Some kinds of bacteria can produce it also.

B. The oxidizing group includes enzymes that promote the addition of oxygen to other substances. This is a very important group of enzymes that play a part in the respiration of all living things. The action of oxidizing enzymes is easily demonstrated by cutting open an apple and noting the browning that results from the rapid oxidation when the cut surface is exposed to the air. Dehydrogenases are oxidizing enzymes in the sense that they function by removing hydrogen from water by aerobic bacteria.

1. Alcoholoxidase is the important enzyme that oxidizes the alcohol produces by yeasts to the acetic acid of vinegar. It is produced chiefly by bacteria of the genus *Acetobacter.* There is some evidence that this is a group of enzymes rather than a single one.

2. Zymases are endoenzymes that change glucose and other monosaccharides into ethyl alcohol and carbon dioxide.

4.3.18 Classification Based on Bacterial Respiration

All living things require oxygen in their metabolism. Part of the oxygen enters into the composition of protoplasm and other constituents of the body, and part combines with carbon, hydrogen, and sometimes other elements or compounds, with the release of chemical energy. The products of this union generally include carbon dioxide and water.

In 1861 Pasteur discovered that certain kinds of bacteria could develop and carry on butyric fermentation in the absence of free oxygen. Since Pasteur's time, our knowledge of this phenomenon of *anaerobiosis* has been greatly extended.

As a result of these studies, bacteria may be grouped, on the basis of their oxygen requirements, as follows:

1. Aerobes are those that require oxygen in the free state.

2. Anaerobes are those that require oxygen in a combined form, as in a sugar. Growth of obligate anaerobes is inhibited in the presence of free oxygen. Three theories have been presented to explain this phenomenon: (a) oxygen is toxic to the cell, (b) hydrogen peroxide is produced by the cells and since the organisms do not secrete the enzyme catalase to decompose it to water and oxygen the hydrogen peroxide is toxic to the anaerobes, and (c) the growth of obligate anaerobes is dependent on a low oxidation-reduction potential, which is not possible in the presence of free oxygen. Probably none of these theories is adequate to explain why obligate anaerobes fail to grow in the presence of free oxygen, but the last reason mentioned seems to be the most satisfactory at present.

3. Facultative anaerobes can use oxygen in the free state if it is available, or they can use it in the combined state as to strict anaerobes.

4. Microaerophiles are organisms that use free oxygen, although their growth is inhibited by the full oxygen content of the atmosphere. In a stab culture made in nutrient agar they grow best at some distance below the surface, where the oxygen tension is low.

Recognize three kinds of respiration. (1) Aerobic respiration—the kind found in most animals and plants. (2) Intermolecular anaerobic respiration, which may take place in either of two ways. Oxygen may be removed from one compound, an oxygen donor, and added to another, an oxygen acceptor, as when a nitrate is reduced to a nitrite and the oxygen thus released is combined with sulfur and water or thiosulfate to form sulfuric acid. Stated more technically, an oxygen donor is oxidized by removal of hydrogen, while another compound serves as a hydrogen acceptor, and is reduced. Reduction of the hydrogen acceptor may involve loss of oxygen, with formation of water. (3) Intramolecular anaerobic respiration, in which an organic compound such as glucose is broken down with partial release of energy and formation of one or more new compounds capable of being oxidized further. The formation of ethyl alcohol from glucose is an example. The complicated series of reactions in the anaerobic decomposition of carbohydrates includes oxidation of both the second and the third types.

Respiration in Autotrophic (Prototrophic) Species. This discussion of respiration has emphasized the release of energy by the oxidation of carbon compounds such as sugars. Something should be added concerning the oxidation of unstable inorganic compounds, which is the kind of respiration carried on by the autotrophic bacteria. In the family Nitrobacteriaceae some members can oxidize hydrogen to water, carbon monoxide to carbon dioxide, and hydrogen sulfide to sulfuric acid. In others, the nitrifying bacteria, oxidize ammonia to nitrites and nitrites to nitrates.

Fermentation. This process has so much in common with respiration that the two can easily be confused. The term "fermentation" was first applied to the evolution of bubbles of the gas, carbon dioxide, in fermenting wine. It was thought of as a sort of cold boiling. The term is still applied to decomposition processes in which gases are evolved in liquids. It is now used, however, to include the formation by microorganisms of organic acids, alcohol, and some other substances by oxidative decomposition of carbohydrates and their derivatives.

Putrefaction. The general conception of putrefaction is the chemical decomposition of proteins and other nitrogenous substances with the production of disagreeable odors. It is usually anaerobic.

Decay. In a somewhat restricted sense of the term, "decay" is used to cover any aerobic decomposition of organic matter, but in a wider sense it is inclusive of putrefaction.

It will be noted that all these processes are brought about by enzymatic action and have much in common with digestion.

4.3.19 Nitrogen Metabolism of Bacteria

It is obvious that nitrogen in some form is needed for the manufacture of protoplasm. Most species of bacteria, like other forms of life, are unable to use free nitrogen but have to be supplied with some nitrogenous compound.

Recent work indicates that some kinds of bacteria, perhaps all, require a supply of the amino acid tryptophan. Some can manufacture it from ammonium salts or from other amino compounds, but others must have it supplied to them. This need may be regarded as a basic principle in the nitrogen metabolism of bacteria.

Proteins. Proteins are widely distributed in plant and animal bodies, both living and nonliving. For saprophytic and parasitic bacteria they are valuable sources of nitrogen. To use them, bacteria must secrete proteases for their digestion, and many of the bacteria in these groups can do this. To be used, the proteins are first broken down by the enzymes into proteoses, peptones, and amino acids. Amino acids may then be synthesized into protoplasm, or may be broken down into a variety of end products.

Amino Acids. If these substances have already been formed by some digestive process before the bacteria receive them, they are ready for use in the synthetic metabolism that goes on within the bacterial cell. Commercial peptone, which is extensively used in artificial culture media for both saprophytic and parasitic species, contains amino acids as well as more complex substances that require digestion. Peptone is not useful to most autotrophic bacteria and is harmful to many of them.

Ammonium Compounds. Many kinds of bacteria in all three of the nutritional groups, autotrophic, saprophytic, and parasitic, can use ammonium compounds. Probably the ability to do this is primitive and, having been acquired by the autotrophic bacteria, was handed down to the others, which still retain it. Except in the autotrophic species, an ammonium compound can be used only in the presence of a carbohydrate, or a similar source of energy. Ammonium compounds seem to be especially valuable as foods for many fungi.

Nitrites. Nitrites have antiseptic properties that make them injurious to most kinds of bacteria. However, the members of one genus, *Nitrobacter,* of the tribe Nitrobacteraceae, can oxidize them to nitrates. Some species of *Actinomyces* can use nitrites in very dilute solution. A few kinds of bacteria can reduce nitrites to ammonia and thus obtain oxygen.

Nitrates. It has been found by actual test that a considerable number of bacterial species can use nitrates and synthesize them into their own proteins. Also, some can use them as a source of oxygen in intermolecular respiration. The special value of nitrates to higher plants is generally recognized.

Free Nitrogen. Very few species of bacteria can use the free nitrogen of the atmosphere and "fix" it into nitrogen compounds. The half dozen species of *Rhizobium* can do this in symbiosis with the roots of leguminous plants in which they live, and the two species of *Azotobacter* and at least one species of *Clostridium,C. butyricum,* can do it nonsymbiotically.

4.3.20 The Mechanism of Infection

Parasitic organisms have the ability to take nourishment from the body of a living animal or plant, either its living protoplasm or secretions. Many bacterial species have never evolved the parasitic habit.

The Virulence of Pathogenic Bacteria. We use the terms *virulence* and *pathogenicity,* although not strictly synonymous, for some pathogens. For example, *Clostridium botulinum* are saprophytes but produce a deadly toxin, while there are few parasites that do very little harm to the bodies of their hosts.

In some cases parasitic organisms have not lost their power of growing saprophytically, as shown by their luxuriant development on artificial culture media, but a few have become strict parasites. Examples of such are *Mycobacterium leprae,* the rickettsias, and the fungi that cause rusts, smuts, and powdery mildews of higher plants.

Virulence must be looked on as variable in degree. Some strains of a pathogenic species cause severe forms of a disease, and other strains cause mild forms. In a given species or strain the virulence may remain fairly constant—as in *Malleomyces mallei,* the cause of glanders in horses, humans, and other animals—or it may vary from time to time. We know that *Salmonella typhosa* freshly removed from a patient has a high virulence, but it loses its virulence by continuous growth on artificial media. In some cases virulence is restored by inoculation into a very susceptible animal.

Virulence of Organism vs. Susceptibility of Host. Susceptibility of the host to disease is also variable in degree, intergrading from practically no resistance to complete resistance to any specific disease. It is obvious, then, that under favorable conditions disease will occur when the virulence of the organism is great enough to overcome the degree of resistance possessed by the host.

Specificity. After it had been suspected, but not yet proved, that some kinds of disease are produced by bacteria, the idea of specificity was expressed by von Plenciz in 1762.

Complete specificity would mean that one species of microorganism could attach only one kind of host and produce only one kind of disease. *Salmonella typhosa,* which causes typhoid fever in humans, is a good example. Actually, specificity is rarely so perfect. Most pathogens are capable of attacking several species of host that may or may not be closely related. The fact that monkeys, rabbits, guinea pigs, and mice may be infected artificially with some human diseases is of great value in experimental medicine.

Specificity expresses itself in the fact that no pathogen is known to attack both a plant and an animal, and very few can attack both a bird and a mammal, or both a warm-blooded and a cold-blooded animal. In the study of any infectious disease the determination of the range of susceptible hosts is important.

4.3.21 Sources of Infection

An extremely important consideration in dealing with infectious diseases is the source from which the germs were obtained.

Sources Outside the Host. Very few species of pathogenic bacteria normally multiply outside the body of the host. Even though they are capable of growing in specially prepared culture media, most of them cannot do so in water, soil, manure, etc. If they occur in such materials it is because they happened to be cast there, and in such places they are diminishing in numbers rather than increasing. Milk and some kinds of cooked foods do, however, offer suitable media for some of them.

Sources Within the Body of the Host. Here is the usual place of reproduction for most pathogens. During the early stages of the disease they increase enormously and are cast off with one or more of the excreta. As the host recovers, the organisms usually become fewer and disappear, but in a few diseases they may continue to inhabit the body after symptoms have disappeared. People and animals harboring such germs are called *carriers.* They are particularly important in diphtheria, typhoid fever, Asiatic cholera, scarlet fever, cerebrospinal meningitis, and pneumonia. As most such individuals are not known to be disease carriers they are not avoided as cases of the disease would be, and hence they are especially dangerous. It is obvious from what has just been said that human diseases are contracted from people more often than from objects or materials.

4.3.22 The Transmission of Disease-Producing Organisms

Bacteria do not pass from the diseased to the well by their own locomotion. Most of those cast off by a patient or a carrier die without reaching a susceptible host, but a small proportion are more fortunate.

Direct Contact Transmission. For many communicable diseases this is the most common method of transmission and with some, such as the venereal disease, it is the exclusive method. It is customary to distinguish between direct contact, in which there is actual touch, and indirect contact, in which a person infects an object that is soon touched by another person. In case the infected object was not touched by another person for some time—weeks or months— the object is called a fomes and the term fomites infection is used. This method is important only for disease caused by very resistant organisms such as *Clostridium tetani* and *Bacillus anthracis* (which are spore formers), *Mycobacterium tuberculosis,* and the virus of smallpox.

Transmission Through the Air. This term is applied to water or food that has become contaminated and is later swallowed by people or animals. It is an important mode of transmission of the different species of Salmonella and is of some importance in a wide range of diseases.

Disease Vectors. These are usually insects, ticks, etc., but may also be other kinds of animals that distribute disease organisms. Vectors offer the exclusive method of transmission of such important diseases as malaria, Rocky Mountain spotted fever, and African sleeping sickness.

4.3.23 Kinds of Immunity

It is convenient and, indeed, highly important to distinguish between the different kinds of immunity. Some of the classifications of this condition are unnecessarily complex and confusing. The following simple classification is well accepted and serves almost all practical purposes.

I. Natural	II. Acquired
(a) Racial	(a) Active
(b) Individual	(b) Passive

Natural immunity is specific. It is the immunity common to a species or race. Because of natural immunity humans do not have blackleg of cattle, and cattle do not have typhoid fever. As a rule all individuals of a species or race are naturally susceptible or naturally immune to a given disease, but occasionally immune individuals are found in a susceptible species.

Acquired immunity is a condition that a person or animal develops during his or her lifetime. He or she may have been susceptible to smallpox when he or she was born, but later developed an acquired immunity to it by having the disease or by having been vaccinated. It is important to recognize that there are two kinds of acquired immunity—that is, immunity may be acquired in the following two different ways:

1. In active immunity the body of the person develops its own immunizing antibodies, which are chemical in nature, as a result of a stimulus received from the entrance of a foreign substance. Called an antigen (e.g., pathogenic bacteria), the living cells of the body in their metabolism produce one or more chemicals that injure the pathogens or neutralize their

products. The fact that the body produces these antibodies through its own activity causes this kind of acquired immunity to be called active.

2. In passive immunity the body that is immunized plays no active part. It passively receives an injection of antitoxin or other protective substance previously formed by a person or animal that had developed active immunity. Some of the antibodies of the animal that produced them by active immunization are deposited in the serum of the blood, and this serum, if injected into a normal person or animal, gives it passive immunity.

4.3.24 Methods of Conferring Immunity

Natural immunity is, in a sense, inherited. Strictly speaking, the offspring inherits from its parents the characteristic of building its body in such a way that it naturally resists certain diseases.

Active immunity is acquired by receiving something into the body that will produce the disease in some form and thus stimulate the body to produce an immunizing substance—antitoxin.

1. Living, fully virulent organisms. Having the disease in the usual way illustrates this method.

2. Living organisms of attenuated virulence. Organisms may be attenuated by heat, by chemicals, or by passage through the body of some particular kind of animal and therefore produce the disease in a mild form. Active immunization against smallpox may be accomplished in this way.

3. Dead organisms. The dead bodies of some pathogenic organisms, when injected into a susceptible host, will stimulate that host to produce active immunity. As the organisms cannot multiply, this is a comparatively safe method. It is used in protecting against typhoid fever, whooping cough, Rocky Mountain spotted fever, and some other diseases.

4. Bacterial products. Bacterial toxins are very poisonous substances, but they can be used in either of two ways to confer active immunity. One way is to inject a very small dose, increasing it for subsequent injections. The other is to treat the toxin first with some chemical that will make it less poisonous. The resulting product is called a toxoid. The toxin of scarlet fever and the toxoid of diphtheria illustrate this method.

Passive immunity can be acquired in only one way—by receiving into the body antitoxin or other protective substance that has been formed by another person or animal and deposited in its blood serum. In comparatively few diseases can passive immunity be conferred. Diphtheria, tetanus, some types of pneumonia, meningitis, and gas gangrene are diseases in which it is used with success.

4.3.25 Vaccines versus Immunizing Serums

There is confusion on the role of vaccines and serums as agents for conferring immunity. The confusion appears to arise partly from the fact that both are, or may be, injected hypodermically with a small syringe, and the person does not know specifically just what is injected.

Vaccines. The term "vaccine," like many others, has both a broad and a restricted meaning. In the broad use of the term it is any biological material injected into the body to stimulate the development of active immunity, such as living or dead microorganisms, toxin, etc. In a more restricted sense, a vaccine is material containing the living organisms, as the virus of a disease, attenuated to make it safer. Smallpox vaccine is the common example. Those who use the term in this way generally call dead bacteria used for the same purpose "bacterins."

Immunizing the body by vaccination is generally done for prevention rather than cure. The vaccine is administered in advance of exposure so as to give the body time to set up active immunity before invasion by the organisms occurs. An exception is found in the use of autogenous vaccines. These are prepared by making cultures of the organisms from the disease lesions of the patient, killing them, and then injecting them back into the same person. They are used for such localized conditions as boils, in which the bacteria are so located that they do not stimulate an active immunity. Such an immunity is, however, set up when they are injected in large numbers under the skin.

As a curative agent the action of the antitoxins is very rapid unless the damage by the toxin has been done already; that is, unless the toxin has already united with the tissue of the nervous system or other vital organs.

4.3.26 The Mechanism of Immunity

The ways by which the body protects itself from disease when pathogens have been introduced, or the way it recovers and rids itself of pathogens that have ravaged it, have been the subject of much study.

It is now generally agreed that more than one mechanism operates in immunity. In some diseases at least two things have to be done to protect the body. (1) The toxins that have been released in the body must be neutralized or they will do harm independently of the organisms that produced them. (2) The organisms themselves must be destroyed or eliminated. These two things require different agents, although they are all considered as antibodies. Antibacterial substances do not destroy toxins and antitoxins do not destroy bacteria.

Opsonins. It has been found that there are antibodies in the blood that make it possible for the phagocyte to engulf bacteria more rapidly than they can without them. These substances are called "opsonins." They are specific, the opsonin of one disease having no effect on the bacteria of a different disease. If serum containing opsonin is added to a bacterial culture, the organisms are not killed or injured by it. They are, however, so affected that if leukocytes are then added, the bacteria are attracted to them and made more susceptible to ingestion. It is possible that the opsonins bring about other changes in the bacterial cells. Experiments have shown that in some diseases the amount of opsonin—that is, the opsonic index—is raised as the patient develops immunity and recovers.

Bacteriolysins. The blood and some other body fluids of normal people have some power of disintegrating or dissolving bacteria. This is called bacteriolysis and is one illustration of the more general phenomenon of cytolysis, or dissolution of foreign cells such as red and white blood corpsucles from other animals. In the case of certain diseases, bacteriolysins that are capable of destroying the causative bacteria have been produced and are present in the blood stream of those who have developed an immunity to them.

This phenomenon has been the subject of extensive researches that have shown that there are two substances in the blood that act jointly in the destruction of bacterial cells. One is a regular constituent of the normal blood of humans and other vertebrates and is known as complement or alexin. It is nonspecific, one kind aiding in the destruction of all kinds of bacteria. It is thermolabile, being destroyed by heat at 56° C for thirty minutes. It does not increase in the blood as the body becomes immune to disease. The other immunizing substance that takes part in bacteriolysis is called amboceptor or sensitizer. It is specific, a particular amboceptor being produced by the body in response to a particular kind of bacteria and reacting only with that kind of bacteria. The amboceptors are thermostable at 56° C for thirty minutes. The normal body has little or no amboceptor but produces it as immunity develops during the course of a disease or following successful vaccination.

Agglutinins. If the blood or serum of an animal containing an antibody is mixed in the presence of an electrolyte such as sodium chloride, with a laboratory culture of an organism of the kind that stimulated its formation, the combination will cause the cells to clump together, or agglutinate, although it will not kill them. This agglutination reaction is used in the diagnosis of typhoid fever, brucellosis in cattle and in humans, and several other diseases. For example, in the Widal test for typhoid fever, if the blood serum of a patient will cause a laboratory culture of *Salmonella typhosa* to agglutinate when tested under proper conditions, it indicates that the patient has formed typhoid agglutinin. In the presence of suggestive symptoms the disease may thus definitely be diagnosed as typhoid fever. An interesting fact is that the cells of a killed culture will be agglutinated as readily as those of a living culture. This shows that the clumping is not brought about by locomotion, but that it is caused by the influence of the antibody on the surface of the cell. More recently the principles of this reaction have been used in determining the potency of influenza virus vaccine as well as the amount of antibody in the serum of an animal previously inoculated with the virus investigations.

Precipitins. The precipitins, which are closely related to or identical with agglutinins, have a similar effect except that they act on molecules of protein or certain other substances and cause these soluble substances to take the form of a fine precipitate. In the agglutination reaction, bacteria are clumped together. The precipitin reaction is thus of value in the serological identification of soluble proteins in medicine, industry, and chemistry.

Antitoxins. Rather early in the study of medical bacteriology it was found that some kinds of bacteria, notably *Corynebacterium diphtheriae* and *Clostridium tetani*, produce deadly toxins, and that the blood serum of convalescents from the diseases produced by these organisms contains a specific antibody, antitoxin, that renders the toxin harmless. Just what the antitoxin does to the toxin has been the subject of some debate, but it is now generally conceded that the union between the two is physical rather than chemical. Certainly the toxin is not irretrievably destroyed, for it can to some extent be separated from a mixture of toxin and antitoxin in which the two are combined. The antitoxins are specific for their respective exotoxins.

Bodily Vigor vs Immunity. One of the most common misconceptions concerning immunity is that, as a rule, a high state of bodily vigor makes one resistant to disease, and a run-down condition makes one susceptible to disease. The facts are these: (1) No perfection of physical condition will protect one against most infectious diseases. People in perfect health readily contract smallpox, measles, or typhoid fever if properly exposed. (2) People in a badly run-down condition will not contract these diseases if they have active immunity against them. (3) A person in poor physical condition is not so likely to recover from prolonged and severe illness as one who is more vigorous. (4) Two infectious diseases, pneumonia and tuberculosis, carry out the popular idea in that people in perfect health do not acquire them so readily as those who are undernourished or otherwise weakened, as by some previous disease. (5) Many noninfectious diseases, such as rickets and scurvy, are direct results of malnutrition and other debilitating conditions.

4.3.27 Hypersensitivity

The bodies of human beings and other mammals are generally tolerant to the introduction of many foreign substances, including most proteins, but under certain conditions they may become extremely sensitive to minute doses taken through the stomach and the respiratory tract.

Two kinds of hypersensitivity, anaphylaxis and allergy, are commonly recognized, but they have much in common, and some authorities consider anaphylaxis as one manifestation of allergy.

Anaphylaxis. This type of hypersensitivity is brought about by introducing into the body a foreign protein of a kind generally regarded as harmless, or certain other substances. A very small dose is sufficient. No unfavorable symptoms are felt, but in about ten days, the body has become so highly sensitive to this protein that another minute dose of it will bring about anaphylactic shock. In the guinea pig, which is particularly responsive, this anaphylactic shock takes place within a few minutes following the second injection. It manifests itself in disturbed respiration—sneezing followed by a spasm in which the animal gasps for breath and usually dies of suffocation in a short time. The symptoms are the same in each kind of animal, regardless of the protein used, but vary in different species of animals. In the guinea pig the shock is due to a persistent contraction of the involuntary muscles of the bronchioles of the lungs; in rabbits there is a dilation of the right side of the heart; in humans these disturbances of the action of the involuntary muscles are less pronounced, and usually there is only a rash on the skin.

An important manifestation of anaphylaxis is serum sickness. As a result of receiving an immunizing serum the body may become sensitized to some protein that is part of the serum—not the antitoxin. A later injection of serum from the same kind of animal, such as a horse, will then cause serum sickness. This may take the form of anaphylactic shock but more often is very different and much milder. After about ten days the patient experiences a rise in temperature, pains similar to mild arthritis, and an extensive rash of the skin that itches and causes much discomfort. The term "serum sickness" is often restricted to these later manifestations, although similar symptoms may occur after initial contact with a foreign serum.

It is generally held that the tuberculin test for the presence of tuberculosis is an anaphylactic reaction. The proteins from Mycobacterium tuberculosis release within the body of the patient and bring about a sensitization.

Allergy. This term is sometimes used to include all kinds of hypersensitivity but is often restricted to those forms in which the body is abnormally sensitive to natural substances such as pollen, feathers, hair, dandruff, insect bites, bee stings, and various kinds of food such as milk, eggs, meats, and vegetable proteins. Some confusion exists between ordinary allergy, in which the person was not hypersensitive until he or she had received the initial dose of the foreign substance, and atopy, in which the person was sensitive from the start. In some cases classed as atopy it is possible that the condition came about through a sensitizing dose that was not realized at the time it was received.

One of the striking things about the allergies is the difference in the reactions of individuals. Toward the same substance some people may be atopic, others may become sensitized by injection, and still others may be immune under all conditions.

Allergy is a phenomenon of tremendous significance to the human race, since it results in such distressing maladies as hay fever, asthma, and many kinds of rashes.

4.3.28 Viruses, Bacteriophages, Rickettsias, and the Pleuropneumonia Group

In this section some of these disease-producing agents are too small to be seen even with a good light microscope. Because many of them readily pass through filters that bacteria cannot pass, they have been called "filterable viruses," but the name "virus" is now preferred. Examples of viral diseases are influenza, smallpox, measles, infantile paralysis, yellow fever, rabies, foot and mouth disease of cattle, dog distemper, mosaic diseases of plants, peach yellows, and curly top of sugar beets.

A number of animal diseases, notably hog cholera, parrot fever, and dog distemper, were once supposed to be of bacterial origin because cultures thought to be pure would cause them when inoculated into susceptible hosts. Later work has shown that the real cause is a virus that contaminated the cultures that would otherwise have been harmless.

Properties of Viruses. There are certain properties that all viruses have in common. (1) In nature they are always associated with diseased plants or animals. No saprophytic viruses are known and hence they are all classed as strict parasites. (2) If a small amount of virus is inoculated into a susceptible host, a great increase takes place as with any other organisms. There is no evidence of the spontaneous generation that has been claimed at various times for animals, bacteria, and finally for viruses. (3) They are specific, each kind of virus attacking only one or a limited number of host species and causing a definite disease with characteristic symptoms. (4) Most of them are antigenic, causing the host, if a person or animal, to produce antibodies that aid in recovery and protect in some measure against later attacks. (5) They are particulate—that is, the virus, as extracted for study, consists of a liquid in which are suspended ultramicroscopic particles. These particles range in size from 10 millimicrons to about 300 millimicrons and the majority of those that cause animal infections are more or less spherical in form. (6) They are somewhat more resistant to injurious conditions such as heat, dryness, and disinfectants than are the vegetative cells of bacteria, but they are less resistant than bacterial spores. Some viruses show a special affinity for certain tissues of the body. Thus in smallpox and measles the skin and mucous membranes are especially damaged, and in rabies and infantile paralysis the central nervous system suffers most and contains the virus in the greatest quantity.

At present the most widely accepted view of the origin of viruses is that presented by Green and Laidlaw. These workers believe that viruses represent degenerate descendants of larger pathogenic microorganisms. the most convincing argument for such an origin is the almost continuous range of forms between typical bacterial pathogens and the smallest viruses. The rickettsias have the appearance and staining characteristics of small bacteria but must be cultivated in a living medium as must the viruses. Some viruses, such as the psittacosis group that causes parrot fever, are relatively large. They stain like bacteria and act more like pathogenic bacteria than typical viruses. On the other hand, they are strict parasites in their nutritional requirements. Vaccinia or cowpox is caused by a medium-sized virus that is relatively complex and might also be a descendant of bacteria. The smaller viruses might equally well be derived from protozoa, spirochaetes, or higher fungi as from bacteria because they have so few characteristic features. Burnet proposes the belief that in the evolution of viruses there has developed an increasing simplicity in structure and a greater dependence on the host for the metabolic needs, until in the smaller viruses there are neither enzymes nor organs, nothing but a self-residuum of genetic mechanism.

It is known that the agent that causes a viral disease may be quite different from that which causes another; but it seems probable that they have much in common.

Inclusion Bodies in Viral Diseases. In many of the viral diseases of humans and animals, visible bodies have been found in the disease cells that are not present in corresponding cells of healthy animals. These are known as "inclusion bodies." In some diseases they are associated with the nucleus, in others with cytoplasm. Their nature is not well understood. Some believe that an inclusion body is a single parasite, others believe that it is a visible collection of the ultramicroscopic particles of the virus, but more regard it as a degeneration product of the diseased cells of the host.

Importance of Viral Diseases. In both the plant and animal kingdom the viral diseases are quite comparable in importance to the bacterial diseases. Plants have more viral diseases than do humans and animals; the number already studied and named is more than two hundred, with others being constantly added to the list. One needs only to glance at the examples given above to realize that some of the worst human and animal diseases belong to this group.

Carriers in Viral Diseases. Knowledge that there are carriers in bacterial diseases is based on finding the organisms in healthy people, either by cultures or by microscopic examination. Obviously such evidence cannot be bad for viral diseases where the causative agent is invisible and will not develop on culture media. There is, however, some epidemiological evidence that carriers occur in some viral diseases, such as influenza and infantile paralysis, where the disease often appears in localities, but there seems to be no alternative to the view that many disease producing viruses survive between epidermic periods in tissues of human carriers.

The uniform behavior of viral diseases from year to year with minor prevalences of extremely high or low virulence has been attributed to the fact that the genetic mechanism itself is a product of evolution. Because of this, the virus is continuously affected by the law of the survival of the fittest. When an extremely virulent form develops it may disappear rapidly if all the hosts are killed and no particles of virus itself may tend to neutralize its virulent activities.

Vaccines for Viral Diseases. The fact that most viral diseases of humans and animals confer a high degree of immunity offers hope that vaccines successful against them will be prepared. It is an interesting fact that two of the earliest vaccines used were for protection against viral diseases, smallpox and rabies. Such vaccines consist of the virus itself, attenuated or weakened so that it is safe to use although still antigenic. Rabies virus is attenuated by drying, and smallpox virus is attenuated by growing in a bovine animal.

The virus of yellow fever is attenuated by passage through the brains of mice and is then cultivated in chick embryos. For this purpose fertilized eggs with live embryos seven days old are used. The egg's shell is disinfected, a small hole is drilled in the end, and the embryo is inoculated with the attenuated virus, using a syringe and needle. The hole is then sealed and the eggs are incubated at 37° C for three to four days, after which they are aseptically opened and the embryos removed. These are pooled, weighed, and ground up in a saline-serum mixture. After centrifuging and filtering, the fluid portion is placed in vials and desiccated. Numerous sterility and potency tests are made before the vaccine is released for use.

In the case of influenza, two types of epidermic influenza virus have been established at present. These are type A and type B strains, each of which produces a specific infection. Recently evidence has accumulated indicating the value of influenza virus vaccine. This vaccine is prepared by inoculating a diluted influenza virus into me embryonic fluid of 10-day incubated fertile hen eggs. After 48 hours of incubation the egg is opened aseptically and the membranes surrounding the embryos, together with the larger blood vessels, are ruptured. The virus is absorbed on the red blood cells. This mixture is removed and by a process involving refrigeration and centrifugation, the virus is finally obtained in a saline solution free of the red blood cells. The purified and concentrated virus is then inactivated with formalin and a preservative is added. Type A and type B vaccine lots are then pooled in equal amounts and immunization and sterility tests are performed before the vaccine is administered.

4.3.29 Bacteriophage

Bacteriophage is a type of virus parasitic on specific bacteria. Literally translated the name means "eater of bacteria." Twort, and later d'Herelle, were the first to observe the lysis of bacteria and this action is often called the Twort-d'Herelle phenomenon. These bacterial viruses are specific and are commonly present in sewage and various types of feces. If these materials are passed through a bacteriological filter, the filtrate will contain material that, upon inoculation into a heavily clouded broth culture of bacteria, will soon cause it to become clear. Similarly, a little of the agent can be added to an actively growing culture and after a few minutes this material is streaked on a Petri dish. After incubation clear spots called plaques will be observed in the streaked areas due to the killing of some of the cells in that area by a specific bacteriophage.

Morphology of Bacteriophage. With the advent of the electron microscope, two strains of coliphage, designated as alpha and gamma but cultured on the same strain of *Escherichia coli*, have been shown to be structurally and differentiated "sperm-shaped" bodies. Both appear to have heads and tails of different sizes. Particles of a micrococcus bacteriophage appear somewhat similar but are of greater dimensions.

Action of Bacteriophage. The lysis of bacteria by bacteriophage is a rapid process in which the bacterium is the host and the virus particle is the parasite. Delbrueck and Luria report that in this phenomenon the first step is the adsorption of the virus on the cell and the next step is the penetration and the multiplication of the bacteriophage within the cell. It appears that only one particle enters the cell, and 21 to 25 minutes later about 135 particles are released as the cell is lysed. These particles may then enter other cells and the lysis continues. Additional study is necessary to understand the mechanism of multiplication of bacterial viruses and the method of bacterial lysis.

4.3.30 The Rickettsia Group

The rickettsias have been described as small, often pleomorphic, gram negative, bacterium-like organisms living and multiplying in arthropod tissues, behaving as obligate intracellular parasites and staining lightly with aniline dyes. These organisms are regarded as intermediate between the true bacteria and the viruses. They resemble bacteria in size, shape, staining characteristics, and nonfilterability. Their obligate intracellular parasitism is similar to that of the viruses. However, the viruses multiply only when the cells in a tissue culture are actively living, while the rickettsial multiplication goes on and is often maximal at a period when the tissue cells are metabolizing slowly or are no longer viable.

There are ten genera in the order Rickettsias, which comprise the pathogenic rickettsias. *Rickettsia prowazekii* is the cause of louse-and-fleaborne typhus fever, a disease that may reach epidemic proportions when a population becomes infected with lice, generally during wars or famines. Rocky Mountain spotted fever and a number of other diseases of this group are caused by Rickettsias ricketsii. All diseases of this group are spread by various species of ticks in which the pathogens have been found in practically every type of cell and in every organ. It is interesting to note that the spotted fever rickettsias multiply well in the cytoplasm as well as in the nuclei of cells in tissue cultures whereas those of the typhus group multiply exclusively in the cytoplasm and are never seen in nuclei.

There are several other rickettsial diseases of importance, such as Q-fever and tsutsugamuchi disease, which may attack humans, and heartwater, a highly fatal and economically important disease in goats, cattle, and sheep. In most cases the human symptoms for the rickettsial diseases are similar, being characterized by fever, skin rashes due to lesions of the blood vessels, and involvement of the brain. The lesions of Rocky Mountain spotted fever first appear on the hands and feet, while in typhus fever their appearance is first noted on the abdomen and back.

In typhus fever and Rocky Mountain spotted fever, recovery from the disease is accompanied by a high degree of active immunity for a long time. A vaccine for each of these diseases has been prepared by a number of interesting methods, some of which were discarded because they called for the use of living cultures. One method still used to some extent involves the cultivation of these strict parasites in the bodies of the vectors. Either the whole vector or certain heavily invaded tissues are ground up, centrifuged, and filtered, and the concentrated rickettsias treated with phenol to disinfect the preparation and inactive the organisms.

At present the yolk sac method developed by Cox, which is similar to the methods described previously for the cultivation of the viruses, is being used most extensively for the preparation of vaccines for rickettsial diseases. In these vaccines it is necessary to inactivate the organisms by a chemical, such as phenol, and to add formalin as a preservative. The active immunity developed for Rocky Mountain spotted fever is not of long duration and the vaccine must be administered annually. One inoculation of the typhus fever vaccine confers active immunity for a long period. Passive immunity against these diseases have not been definitely established.

4.3.31 Skills to Review Bacteria and Viruses

Review the following terms and concepts using the D-E-F-IN-E model shown earlier. (See chapter 1.)

_____ Bacteria
_____ Bacteriophage
_____ Virus
_____ Rickettsiae
_____ Immunity
_____ Types of Bacteria
_____ Classification of Bacteria
_____ Hypersensitivity
_____ Sources of Infection
_____ Class Schizomycetes
_____ Vaccine
_____ Nonvirulent
_____ Nutritional Grouping of Bacteria
_____ Bacteria and Enzymes Relationship

_____ Characteristics of Class Schizomycetes
_____ Key to the Orders and Suborders of the Class Schizomycetes
_____ The Order Eubacteriales
_____ The Suborder Eubacteriineae
_____ Families in Eubacteriineae
_____ The Suborder Caulobacteriineae
_____ The Suborder Rhodobacteriineae
_____ The Order Actinomycetales
_____ The Order Chlamydobacteriales
_____ The Order Myxobacteriales
_____ The Order Spirochaetales
_____ Bacterial Respiration
_____ Nitrogen Metabolism of Bacteria
_____ The Mechanism of Infection
_____ Sources of Infection
_____ The Transmission of Disease-Producing Organisms
_____ Kinds of Immunity
_____ Methods of Conferring Immunity
_____ Vaccines vs. Immunizing Serums
_____ The Mechanism of Immunity
_____ Hypersensitivity
_____ Viruses, Bacteriophages, Rickettsias, and the Pleuropneumonia Group

4.4 REFERENCES

Hoar, William S. *General and Comparative Physiology*, 3rd ed. (Prentice-Hall, Inc., 1983).

Jackson, John D., and Jane B. Taylor. *Study Guide for Starr's Biology Concepts and Applications* (Wadsworth Publishing Company, 1991).

Kaufman, Peter B., et. al., *Practical Botany* (Reston, 1983).

Kaufman, Peter B. *Plants: Their Biology and Importance* (Harper and Row, 1989).

Noggle, G. Ray, and George J. Fritz. *Introductory Plant Physiology*, 2nd ed. (Prentice-Hall, Inc., 1983).

Rayle, David L., and Hale L. Wedberg. *Botany: A Human Concern*, 2nd ed. (Holt, Rinehart and Winston, 1980).

Schmidt-Nielsen, Knut. *Animal Physiology* , 3rd ed. (Prentice-Hall, Inc., 1970).

_____*Animal Physiology: Adaptations and Environment*, 4th ed. (Cambridge University Press, 1990).

Starr, Cecie. *Biology: Concepts and Applications* (Wadsworth Publishing Company, 1991).

Villee, Claude A., and Solomon, Eldra. *Biology*, 2nd ed. (Saunders College Publishing, 1989).

Wilkins, Malcom. *Plantwatching: How Plants Remember, Tell Time, Form Partnerships and More* (Facts on File, Inc., 1988).

Chapter 5:
Developing Quantitative Reasoning and Ability

5.0 INTRODUCTION TO QUANTITATIVE ABILITY

The Quantitative Ability examination is forty-five minutes long and contains sixty-five items. To prepare successfully for the quantitative ability section, you need to develop your ability to reason with numbers, manipulate numerical relationships, and apply information appropriately in situations involving quantitative material.

This chapter follows the PCAT test booklet outline. It presents mathematical concepts and exercises in various topics. Speed and accuracy are necessary for proficiency on this section. No mathematical tables, ruler, measuring devices, calculating devices, calculators, slide rules, etc., are allowed inside the testing center. Therefore, it is recommended that you prepare for the PCAT without such aids. The Quantitative Ability examination has items that are divided into two groups: mathematical operations and applied mathematics problems. Mathematical operations test your knowledge of arithmetic, algebra, and geometry. The applied mathematics problems consist of practical word problems.

5.1 QUANTITATIVE APPROXIMATION SKILLS

The ability to approximate, estimate, and round off numbers in mathematical calculations are useful skills for the PCAT. Regarding approximation and estimation, work with these skills carefully because alternative answer choices may be very close. During practice compare your estimated answer to the actual answer. Experience and practice will make you a better estimator. Review section 5.7.2 to understand precision and accuracy in measurements.

Learn to express a decimal in fewer digits, an approximation called rounding. In some cases doing mental arithmetic by changing an arithmetic problem to an equivalent problem can be done easily (without pencil or paper). This type of approximation is called number rounding.

(a) Rounding down:
Round off 3.1416 to two decimal places. (Answer: 3.14)
If the first digit to be dropped is less than five, then the last retained digit is unchanged (rounding down).

(b) Rounding up:
Round 0.4536 to three decimal places. (Answer: 0.454)
If the first digit to be dropped is greater than five, then the last retained digit is increased by one.

(c) Number rounding:
Numbers may be rounded to the nearest ten, hundred, thousand, etc.
246 → Rounded to nearest ten is 250.
→ Rounded to nearest 100 is 200.

(d) Sum estimation:

(i) Estimate sums by rounding to the nearest ten.
$789 + 42 = 831
790 + 40 = 830

(ii) Estimate sums by rounding to the nearest 100.
428 + 583 = 1,011
400 + 600 = 1,000

(iii) Numbers can be added by conversion to simpler numbers.
789 + 42 = (700 + 89) + (40 + 2)
= (700 + 40) + (89 + 2)
= (740 + 80) + 9 + 2
= 820 + 11 = 831

(e) Multiplication by rounding numbers:
Simplification is made easier by taking each number and rewriting it as a sum or difference of equivalent numbers, i.e., 58 = 50 + 8 and 66 = 60 + 6, therefore using the form $(a + b)(a + b) = a^2 + 2ab + b^2$, the result is as follows:

(i) 58 × 66 = (50 + 8) (60 + 6)
= 3,000 + 300 + 480 + 48
= 3,000 + 300 + 400 + 80 + 40 + 8
= 3,700 + 128
= 3,828 (exact answer)

Approximate answer:
58 × 66 = 60 × 65
= 3,900

(ii) Find the approximate quotients:
$\frac{89}{58} \cong \frac{90}{60} \cong 1.50$
$\frac{89}{58} = 1.53$ (exact answer)

5.2 FRACTION SIMPLIFICATIONS AND FACTOR DETERMINATION SKILLS

A fractional number is a ratio of two numbers expressed as a/b in which *a* can be any positive or negative number and *b* can be any positive or negative number except 0. The fraction is made up of two parts, the numerator and the denominator. In $\frac{3}{7}$ the numerator is 3, which indicates how many of the 7 equal parts are considered. In $\frac{5}{6}$ the number 6 is the denominator that indicates the number of equal parts. Factors are associated with fractional operations and interpretations.

5.2.1 Concepts Related to Simplification of Fractions

(a) When the numerator is less than the denominator, the fraction is called a *proper fraction,* otherwise the fraction is called an *improper fraction.*

Proper fractions: $\frac{1}{2}$ $\frac{3}{4}$ $\frac{7}{9}$ $\frac{11}{13}$

Improper fractions: $\frac{5}{3}$ $\frac{6}{6}$ $\frac{10}{5}$ $\frac{8}{5}$

(b) A *mixed number* has a whole number part and a fraction part.

$3\frac{1}{4}$ 3 = whole number part +

$\frac{1}{4}$ = fractional part

(c) Reduction of equivalent fractions:
Equivalent fractions are fractions with the same value but different numerators and denominators.

Examples: $\left(\frac{2}{6} \text{ and } \frac{1}{3}\right)$, $\left(\frac{3}{4} \text{ and } \frac{9}{12}\right)$, $\left(\frac{1}{2} \text{ and } \frac{3}{6}\right)$

(d) Fraction multiplication:
Multiplying a numerator and denominator by the same whole number can produce equal fractions:

$\frac{1}{2} = \frac{3}{6}$ because $\frac{3}{3} \times \frac{1}{2} = \frac{3}{6}$

$\frac{3}{4} = \frac{9}{12}$ because $\frac{3}{3} \times \frac{3}{4} = \frac{9}{12}$

(e) Reciprocal fractions:
Reciprocal fractions are two fractions whose numerators and denominators are reversed. Their product is always equal to 1.

$\frac{1}{5}$ and $\frac{5}{1}$ are reciprocals, $\frac{1}{5} \times \frac{5}{1} = 1$

$\frac{3}{4}$ and $\frac{4}{3}$ are reciprocals because $\frac{3}{4} \times \frac{4}{3} = 1$

5.2.2 Concepts Related to Determining Factors

The factors of a whole number are those whole numbers that divide *evenly* into the given number. A whole number is even if it can be divided evenly by 2, otherwise it is odd.

Example: Write the factors of 8
8: 1, 2, 4, 8
Example: Write the factors of 28
28: 1, 2, 4, 7, 14, 28

(a) Divisibility skills:

When is 2 a factor? 2 is a factor of a number if the last digit in the number is even.

When is 3 a factor? 3 is a factor of a number if the sum of the number's digits is divisible by 3.

When is 4 a factor? 4 is a factor of a number if the sum of the number's last 2 digits is divisible by 4.

When is 5 a factor? 5 is a factor of a number if the last digit in the number is 0 or 5.

When is 6 a factor? 6 is a factor of a number if the last digit is even and the sum of the digits is divisible by 3.

(b) Common (c) factors and how to find them:
Common (c) factors are identical factors that are common (c) and contained in two or more numbers.

Example: Write all the factors of 8 and 28
8: 1, 2, 4, 8
c c c
28: 1, 2, 4, 7, 14, 28
Common factors: 1, 2, and 4

(c) Finding the GCF:
The greatest common factor (GCF) is the greatest or largest of the common factors found in two or more numbers.

Example: Write the GCF of 24 and 32
Factors of 24: 1, 2, 3, 4, 6, 8, 12, 24
Factors of 32: 1, 2, 4, 8, 16, 32
Common factors: 1, 2, 4, 8
GCF: 8
A fraction is said to be in simplest form when the GCF of the numerator and denominator is 1.

(d) GCF simplification:
Dividing the numerator and denominator of a fraction by the GCF does not change the value of a fraction. It simply reduces the fraction to a simpler form.

Example: $\frac{6}{8} = \frac{6}{8} \div \frac{2}{2} = \frac{3}{4}$
GCF of 6 and 8 is 2
6 = 1, 2, 3, 6
8 = 1, 2, 4, 8
GCF = 2

Example: Reduce $6\frac{8}{12}$ to lowest term

$$6 + \frac{8}{12} \div \frac{4}{4} = 6 + \frac{2}{3} = 6\frac{2}{3}$$

(e) Finding the common multiple:
The multiple is the product of a given number and a whole number. To find the multiples of a number, multiply it by each integer number, e.g., 1, 2, 3, 4, etc.

Example:
Multiples of 3 are 3, 6, 9, 12, 15...
Multiples of 4 are 4, 8, 12, 16, 20...
If one number is divisible by another, it is a multiple of that number. When the multiples of two or more numbers have a value in common, this value is called a *common multiple* of the numbers.
3: 6, 9, 12, 15
5: 10, 15
15 is a common multiple of 3 and 5

(f) Finding the least common multiple finding:
The smallest common multiple of two or more numbers is called the Least Common Multiple (LCM).

2 = 2, 4, 6, 8, 10, 12
3 = 3, 6, 9, 12
4 = 4, 8, 12
LCM = 12

The Least Common Denominator of two or more fractions is the LCM of the denominators of the fractions.

Example: Find the LCD of $\frac{1}{4}$ and $\frac{1}{5}$

$\frac{1}{4}$ = 4, 8, 12, 16, 20, 24

$\frac{1}{5}$ = 5, 10, 15, 20, 25

LCD = 20

5.3 OPERATIONAL MATH WITH FRACTIONS

5.3.1 Addition of Fractions

(a) Adding like denominators:
To add fractions that have common denominators, add their numerators and keep the same common denominator.

Example: Determine the sum of $\frac{1}{4}+\frac{5}{4}+\frac{3}{4}$ by adding the numerators: 1 + 5 + 3 = 9 keeping the same common denominator, 4.

$$\frac{1}{4}+\frac{5}{4}+\frac{3}{4}=\frac{9}{4}=2\frac{1}{4}$$

(b) Adding unlike denominators:
To add fractions with unlike denominators, determine the least common denominator. Express each fraction in equivalent form with the LCD. Then perform the addition.

Example: Determine $\frac{1}{2}+\frac{3}{4}+\frac{2}{8}$
LCD = 8

The sum with the fractions in equivalent form is $\frac{4}{8}+\frac{6}{8}+\frac{2}{8}=\frac{12}{8}$ or $\frac{3}{2}$ or $1\frac{1}{2}$.

(c) Adding mixed numbers:
To add mixed numbers calculate the sum of the integers separately from the sum of the fractions. Then add the sums.

Example: Add the mixed numbers $7\frac{1}{6}$ and $2\frac{3}{4}$
First, add the integers: $7 + 2 = 9$
then add the fractions, $\frac{1}{6}+\frac{3}{4}=\ ?$
The LCM = 12: $\frac{1}{6}+\frac{3}{4}=\frac{2}{12}+\frac{9}{12}=\frac{11}{12}$
$$7\frac{1}{6}+2\frac{3}{4}=9\frac{2+9}{12}=9\frac{11}{12}$$

5.3.2 Subtraction of Fractions

As with addition, before two fractions can be subtracted they must have a common denominator.

Example: $\frac{3}{4}-\frac{2}{3}$
The LCD is 12. The subtraction with the fraction in equivalent form gives:
$$\frac{3}{4}\times\frac{3}{3}-\frac{2}{3}\times\frac{4}{4}=\frac{9}{12}-\frac{8}{12}=\frac{1}{12}$$

5.3.3 Multiplication of Fractions

(a) Multiplication:
To multiply two or more fractions multiply their numerators to obtain the numerator of the product. Multiply the denominators to obtain the denominators of the product.

Example: Multiply $\frac{3}{7}\times\frac{2}{5}$
The desired product is $\frac{3\times 2}{7\times 5}=\frac{6}{35}$

(b) Cancelling common factors:
Calculations are greatly simplified and the product put in simplest terms by cancellation of common factors.

Example: $\frac{2}{5} \times \frac{10}{3} \times \frac{6}{7}$

Express all the numerators and denominators in factored form, cancel the common factors, and carry out the multiplication of the remaining factors. Cancellation lets you work with smaller rather than larger numbers in the numerator and denominator, which decreases the chances of error.

$$\frac{2}{5} \times \frac{2 \times 5}{3} \times \frac{2 \times 3}{7} = \frac{8}{7}$$
$$= 1\frac{1}{7}$$

(c) Mixed number multiplication skill:

Every integer, $\frac{a}{b}$ where $b \neq 0$, can be written as a fraction. An integer divided by 1 is equal to the integer.

Example: $\frac{3}{5} \times 6 \Rightarrow \frac{3}{5} \times \frac{6}{1} = \frac{3 \times 6}{5} = \frac{18}{5} = 3\frac{3}{5}$

To multiply mixed numbers, convert them first into fractions and then apply the rule for multiplication of fractions.

Example: Multiply $1\frac{3}{4}$ by $3\frac{1}{7}$

Convert $1\frac{3}{4}$ and $3\frac{1}{7}$ into common or improper fractions (an improper fraction is one in which the numerator is larger than the denominator, otherwise it is a proper fraction) and multiply:

$$1\frac{3}{4} = \frac{4}{4} + \frac{3}{4} = \frac{7}{4}$$
$$3\frac{1}{7} = \frac{21}{7} + \frac{1}{7} = \frac{22}{7}$$
$$\frac{7}{4} \times \frac{22}{7} = \frac{7}{2 \times 2} \times \frac{2 \times 11}{7} = \frac{11}{2} = 5\frac{1}{2}$$

5.3.4 Division of Fractions

(a) Division:

To divide one fraction by another, invert the second fraction after the division sign and multiply the fraction, which is the process of interchanging the numerator and denominator of the second fraction. This gives the reciprocal of a fraction.

The reciprocal of $\frac{a}{b}$ is $\frac{b}{a}$, where, $a \neq 0$, and $b \neq 0$. For example, the reciprocal of $\frac{3}{2}$ is $\frac{2}{3}$.

(b) Finding the reciprocal:
To find the reciprocal of a whole number, first write the whole number as a fraction with a denominator of 1; then find the reciprocal of that fraction:
The reciprocal of 5 is $\frac{1}{5}$, because $5 = \frac{5}{1}$
The reciprocal of a number is 1 divided by the number. It follows from the definition that the product of a number and its reciprocal is 1.

Example: the reciprocal of $\frac{a}{b}$ is $\frac{b}{a}$, therefore $\frac{a}{b} \times \frac{b}{a} = \frac{ab}{ab} = 1$

Example: Divide $\frac{3}{5}$ by 7

Division by Zero
It is important to emphasize that division by zero is impossible, therefore a fraction cannot have zero as a denominator.

The division operation can be obtained by $\frac{3}{5} \div \frac{7}{1}$, rewriting 7 as $\frac{7}{1}$.
Applying the rule for division of fractions, the result is:
$\frac{3}{5} \div \frac{7}{1} = \frac{3}{5} \times \frac{1}{7} = \frac{3}{35}$.

(c) Dividing mixed numbers:
To divide mixed numbers, convert them first to fractions and apply the rule for division.

(d) Miscellaneous examples:
Example: What is the value of $\frac{1}{6} - \frac{3}{8} - \frac{2}{3} + \frac{3}{4}$?

A. $\frac{1}{24}$

B. $\frac{-3}{24}$

C. $\frac{21}{24}$

D. $\frac{-1}{24}$

The correct answer is **B.**

Solution: Find the LCD of 6, 8, 3, 4.
6 = 6, 12, 18, 24 (multiples)
8 = 8, 16, 24 (multiples)
3 = 3, 6, 9, 12, 15, 18, 21, 24 (multiples)
4 = 4, 8, 12, 16, 20, 24 (multiples)
LCD = 24

$$\frac{1}{6}-\frac{3}{8}-\frac{2}{3}+\frac{3}{4}=\frac{4(1)-3(3)-8(2)+6(3)}{24}$$
$$=\frac{4-9-16+18}{24}$$
$$=\frac{-5-16+18}{24}$$
$$=\frac{-21+18}{24}$$
$$=\frac{-3}{24}$$

Example: Multiply $5\frac{3}{7} \times 3\frac{1}{2}$:

A. $\frac{2}{7}$

B. $\frac{19}{7}$

C. 19

D. $\frac{7}{2}$

The correct answer is **C.**

Solution: Change both mixed numbers to improper fractions.

$$5\frac{3}{7}=\left(\frac{35+3}{7}\right);\ 3\frac{1}{2}=\frac{6}{2}+\frac{1}{2}=\frac{7}{2}$$

Multiply using the rule for multiplying fractions: $\frac{38}{7}\times\frac{7}{2}=\frac{2\times 19}{7}\times\frac{7}{2}=19$

5.4 PERCENTS, DECIMALS, AND FRACTIONS

Remember the following conversion model for percents, decimals, and fractions:

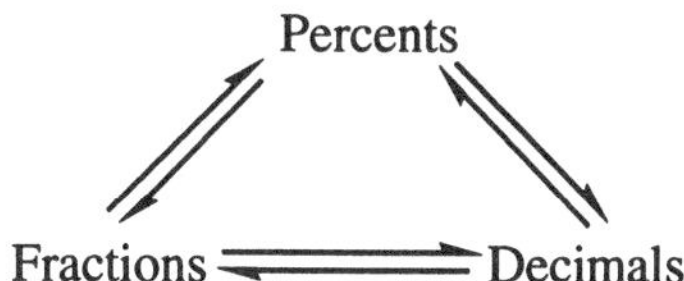

Fig. 5.1 — Conversion Model for Percents, Decimals, and Fractions

Percent means "part of 100," one one-hundredth. If you consider that a quantity is subdivided into 100 equal parts, a certain percent of the quantity is the number of these hundredth parts involved. The word *rate* is sometimes used for percent.

Thus, a percent is really a fraction: 25% is 25 parts of 100, or $\frac{25}{100}$, or $\frac{1}{4}$.

Percentage results from taking a specified percent of a quantity. The process of using percent in calculations is called percentage operations. *Base* is the number of which a given percent is calculated. When percent is involved, it is the quantity that is divided into 100 parts.

5.4.1 Conversion Skills for Percents, Decimals, and Fractions

Percent is a special type of fraction with 100 as a denominator. The symbol for percent is %. Thus, 20 percent (20%) means 20 hundredths or $\frac{20}{100}$, 60 percent (60%) 60 hundredths or $\frac{60}{100}$. A percent may always be reduced to a fraction and then this fraction may in turn be expressed in decimal form. Thus, 25 percent represents the same fractional measure as $\frac{25}{100}$ or $\frac{1}{4}$ or the same decimal measure as 0.25. A fractional measure can always be expressed as a percent by writing an equivalent fraction with 100 as its denominator.

Thus, $0.24 = \frac{24}{100} = 24\%$ and $1.15 = \frac{115}{100} = 115\%$

Skills for converting a decimal fraction to a percent and vice versa are as follows:

(a) Decimal to percent conversion:
To convert a decimal fraction to equivalent percent, multiply the decimal fraction by 100. This means that the decimal point has to be moved two places to the right. For example, express 2.15 as a percent. Multiply by 100, which means moving the decimal point two places to the right.

$2.15 \times 100 = 215\%$.

(b) Fraction to decimal conversion:

To convert a percent to a decimal fraction, divide the numerator by the denominator using long division, e.g., express $\frac{1}{4}$ as a decimal by dividing 1 into 4. One does not divide into 4, hence add a zero and put a decimal point in the quotient, $\frac{1.0}{4}$ = 0.2. Add another zero to get $\frac{1.00}{4}$ = 0.25 to two decimal places. Memorize a few common conversions for the PCAT: $\frac{1}{4}$ = 0.25; $\frac{1}{2}$ = 0.50; $\frac{3}{4}$ = 0.75; $\frac{1}{8}$ = 0.125; $\frac{3}{16}$ = 0.1875; $\frac{3}{8}$ = 0.375.

(c) Fraction to percent conversion:
To convert a fraction to percent, convert the fraction so that its denominator is 100. The numerator of the new fraction is the percent. The fraction also may be converted into its decimal equivalent using long division.
Example: Express $\frac{6}{25}$ as a percent by multiplying the fraction by $\frac{4}{4}$, $\frac{6}{25} \times \frac{4}{4} = \frac{24}{100} = 24\%$.

Example: Express $\frac{3}{7}$ as a percent by converting $\frac{3}{7}$ to its decimal equivalent,

$\frac{3}{7} = 3 \div 7 = 0.42857.... \cong 42.86\%$.

5.4.2 Word Problems Using Percent Rate, Percentage Change

All percentage problems can be reduced to three types.

1. Calculating the percent of a given quantity, = percentage.
2. Determine the rate or percent rate, = rate.
3. Calculating the base or the quantity, = base.

Most percent problems involve three quantities:

The rate, **R**, which is followed by a percent (%) sign.
The base, **B**, which follows the word "of" or a preposition.
The amount of percentage, **P**, which usual follows the word "is" or a verb.

Thus a basic equation or formula can be used to solve most types of percentage problems.

$\frac{R}{100} = \frac{P}{B}$, where
R = Rate or %
B = Base
P = Percentage

Example: What is 5.7% of 160?

Using the formula $\frac{R}{100} = \frac{P}{B}$, noting R = 5.7%, P = unknown, and B = 160

$$\frac{5.7}{100} = \frac{P}{160}$$
$$100\,P = 160\,(5.7)$$
$$P = \frac{10 \times 16\,(5.7)}{10 \times 10} = \frac{91.2(10)}{10 \times 10}$$
$$= 9.12$$

Answer: P = 9.12

Example: 72 is what percent (%) of 120?

Using the formula $\frac{R}{100} = \frac{P}{B}$
R = unknown
P = 72
B = 120

$$\frac{R}{100} = \frac{72}{120}$$
$$120\,R = 72\,(100)$$
$$R = \frac{72\,(10)\,(10)}{12\,(10)} = \frac{720}{12} = 60$$

Answer: R = 60%

Example: A copper compound contains 80% copper by weight. How much copper is there in a 1.95 g sample of the compound?

A. 15.60
B. 156
C. 1.56
D 15.0

The correct answer is **C.**

Solution: Using the formula $\frac{R}{100} = \frac{P}{B}$,

R = 80%
P = Unknown
B = 1.95

$$\frac{80}{100} = \frac{P}{1.95}$$
$$100\,P = 80\,(1.95)$$
$$P = \frac{(10)\,(8)\,(1.95)}{(10)\,(10)}$$
$$P = \frac{15.60}{10} = 1.56$$

Therefore, the given sample contains 1.56g of copper.

Special Percent Skills

(a) Percent change, percent increase, and percent decrease are special types of percent problems in which the difficulty is in making sure to use the right numbers to calculate the percent. The full formula is:

$$\frac{\text{(New Amount)} - \text{(Original Amount)}}{\text{(Original Amount)}} \times 100 = \text{Percent change}$$

(b) Where the new amount is less than the original amount, the number on top will be a negative number and the result will be a *percent decrease.* When a percent decrease is asked for, the negative sign is omitted.

(c) Where the new amount is greater than the original amount, the percent change is positive and is called a *percent increase.* The percent of increase or decrease is found by putting the amount of increase or decrease over the original amount and changing this fraction by multiplying with 100.

Example: Mrs. Morris receives a salary increase from $25,000 to $27,000. Find the percent increase.

Using the formula,

$$\frac{\text{(New Amount)} - \text{(Original Amount)}}{\text{(Original Amount)}} \times 100$$

$$\frac{\$27000 - \$25000}{\$25000} \times 100 = \frac{2000}{\$25000} \times 100 = \frac{20}{250} \times 100 = \frac{200}{25} = 8\%$$

The percent increase is 8%.

(d) A percentage is just an alternative way of representing a fraction or ratio as explained earlier. The statement "x is P percent (P%) of y" means that:

$$x = \frac{P}{100} \bullet y \quad \text{or, equivalently,} \quad P = \frac{x}{y} \bullet 100$$

Important: A percentage is a fraction with a denominator of 100, e.g., a nickel is 5% of a dollar. Percentages are typically used to express the fractional part that one quantity is of another; for example, if there are 16 women in a class of 25 students, then alternatively one can say that P = (16/25)(100) = 64% of the students in the class are women. Percentages are also used to express a change in a quantity in terms of its percent increase or decrease. By definition, if x_2 is the result when x_1 is increased by P%, then:

$$x_2 = x_1 + \frac{P}{100} \bullet x_1 = x_1 \bullet (1 + \frac{P}{100});$$

if x_2 is the result when x_1 is decreased by P%, then:

$$x_2 = x_1 - \frac{P}{100} \bullet x_1 = x_1 \bullet \left(1 - \frac{P}{100}\right).$$

It is important to note that in both of these definitions the change in the variable is expressed as a percentage of its original value (x_1), not its final value (x_2).

Example: What is the percent increase or decrease in a quantity x when its value is: a) doubled, b) halved, c) reduced by a third, d) reduced to a third of its original value, and e) reduced to a fifth of its original value?

(a) $x_2 = 2x_1$; $2x_1 = x_1\left(1 + \frac{P}{100}\right)$, P = 100% increase

(b) $x_2 = \frac{1}{2}x_1$; $\frac{1}{2}x_1 = x_1\left(1 - \frac{P}{100}\right)$, P = 50% decrease

(c) $x_2 = \frac{2}{3}x_1$; $\frac{2}{3}x_1 = x_1\left(1 - \frac{P}{100}\right)$, P= $33\frac{1}{3}$% decrease

(d) $x_2 = \frac{1}{3}x_1$; $\frac{1}{3}x_1 = x_1\left(1 - \frac{P}{100}\right)$, P = $66\frac{2}{3}$% decrease

(e) $x_2 = \frac{1}{5}x_1$; $\frac{1}{5}x_1 = x_1\left(1 - \frac{P}{100}\right)$, P = 80% decrease

5.5 SCIENTIFIC (EXPONENTIAL) OPERATIONAL SKILLS

5.5.1 Scientific Notation

A number is said to be in scientific notation if it is expressed as the product of a number between 1 and 10 and some integral power of 10. For example, 1,000 is written in scientific notation as 1×10^3 or more simply, 10^3; 0.0001 is written as 10^{-4}; $1247 = 1.247 \times 10^3$; and finally, $0.000786 = 7.86 \times 10^{-4}$.

5.5.2 Conversion to and from Scientific Notation

Since the decimal point of any number can be shifted at will to the left or to the right by multiplying by an appropriate power of 10, any number can be expressed in scientific notation. In general, if **n** is any number, we write $n = a \times 10^z$, where **a** is a number between 1 and 10 and **z** is an integer, positive or negative.

Example: Write 10,000,000 in scientific notation. The decimal point in 10,000,000 is after the last zero. The first significant digit is 1. Move the decimal point to the left seven places (1.000 000 0) multiplying by 10^7 gives the number in scientific notation as: 10,000,000 = 1×10^7, usually written 10^7.

Example: Write 0.005329 in scientific notation. The decimal point is moved to the right three places. The resulting number is $0.005329 = 5.329 \times 10^{-3}$.

5.6 CONVERSION OF UNITS OF MEASUREMENT

Measurement includes a number and a stated unit of measurement, i.e., 7 miles. The three practical units are length, mass, and volume. One unit of measure can be converted to another unit of measure provided they belong to the same unit of measurement. The units of length are inch, foot, yard, and mile.

Equivalence between units can be used to form conversion rates to change one unit of measure to another.

12 inches (in.)	=	1 foot (ft.)
3 feet (ft.)	=	1 yard (yd.)
36 in.	=	1 yd.
5280 ft.	=	1 mile (mi.)
16 ounces (oz.)	=	1 pound (lb.)
4 quarts (qts.)	=	1 gallon (gal.)

Example: Thirty-two bricks, each 8 inches long, are laid end-to-end to make the base of a wall. Find the length of the wall in feet.

1. First find or change 8 inches to feet.
   12 in. = 1 ft.
   $8 \text{ in.} = \frac{8}{12} = \frac{2}{3} \text{ ft.}$

2. Multiply: $\frac{2}{3}$ ft. $\times 32 = \frac{2}{3} \times \frac{32}{1} = \frac{64}{3}$
$= 21$ ft. 4 in.

5.7 PROBABILITY AND STATISTICS CONCEPTS

Probability values range from one to zero. A value of 1 stands for absolute certainty, and zero indicates there is no chance at all that the event will occur. There are very few things in life about which we can be absolutely certain. Most things in life, however, have probability values of their occurrence somewhere between 1 and zero.

If you take a new coin that has not been mutilated and toss it, we can state that the probability of obtaining a head is one out of two. This can be written as $P = \frac{1}{2}$, or 0.5.

It is also true that the probability of obtaining a tail is $\frac{1}{2}$, or 0.5.

In this situation, only one of these two outcomes can occur. Notice that the sum of the two probabilities is equal to 1. We designate the probability of an event occurring by use of the symbol **p** and the probability of it not occurring by the **q**. The sum of **p + q** is always equal to 1.

Example: Take a die with six sides and toss it into the air. What is the probability of any single side coming up? The probability of any single side coming up is $\frac{1}{6}$ or 0.167. That is when we toss a die, the chance of throwing a six spot is one in six. There are five chances in six chances of some other number appearing on the upturned face.

In this case, $\mathbf{p} = \frac{1}{6}$ and $\mathbf{q} = \frac{5}{6}$, therefore $\mathbf{p} + \mathbf{q} = \frac{1}{6} + \frac{5}{6} = \frac{6}{6} = 1$

Example: There are 6 yellow marbles and 2 blue marbles in a bag. If Sara draws a marble out of the bag without looking, what are the chances that it will be blue?

A. $\frac{2}{8}$

B. $\frac{6}{8}$

C. $\frac{2}{6}$

D. $\frac{6}{2}$

The correct answer is **A.**

Solution: Let **p** = number of favorable outcomes, which is 2
q = number of unfavorable outcomes, which is 6
p + q = total outcomes, which is 2 + 6 = 8

$$\frac{\mathbf{p}}{\mathbf{p+q}} = \frac{2}{8}$$

5.7.1 Statistical Data Analysis Skills

Data from two experiments are presented and analyzed. Applied statistical analysis is being illustrated.

Experiment A: A psychology experiment designed to test the difficulty of a particular maze for rats is done by having ten rats run the maze. The results for their solution times to the nearest 0.1 seconds are:

8.3, 7.1, 8.8, 11.1, 7.0, 13.7, 9.5, 10.3, 10.8, 9.9

Experiment B: Two groups of 35-year-old subjects, one of men and one of women, have their blood cholesterol levels (mg/100 ml) measured. The data obtained (rounded to the nearest 1 mg/100 ml) are:

Group I (men): 195, 198, 199, 196, 195, 196, 191, 194, 195, 196
Group II (women): 196, 193, 194, 201, 202, 205, 204, 202, 199, 204

Having this data, the problem now becomes one of how to organize and analyze them so that they can be interpreted/presented to someone else clearly and meaningfully. The information above reflects two types of data that are commonly encountered in raw form (as taken during an experiment and not manipulated into graphs, means, ranges, etc.). In Experiment A, the data are of a **continuous** nature because all decimal values of time are possible (e.g., 8.003, 9.1083, etc.) even though they are not recorded. **Count** data is important for integer values such as age of a person, or number of times teeth are brushed each day. In experiment B, cholesterol level is a continuous variable but it is being rounded to compare cholesterol count of two groups.

Problem 1: Are the data in Experiment A count data or continuous data?

5.7.1.1 SIMPLE DATA ANALYSIS

Often it is a good idea, when presented a set of data, to make some simple observations. The easiest way to do this is to organize the data in ascending or descending order (or groups). Experiment A's data will be organized into an ascending order:

7.0, 7.1, 8.3, 8.8, 9.5, 9.9, 10.3, 10.8, 11.1, 13.7

Next, get a feeling for the data in Experiment A by using the simple steps below:

Experiment A:
(1) smallest value = 7.0
(2) largest value = 13.7
(3) range is 7.0 to 13.7: 13.7 – 7.0 = 6.7
(4) average might be about 10: $\frac{13.7 + 7.0}{2} \cong 10$

These simple observations, which can be made rapidly, gives you an idea about the limits of the data, the average value of the data, the variability of the data, and the distribution of the data over its possible values.

Problem 2: Do the same type of simple analysis on the data for Groups I and II in Experiment B as was done for Experiment A.

Structuring the Data

If it has not already been done, the next steps in the analysis will probably be to construct graphs and/or tables from the data; our concern now is mostly with tables. When interpreting **tables**, like interpreting graphs, it is essential to read the headings at the tops and sides of the tables to determine what is being presented. Then, survey the whole table to get a feel for the data and any noticeable general trends there. Next, look for more specific points or regions of data that may be of interest. Whether or not in conjunction with a table, another simple way to structure a set of data is to determine what **percentages** (or proportions) of it meet specified classifications. This is best illustrated by **examples**:

Experiment A:

(i) For some reason, you are interested in the percentage of rats with times less than 9.0 seconds:

$$\% \text{ with times less than 9.0 seconds} = \frac{4}{10} \times 100 = 40\%$$

(ii) You are told that 40% of the rats ran the maze in times greater than 10.0 seconds. How many rats, T, ran the maze in times greater than 10.0 seconds?

$$T = \frac{40}{100} \times 10 = 4$$

Problem 3: What are the respective percentages of subjects in Groups I and II of Experiment B who had blood cholesterol levels of 196 or lower?

Statistical Analysis

Once a set of data is structured in a desired format and preliminary analysis has been done, more formal statistical calculations can be made to describe it. Statistically, the two key features of a set of data are its central tendency and its variation.

Central Tendency

The central tendency of a set of data is the value it seems to approach. It is also called the "expected value." It is the one value that is taken to be representative of the whole set of data. The common measures of central tendency are the mode, the median, and the average (or mean). Only the computation of averages is required for the PCAT. The mode and the median are not required; however, their definitions will be given if they are needed on the PCAT. For this reason, you should be familiar with them beforehand.

The **average** takes into account directly the value of each piece of data. It is calculated by adding together each piece of data and then dividing the sum by the total number of pieces of data:

$$\text{The average} = x = \frac{x_1 + x_2 + \ldots + x_n}{n},$$

where $x_1, x_2, \ldots, x_n$ = the individual pieces of data and n = the total number of pieces of data.

For example:

$$\text{Experiment A: The average} = \frac{7.0 + 7.1 + 8.3 + 8.8 + 9.5 + 9.9 + 10.3 + 10.8 + 11.1 + 13.7}{10}$$

$$= (9.65) \approx 9.7$$

(remember that the eyeballed average was about 10)

The **median** is the value in a set of data that is positionally halfway between the lowest and highest values in the set. It is determined by listing all the values in the set of data in ascending order and then identifying the one that is positionally in the middle. In general, when there is an even number of values in a set of data, the median is calculated by taking the average of the middle two numbers. Examples of medians are:

Experiment A: The values in ascending order are:

7.0, 7.1, 8.3, 8.8, 9.5, 9.9, 10.3, 10.8, 11.1, 13.7

Since there is an even number of values (10), the two middle values are 9.5 and 9.9.

$$\text{The median} = \frac{9.5 + 9.9}{2} = 9.7$$

The **mode** is the most frequent value that appears in a set of data. It exists only if one value occurs more often than any of the other values. Examples are:

Experiment A: None exists—each value occurs only once.

The question naturally arises as to which measure of central tendency is the best; the answer is that it depends on the distribution of the data. Consider three sets of data, which are presented graphically in histograms, where N = the frequency of a particular value of the variable x:

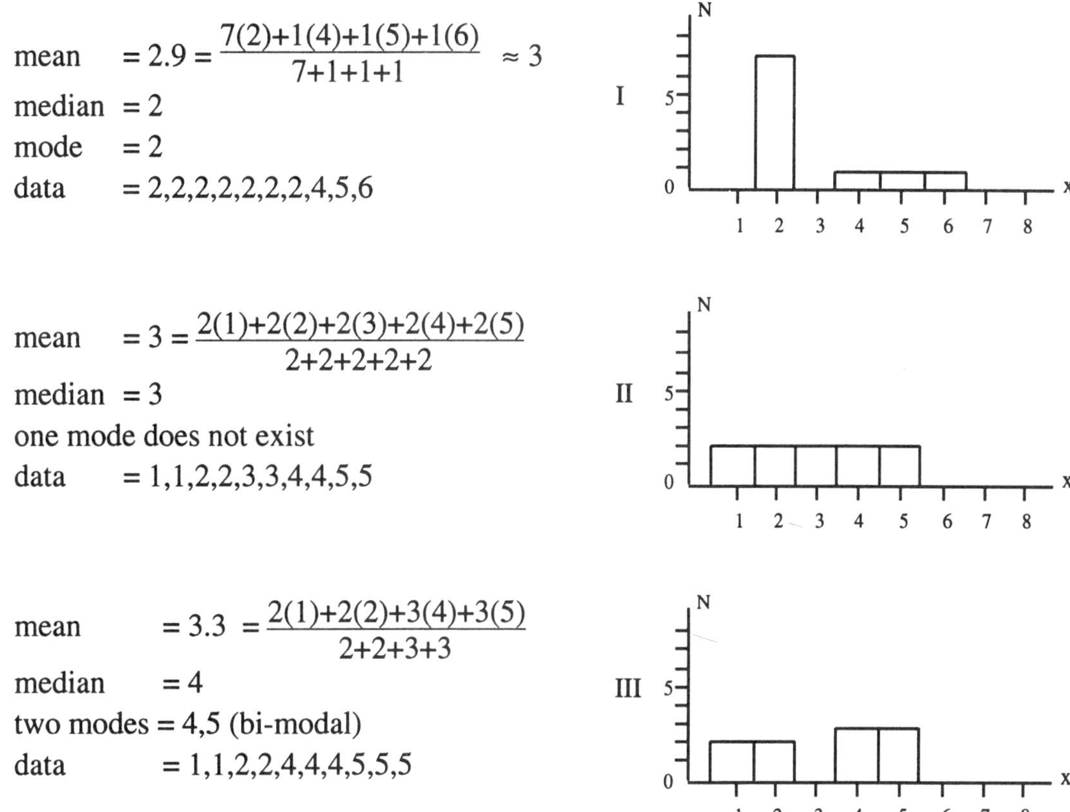

Fig. 5.2 — Histograms Illustrating Mean, Median, and Mode

For the data in histogram I, both the mode and the median are good measures of central tendency; the average (mean) is probably not. Whenever the frequency of one value predominates in a set of data, the mode is usually a good measure of central tendency. Unique modes do not exist for the data in histograms II and III. For the data in histogram II, both the average and the median are good measures of central tendency. When the values of a set of data are distributed fairly evenly over the range of the data (as in this case), the average is sometimes considered better because it takes into account directly the value of each piece of data. The median is probably a better measure of central tendency than the average for the data in histogram III. Typically, the median is preferable to the average in cases where the values in a set of data are clustered toward one end of the range, but not in a way where the mode would become a good measure of central tendency as in histogram I.

Problem 4: Calculate the mode, the median, and the average for each group in Experiment B; identify, if possible, which of the three measures of central tendency is probably best for each group.

Variation or Dispersion Around Average

The measures of central tendency discussed above each give one value to describe a whole set of data. This one value is inadequate to "completely" describe the data because it gives no sense of the variation (or the dispersion) of the data about this value. In other words, we need a knowledge of the variation in a set of data to complement our knowledge of its central tendency. The common measures of variation are the range, the variance, and the standard deviation.

The **range** is simply the difference between the highest and lowest values in a set of data. For example:

Experiment A: Range = 13.7 – 7.0 = 6.7

Experiment B: Range = 90 – 50 = 40

Because the range takes into account only the highest and lowest values in a set of data, it is a rough measure of variation. In some cases, it is really not a reasonable measure of variation. When either or both of the extreme values in a set of data are far out of line with the rest of the data, the range is a questionable measure of variation. For example, consider the data presented in the histograms below (N = the frequency of a particular value of the variable x):

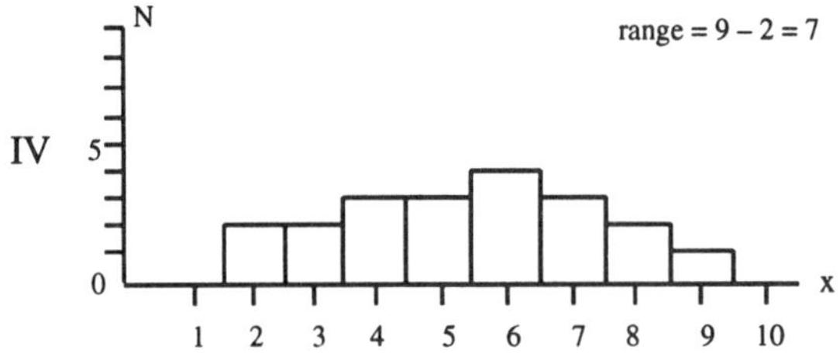

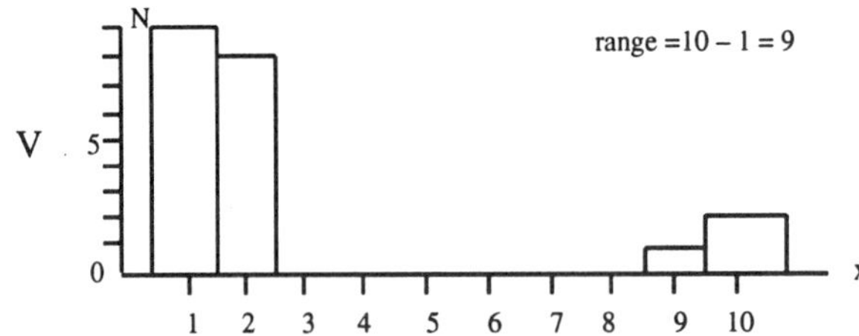

Fig. 5.3 — Histograms Illustrating Range and Variation in Data

The range of the data in histogram IV gives a good idea of that data's variability. On the other hand, the range of the data in histogram V does not really give a good idea of that data's variability.

5.7.2 Precision and Accuracy in Measurements

So far, we have been concerned with characterizing the distribution of the values in a set of data using complementary measures of central tendency and variation. When analyzing data, we are also interested in examining the nature (e.g., the limitations) of the measurements that a set of data comprises. These considerations lead to the notion of measurement error which stems from a desire to know the possible difference between the exact, true value of a quantity and our measured (or calculated) value of it. Review section 5.1 to understand how "rounding" of numbers is related to significant digits.

Before embarking on a discussion of precision and accuracy, the **significant digits** of a number must be understood. A digit is significant when it has been measured exactly. Examples of determining the number of significant digits are:

(1) 7.000 four (4) significant digits; digits listed after a decimal point are assumed to be accurately measured.

(2) 7000 one (1) significant digit; no decimal point—see (3) below.

(3) 7000 four (4) significant digits; no decimal point (the decimal point implies that all zeros are accurately measured).

(4) 7001 4 significant digits; all zeros between nonzero digits are significant.

When adding, multiplying, etc., the number of significant digits in the result cannot be such that it is any more precise than the least precise number involved in its calculation (see discussion of precision below). Consider as examples:

Experiment A: Each piece of data in this experiment has two (e.g., 8.3) or three (e.g., 10.3) significant digits. When the mean for these data is calculated, it comes out initially as 9.65 but is rounded off to 9.7 because some of the numbers used to calculate this mean have only two significant digits.

Likewise, the variance of these data is initially calculated as 3.643 but has to be rounded off to 3.6 (two significant digits). See these calculations in examples above.

Problem 5: Check in your calculations for the five data analysis problems above that you kept track of significant digits.

Measurement errors occur in data because it is not possible to get exact numbers from experiments. In any experiment, there is a limit to how close we can get to knowing the true value of the quantity being measured. Consequently, there are several definitions/concepts with which you should be familiar that are used to describe and assess the error in a measurement or calculation.

The **precision** of a number or an experimental value is the smallest unit of measurement and is therefore closely related to the significant digits in a measured number. Consider as examples:

Experiment A: The solution times for the rats running the maze are recorded to the nearest 0.1 seconds; therefore, the precision of these time measurements is 0.1 seconds. It is also called the "least count" of the measuring instrument.

The **accuracy** of a number is how far the measured value of a variable may be from its true value. The true value is normally considered as an "average" obtained from a large set of data values. Consider as examples:

Experiment A: The precision of the watch used to measure each maze solution time is 0.1 seconds. Neglecting any other possible sources of error, the accuracy of each time measurement is ± 0.05 seconds. Specifically, when a rat's measured solution time is 8.8 seconds, the true solution time is 8.8 ± 0.05 seconds, i.e., it is known to be between 8.75 and 8.85 seconds.

Experiment B: The precision in the blood cholesterol level experiments is 1 mg/100 ml; therefore, their accuracy is ± 0.5 mg/100 ml. A measured value of 196 corresponds to a true value that is somewhere between 195.5 and 196.5.

However, when error results from sources other than the limitations of the measuring device, the accuracy and the precision are not usually so simply related. In many experiments, there may be factors other than the precision of the measurements involved which decrease the accuracy of their results.

Measurement errors can be classified under three headings: mistakes, systematic errors, and random errors. **Mistakes** are usually nonrepetitive errors that might result from human errors such as misreading an instrument or occasions of performing a step wrong in an experimental procedure. The error that results from a mistake is largely unpredictable and unless caught will probably affect the data in some unknown way. A **systematic error** is a repetitive error caused by human error, instrument error, or experimental design error. It is repeated in every measurement, usually, to the same extent. If a systematic error is detected, there is a possibility that it can be corrected to some extent. An example of a systematic error would be a case where we are measuring a series of temperatures in an experiment and the thermometer being used to make these measurements is miscalibrated 2°C too high. In this case, the set of temperature measurements would have a systematic error of 2°C (too high).

We always attempt to do experiments under uniform conditions. Nevertheless, in practice, there is always some variability in these "uniform" conditions that cannot be removed. Thus, even if all human, instrument, and experimental design errors are corrected in an experiment, a variability that is called **random error** will still probably exist in its measurements. Consider as an example of random error:

Example: We perform an experiment to determine the temperature dependence of the solubility of a particular organic salt in water. Our experimental apparatus is capable of maintaining a constant temperature of ± 1°C. Say we are particularly interested in measuring the salt's solubility at 37°C. Although we take it to be 37°C, each time we take a solubility measurement the true temperature is actually somewhere between 36°C and 38°C. Since the salt's solubility is temperature dependent, this variability in the true temperature results in a random error in the solubility measurements at 37°C. This random error, of course, directly affects the accuracy of these solubility measurements.

5.7.3 Solutions to Data Analysis Problems

(1) The data in Experiment A are continuous data.

(2) <u>Group I:</u> Put the data in ascending order: 191, 194, 195, 195, 195, 196, 196, 198, 199; then:

(1) smallest value = 191
(2) largest value = 199
(3) range is 199 – 191 = 8
(4) most values are around 195 or 196, so the average is probably about 195 or 196
(5) there are few values at the ends of the range (191 and 199), but many at the middle (195 to 196)

(3) Group II: Put the data in ascending order: 193, 194, 196, 199, 201, 202, 202, 204, 204, 205; then:

(1) smallest value = 193
(2) largest vale = 205
(3) range is 205 – 193 = 12
(4) average might be about 199: $\frac{193 + 205}{2} = 199$
(5) the values cluster toward the higher end of the range

(4) Group I: Percentage with blood cholesterol levels of 196 or lower = $\frac{8}{10} \times 100 = 80\%$

Group II: Percentage with blood cholesterol levels of 196 or lower = $\frac{3}{10} \times 100 = 30\%$

(5) Group I: A unique mode does not exist, as 195 and 196 both appear three times.

The median $= \frac{195 + 196}{2} = 196 = (195.5)$

The average $= \frac{191 + 194 + 3(195) + 3(196) + 198 + 199}{10}$

$= 196 = (195.5)$

Both the average and the median are good measures of the central tendency of Group I's data.

Group II: A unique mode does not exist, as 202 and 204 both appear twice.

The median $= \frac{201 + 202}{2} = 202 = (201.5)$

The average $= \frac{193 + 194 + 196 + 199 + 201 + 2(202) + 2(204) + 205}{10}$

$= 200$

It is a toss-up as to which measure of central tendency, the median or the average, is probably better. Qualitatively, the average tends to reflect the spread of data at the lower end of the range more than the median does, while the median tends to reflect the cluster of data at the high end of the range more than the average does.

(6) See solutions to problems 1 through 5.

5.8 PLANE GEOMETRY CONCEPTS

Geometry deals with measurements of sides, angles, areas, and perimeters and volumes. It can be divided into two branches: plane and solid. Plane and solid geometry are inseparable from two-dimensional and three-dimensional perceptual abilities. You should spend considerable time reviewing principles in plane and solid geometry before studying chapter 6. For example, learn the difference between plane angles and dihedral angles by looking at real-life examples. Angles in two dimensions (between two lines or rays) are plane angles. Angles in three dimensions (between two or three surfaces) are dihedral or solid angles. Look at various corners in your room. Each corner forms dihedral or solid angles. Learn to connect dihedral angles to isometric and perspective views of a solid object, such as wings of an airplane.

Angles:

An **angle** is formed by two lines meeting at a point.
Right Angle—an angle that measures 90°
Complementary Angles —the sum of two angles whose measure is 90°
Supplementary Angles—the sum of two angles whose measure is 180°
Acute Angle—an angle whose measurement is less than 90°
Obtuse Angle—an angle whose measurement is greater than 90°
Straight Angle—an angle whose measurement is equal to 180°
Perimeter—the distance around a plane figure.

5.8.1 Rules and Formulas

1. The sum of the measure of the angles in a triangle is 180°.

2. Perimeter is the distance around a figure. To find the perimeter, add the length of the sides: Perimeter = p; and p = a + b + c

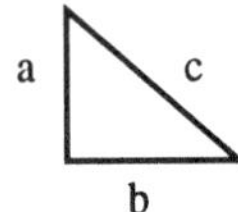

3. Square Perimeter :
$p = s + s + s + s$
$p = 4s$

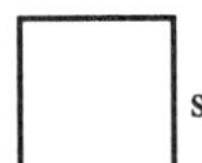

4. Rectangle Perimeter:
$p = 2 \times \text{length} + 2 \times \text{width}$
$p = 2L + 2W$

W L

5. Circumference (c) of a circle is the distance around the circle. The diameter is twice the radius times π(pi) or π times the diameter.

$c = 2 \times \pi \times \text{radius}$
$c = 2 \pi r$
$c = \pi \times \text{diamete}$
$c = \pi d$
$\pi \approx 3.14, \frac{22}{7}$

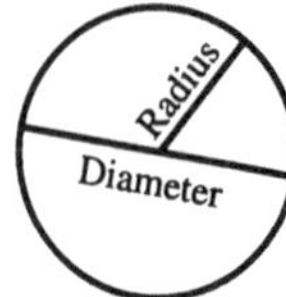

6. Composite geometric figures are made of two or more simple geometric figures:

Composite figure = 3 sides of a rectangle + $\frac{1}{2}$ the circumference of a circle

Perimeter of the composite figure = (2 × length) + width + $\frac{1}{2} \times \pi \times$ diameter

5.8.2 Similar Triangle Concepts

Similar figures are figures that have the same shape but not necessarily the same size. Similar figures have corresponding sides and angles. The relationship between the sizes of each of the corresponding sides or angles can be written as a ratio, and each ratio will be the same.

The two triangles below, ABC and DEF, are similar. The ratios of corresponding sides are equal.

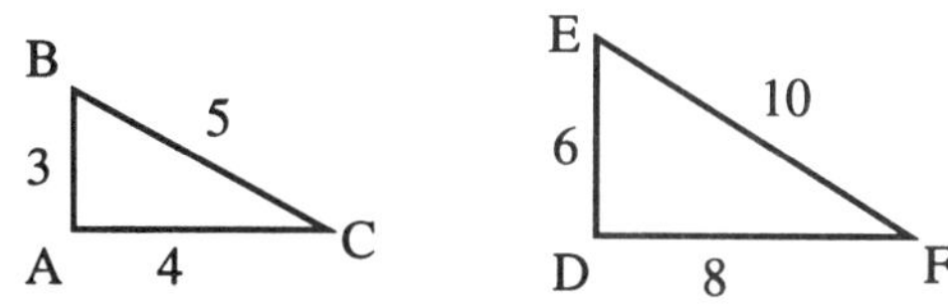

$\frac{AB}{DE} = \frac{3}{6} = \frac{1}{2}$; $\frac{BC}{EF} = \frac{5}{10} = \frac{1}{2}$; and $\frac{AC}{DF} = \frac{4}{8} = \frac{1}{2}$

The ratio of the corresponding sides = $\frac{1}{2}$

Since the ratios of corresponding sides are equal, three proportions can be formed:

$\frac{AB}{DE} = \frac{BC}{EF}$; $\frac{AC}{DF} = \frac{BC}{EF}$ and $\frac{AB}{DE} = \frac{AC}{DF}$

Example: Triangles ABC and DEF are similar. Find the perimeter of Δ ABC.

A. 11
B. 12
C. 14
D. 13

The correct answer is **B.**

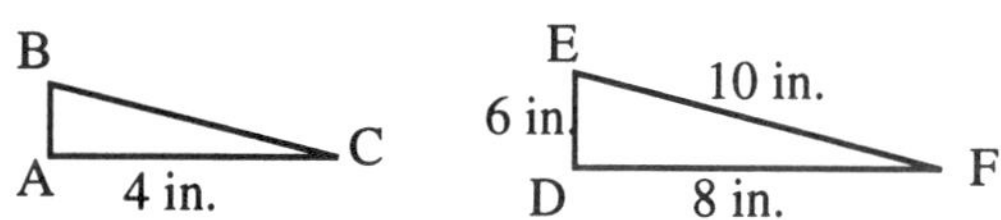

Find the length of BC by using proportion

$$\frac{AC}{DF} = \frac{BC}{EF}$$

$$\frac{4 \text{ in.}}{8 \text{ in.}} = \frac{BC}{EF}$$

$$8\,BC = 40 \text{ in.}$$

$$BC = 5 \text{ in.}$$

$$\frac{BC}{EF} = \frac{AB}{DE}$$

$$\frac{5 \text{ in.}}{10 \text{ in.}} = \frac{AB}{6 \text{ in.}}$$

$$10AB = 30 \text{ in.}$$

$$AB = 3 \text{ in.}$$

The perimeter of $\Delta ABC = 4 + 3 + 5$
$= 12$

5.8.3 Cartesian or Analytic Geometry

All graphical representations of data and functions are based on some sort of coordinate system. Even bar graphs (histograms) and pie graphs have an implicit coordinate system in their construction. By far the most commonly used graphs are based on the rectangular (Cartesian) coordinate system that consists of two perpendicular axes, each representing a variable:

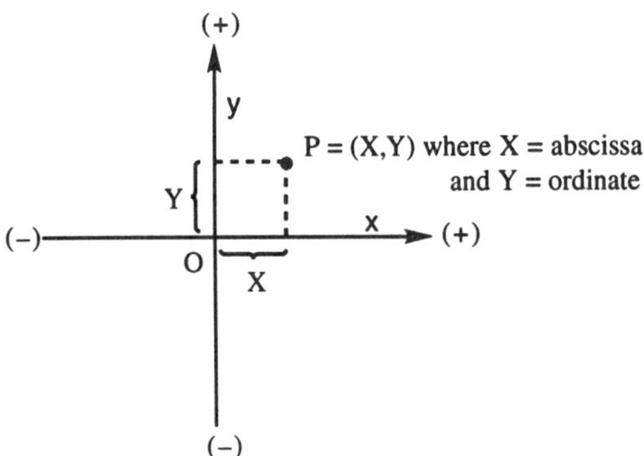

Fig. 5.4 — Cartesian Coordinate System

The intersection of the two axes in the Cartesian plane is called the origin (O). The origin splits each axis into two segments that respectively represent positive and negative values of that axis' variable. Usually the ordinate represents the dependent variable (y) and the abscissa represents the independent variable (x). The standard positive and negative segments of each axis are labeled on the graph above; this is also shown by the arrows that indicate the directions of positive change for each axis' variable. Each point in the Cartesian plane is represented by a pair of coordinates (called an ordered pair), each of which represents a distance from the origin along one of the axes [e.g., the point P = (x,y) on the graph above and the origin O = (0,0)].

Slope or Rate of Change:

Probably the most important parameter in interpreting the relationship between the two variables in a graph is the slope. The slope of the line segment between two points is defined as the ratio of the change in the ordinate to the change in the abscissa:

$$\text{slope} = \frac{\text{change in ordinate}}{\text{change in abscissa}} = \frac{\Delta y}{\Delta x} = \frac{\text{Rise}}{\text{Run}} = \frac{\text{change in dependent variable}}{\text{change in independent variable}}$$

A slope exists for every point on a graph whether it is a straight line or a curved line. For each point on a graph, the slope is the rate of change (positive or negative) in the ordinate with respect to the change in the abscissa. It may be constant as for straight lines or portions of curves that are straight, or it may be constantly changing as for curved lines. In practice, the slope is calculated as follows:

For straight lines:

$$\text{slope} = m = \frac{y_2 - y_1}{x_2 - x_1} = \frac{\Delta y}{\Delta x} = \text{constant}$$

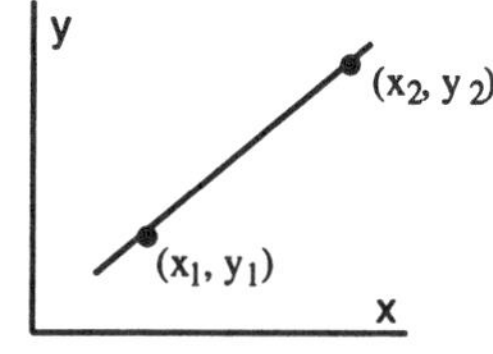

For curved lines:

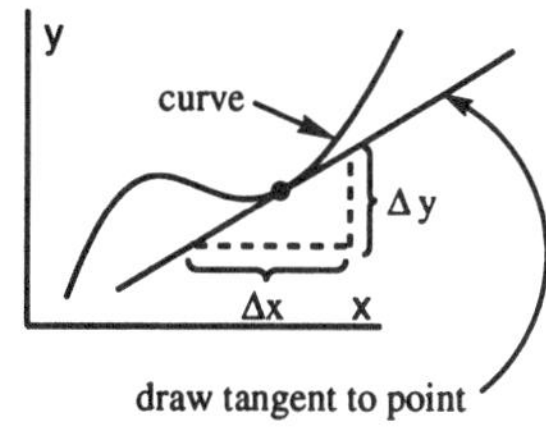

measure Δx,Δy for any two points on tangent

$$\text{slope} = m = \frac{\Delta y}{\Delta x} \neq \text{constant (changes along the curve)}$$

Fig. 5.5 — Definition Sketch for Slope

Example 1.
Calculate the slope of the line graphed below:

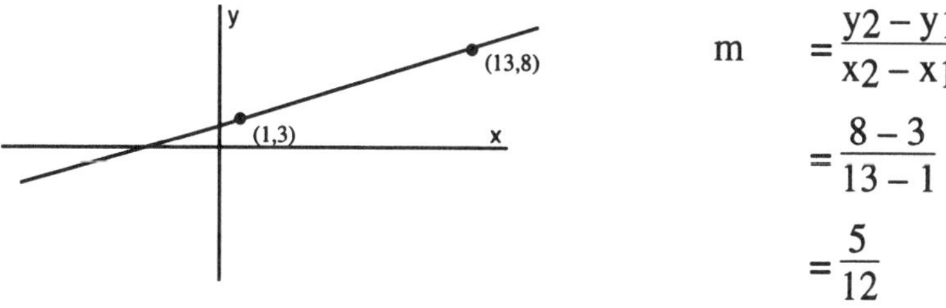

$$m = \frac{y2 - y1}{x2 - x1} = \frac{8 - 3}{13 - 1} = \frac{5}{12}$$

5.9 ALGEBRAIC EQUATIONS AND PROPORTIONALITY PROBLEMS

The solution of a simple equation in one variable usually amounts to the isolation of an "**unknown quantity**" or variable on one side of the equation. Any operation, except multiplication or division by zero, can be used to achieve this "isolation" as long as it is done to both sides of the equation. More generally, the basic rule for solving equations is that whatever is done to one side must be done to the other side so that the equality of the sides is not affected. It is like a weighing scale with two balanced sides or pans. Before considering some examples of solving equations, first it is important to recall that, when manipulating an expression (whether or not it is part of an equation), the order of operations is as follows:

Order of Operations

(1) parentheses
(2) powers or exponents
(3) multiplication and division (whichever comes first from the left side of the expression)
(4) addition and subtraction (whichever comes first from the left side of the expression)

Example 1: Solve for a: $4a + 5 = 13$

$$\begin{aligned} 4a + 5 - 5 &= 13 - 5 \\ 4a &= 8 \\ \frac{4a}{4} &= \frac{8}{4} \\ a &= 2 \end{aligned}$$

Example 2: Solve for m: $\frac{10}{m} - 8 = \frac{5}{3}$

$$\begin{aligned} \frac{10}{m}(3m) - 8(3m) &= \frac{5}{3}(3m) \\ 30 - 24m &= 5m \\ 30 &= 29m \\ m &= \frac{30}{29} \end{aligned}$$

Example 3: Solve for c: $3c^2 = 75d^4$

$$\begin{aligned} c^2 &= 25d^4 \\ \sqrt{c^2} &= \sqrt{25d^4} \\ c &= \pm 5d^2 \end{aligned}$$

Example 4: Solve for q:

$$\begin{aligned} 3[(q+2)^2 - 4q] &= 2q^2 + 13 \\ 3[(q+2)(q+2) - 4q] &= 2q^2 + 13 \\ 3[q^2 + 4q + 4 - 4q] &= 2q^2 + 13 \\ 3q^2 + 12 &= 2q^2 + 13 \\ q^2 &= 1 \\ q &= \pm 1 \end{aligned}$$

Problem 1: Solve for a: $s(a - p) + q = ta + r^2$

Problem 2: Solve for d: $\frac{1}{d-2} + \frac{2}{d+3} = \frac{4}{d-2}$

Problem 3: Solve for x: $3(4x - 2[1 - (x + 5) + 3]) = 13x + 19$

5.9.1 Proportionality

(a) Some problems will be solvable by recognizing that the quantities in question are directly or inversely proportional to each other. Two variables, x and y, are **directly proportional** if their ratio has a constant value, a:

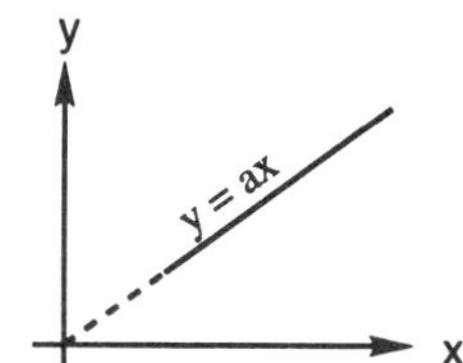

$$\frac{y}{x} = a \quad \text{or} \quad y = ax.$$

(Linear variation)

Figure 5.6 — Linear Variation

Consequently, for any distinct values of x, x_1, and x_2, there are corresponding values of y, y_1, and y_2, such that:

$$\frac{y_1}{x_1} = \frac{y_2}{x_2}. \qquad \text{(x, y directly proportional)}$$

If we know three of the terms in this proportion, then we can always determine the fourth term.

Example 5: If two moles of compound A react with 5 moles of compound B to form 3 moles of compound C, then how many moles of A are required to react completely with 7 moles of B?

In a chemical reaction, the quantities of reactants/products are directly proportional. (Why?)

Let x_1 = 2 moles of A and $y_1 = 5$ moles of B.
Then, x_2 = number of moles of A and $y_2 = 7$ moles of B such that:
$\frac{5}{2} = \frac{7}{x_2}$; x_2 = 2.8 moles of A.

Problem 4: In Example 5, how many moles of C are formed?

(b) Two variables, x and y, are **inversely proportional** if their product has a constant value, b:

$$xy = b \quad \text{or} \quad y = \frac{b}{x}.$$

(Nonlinear or hyperbolic variation)

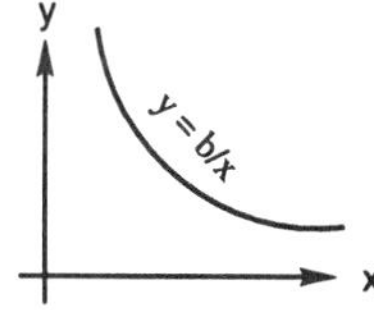

Fig. 5.7 — Nonlinear Variation

Consequently, for any distinct values of x, x_1, and x_2, there are corresponding values of y, y_1, and y_2, such that:

$$x_1y_1 = x_2y_2 \quad \text{or} \quad \frac{y_1}{x_2} = \frac{y_2}{x_1} \qquad \text{(x,y inversely proportional)}$$

If we know three of the terms in this equation, $x_1y_1 = x_2y_2$, then we can always determine the fourth term.

Example 6: A car traveling at x mph takes 5 hours to go from city A to city B. Traveling at x – 15 mph, the car makes the return trip in six and two-thirds hours. What was the speed of the car on the return trip?

Since displacement = (speed)(time), d = vt, speed and time are inversely proportional for a constant displacement. Let $v_1 = x$ mph and $t_1 = 5$ hours; $v_2 = x - 15$ mph and $t_2 = 6\frac{2}{3}$ hours $= \frac{20}{3}$ hours. Then:

$$\begin{aligned} 5x &= (x - 15)\frac{20}{3} \\ 15x &= 20x - 300 \\ 5x &= 300 \\ x &= 60 \ ; \ v_2 = x - 15 = 45 \text{ mph.} \end{aligned}$$

Problem 5: Before an engine tune-up, a car with a gas consumption rate of r gallons/mile can go 400 miles on a full tank of gas. After a tune-up, the same car has a gas consumption rate of r – .01 gallons/mile and can go 500 miles on a full tank of gas. What was the gas consumption rate of the car before it had an engine tune-up?

Problem 6: The ideal-gas law for 1 mole of any gas is pV = RT. Thus, two different macroscopic states of a mole of a particular gas are respectively described by

$$p_1V_1 = RT_1 \text{ and } p_2V_2 = RT_2.$$

Write an equation that shows the relationship between these two states. According to this equation, the pressure p is inversely proportional to what quantity?

An important application of proportionality is to use it to find proportional changes in variables that occur when other related variables change. This is called "sensitivity analysis" and is an important part of the PCAT on all subjects being tested. It teaches how to think proportionally.

Problem 7: In 1984, a particular item A cost $2,500. In 1986, the price of A rose 20% due to scarcity while in early 1987 there was 10% increase in the price of A over its 1986 price. At the end of 1987, A was put on sale with a 30% decrease in price. What was the sale price of A?

5.9.2 Solutions to Algebra Problems

(1) $a = \frac{r^2 + sp - q}{s - t}$; $\quad s(a - p) + q = ta + r^2$

$$\begin{aligned} sa - sp + q &= ta + r^2 \\ a(s-t) &= r^2 + sp - q \\ a &= \frac{r^2 + sp - q}{s - t} \end{aligned}$$

(2) $d = -13$;

$$\begin{aligned} \frac{1}{d-2} + \frac{2}{d+3} &= \frac{4}{d-2} \\ d + 3 + 2(d-2) &= 4(d+3) \\ 3d - 1 &= 4d + 12 \\ d &= -13 \end{aligned}$$

[Multiply through by (d–2)(d+3)]

(3) $x = \frac{13}{5}$;

$$\begin{aligned} 3(4x - 2[1 - (x+5) + 3]) &= 13x + 19 \\ 3[4x - 2(4 - x - 5)] &= 13x + 19 \\ 3(4x + 2x + 2) &= 13x + 19 \\ 18x + 6 &= 13x + 19 \\ x &= \frac{13}{5} \end{aligned}$$

(4) $C = \frac{21}{5}$ moles

Let $x_1 = 5$ moles of B and $y_1 = 3$ moles of C;
then $x_2 = 7$ moles of B and y_2 = number of moles of C.

Since B and C are directly proportional:

$$\frac{y_2}{7} = \frac{3}{5}; \quad y_2 = \frac{21}{5} \text{ moles of C}$$

(5) $r = .05$ gallons/mile

From the problem, $xy = a$, where:
x = gas consumption rate (gallons/mile),
y = number of miles that the car can go on a full tank of gas,
a = number of gallons in full tank of gas (constant).
Thus, x and y are inversely proportional with $x_1 = r$,

$$\begin{aligned} y_1 &= 400, \quad x_2 = r - .01, \text{ and } y_2 = 500; \\ r(400) &= (r - .01)500 \\ 400r &= 500r - 5 \\ r &= .05 \text{ gallons/mile} \end{aligned}$$

(6) $\frac{p_1V_1}{T_1} = \frac{p_2V_2}{T_2}$; $\frac{V}{T}$

$p_1V_1 = RT_1$ and $p_2V_2 = RT_2$ can be rewritten

as: $\frac{p_1V_1}{T_1} = R$ and $\frac{p_2V_2}{T_2} = R$.

Therefore, the two states are related by:

$$\frac{p_1V_1}{T_1} = \frac{p_2V_2}{T_2}.$$

From the definition of inversely proportional variables, if p is one of the variables, then the other variable is V/T.

(7) Sale price (1987) = \$2,310

$$
\begin{aligned}
\text{1984: cost of A} &= \$2{,}500 \\
\text{1986: cost of A} &= \$2{,}500 + \frac{20}{100} \times \$2{,}500 \\
&= \$3{,}000 \\
\text{1987: cost of A} &= \$3{,}000 + \frac{10}{100} \times \$3{,}000 \\
&= \$3{,}300 \\
\text{Sale price (1987)} &= \$3{,}300 - \frac{30}{100} \times \$3{,}300 \\
&= \$2{,}310
\end{aligned}
$$

5.10 APPLIED MATHEMATICS PROBLEMS

When word problems or applications are used on standardized tests such as the PCAT, they often introduce an element of anxiety. The diversity and depth of appropriate applications generate a feeling of uneasiness for many students. Furthermore, applied problems are often more difficult and require multiple steps. To work these problems you must understand more than just the mathematics related to a problem situation; you need also to understand certain facts about the situation. To solve science-related problems, you must know basic information about force, weight, measures, and other concepts of science.

There are many different types of applied word problems, including percents, ratio and proportion, distance problems, and motion problems. Each of these types is discussed later in this section, but now it is time for practice.

Work the following problem NOW and complete it before you read further. As you work the problem, write out ALL the steps.

Problem: A man 2 meters tall stands 3 meters from an intense source of light at the level of his feet. The man's shadow appears on a wall 15 meters from the source of light. How tall is the shadow?

A. 6 meters
B. 10 meters
C. 12.5 meters
D. 17.5 meters

A FORMULA FOR PROBLEM SOLVING

1. Careful reading. Read to fully understand the problem, including both the *question asked* and the *situation described* (context). Most students spend too little time making sense of the problem situation. Here it is often helpful to draw a rough diagram. When complex data are presented you will need to use the techniques described in section 5.6.1 on data analysis.

2. Gather your facts. Decide what things YOU must bring to the problem. These may include facts you have learned, mathematical formulas, or patterns of reasoning. These are the tools you will need to get from the situation that has been described to a point from which you can answer the questions that have been asked.

3. Use the tools you selected in step 2 above to manipulate the problem situation and thereby produce answers to the questions asked. Here you may find that your tools are inadequate and your knowledge of the problem is inaccurate or vague. Care and attention to steps 1 and 2 can stop you from wasting time on a series of dead ends.

4. Check everything. Is your answer reasonable within the scope of the problem?

In the shadow problem, if you recognize that the data forms two similar triangles, solving the problem becomes easy. To solve it, *carefully* make a ratio according to the rule that allows you to compare similar triangles: $3/15 = 2/x$.

We emphasized the word *carefully* in the paragraph above because the test-maker, who knows that some students will do this step carelessly, has included a distracter that fits. For example, if your answer was 6, you probably put 12 in place of the 15 in the ratio.

Many students lack the patience or confidence to work through all the steps to solve the problem; they take short-cuts and make errors. For example, some students draw the picture accurately and then try to solve for the hypotenuse—a complicated and time-consuming task that fails to yield the correct answer—although, once again, the test-maker included a distracter that fits.

The third step, solving the problem, is elementary only if you have correctly completed the first two steps. This problem is not especially difficult either in content or mathematics, but in order to solve it correctly you must think carefully and be precise. These are the qualities of a good problem solver. If you think about it, these are the qualities we want in our pharmacists as well.

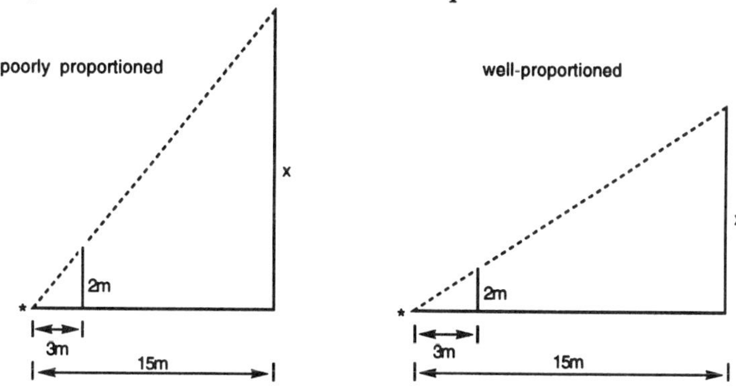

Fig. 5.8— Shadow Problem Data

5.10.1 Word Problems Using Percents

Problems involving percents were explained and illustrated in section 5.4 and therefore will not be discussed here.

5.10.2 Word Problems Using Ratios and Proportions

A *ratio* is the comparison by division of two quantities expressed in the same units. For example, the heights of two poles may be in the ratio of 3 to 7, which means that the height of the first pole could be 3 feet and the height of the second could be 7 feet. The colon (:) is used to indicate ratio and is written 3:7, which means 3 to 7. The ratio is often written as a fraction, 3/7.

Example: Ann has $300. Bob has $1,200. Compare Ann's amount to Bob's amount.

$$\frac{\text{Ann}}{\text{Bob}} = \frac{3}{12} = \frac{1}{4}$$

A *proportion* states that two ratios are equal. For example, the ratios 2:3 and 4:6 are equal and form a proportion, which may be written as 2:3 = 4:6, or 2:3::4:6.

The proportion 2:3::4:6 is read "2 is to 3 as 4 is to 6." The inside numbers 3 and 4 are called the means, and the outside numbers 2 and 6 are called the extremes.

Any proportion can be written in fractional form: 2/3 = 4/6.

In any proportion, the product of the means is equal to the product of the extremes, i.e., 3:4 = 6:8 is a proportion and the product of the means (4) (6) = 24 and the product of the extremes (3) (8) = 24.

Example: Determine a if 3:5 = a:15

$$\begin{aligned} \frac{3}{5} &= \frac{a}{15} \\ 5a &= 3(15) \\ a &= \frac{45}{5} \\ a &= 9 \end{aligned}$$

Example: If 3 cups of beans will serve 12 people, how many people will 6 cups serve (assuming equal serving size)?

Solution: $$\begin{aligned} \frac{3\text{ cups}}{12\text{ people}} &= \frac{6\text{ cups}}{x\text{ people}} \\ 3x &= 6(12) \\ 3x &= 72 \\ x &= 24 \end{aligned}$$

Answer: 6 cups will serve 24 people.

5.10.3 Word Problems Using Distance, Rate, and Time

The solution of distance problems is based on the equation d = rt, where d is the distance traveled, r is the rate of travel, and t is the time spent traveling.

(a) Distance determination skill

Example: A car travels an average speed of 60 miles per hour for 5 hours. How far does it travel in that time?
The distance is the rate traveled multiplied by the time.
60 miles × 5 hours = 300 miles per hour.

(b) Rate determination skill

Example: A train travels 400 miles in 8 hours. What is the train's average speed?
The rate is the distance traveled divided by the time.
400 miles ÷ 8 hours = 50 miles per hour.

5.10.3.1 RELATING MOTION OF TWO OBJECTS

Combined quantities involve more than one distance, rate, or time.

Example: The rate at which two objects approach each other when traveling toward each other or in directly opposite directions, and the rate at which they approach each other or separate, is the sum of their respective rates.

Skills involved in solving a combined quantity problem:

Example: A car leaves a town traveling 30 miles per hour. Two hours later, a second car leaves the same town, on the same road, traveling at 50 miles per hour. In how many hours will the second car be passing the first car?

(a) Draw a diagram to illustrate

d = 30 (t + 2)
first car
second car
d = 50t

(b) For each object, write a numerical or variable expression for the distance, rate, and time. The results can be recorded in a table.

The first car traveled two hours longer than the second car.

	Rate, r	×	Time, t	=	Distance, d
First car	30	×	t + 2	=	30 (t + 2)
Second car	50	×	t	=	50t

(c) Determine how the distances traveled by each object are related.

Example: The total distance traveled by both objects may be known or it may be known that the two objects traveled the same distance.

$$30(t+2) = 50t$$
$$30t + 60 = 50t$$
$$60 = 50t - 30t$$
$$60 = 20t$$
$$3 = t$$

The second car will be passing the first car after 3 hours.

Example: Two long distance runners, Beth and Paul, ran the same course. Paul traveled 2 miles per hour slower than Beth. Beth finishes the course in 4 hours and Paul finishes in 6 hours. What is the speed of each runner and what is the length of the course?

Solution: Let r represent Beth's rate. Then r – 2 represents Paul's rate. Since d = rt, Beth's distance is r•4, and Paul's distance is (r – 2)6.

	Rate	×	Time	=	Distance
Beth	r	×	4	=	4r
Paul	r – 2	×	6	=	6(r – 2)

$$4r = 6r - 12$$
$$12 = 2r$$
$$6 = r$$

Beth's rate is 6 miles per hour, and Paul's rate is 4 miles per hour.

The length of the course can be determined by applying d = rt to either runner.

Using Beth's rate, we obtain
$d = rt$
$d = 6(4)$
$d = 24$

Therefore, the length of the course is 24 miles.

5.10.3.2 DETERMINING AVERAGE RATE

(a) To average two or more different rates when the time is the same for both rates, add the rates and divide by the number of rates.

Example: If a woman travels for 4 hours at 40 miles per hour, at 50 miles per hour for the next 4 hours, and 60 miles per hour for the next 4 hours, then her average rate for the 12 hours is (40 + 50 + 60) ÷ 3 = 50 miles per hour.

(b) To average two or more different rates when the times are not the same but the distances are the same,
1. assume the distance to be a convenient length,
2. find the time at each given rate, and
3. find the sum of the distances and divide by the total time to find the average rate.

Example: Two boys travel a certain distance at the rate of 40 miles per hour and return at the rate of 20 miles per hour. What is the average rate for both trips?

Solution: Assume the distance is the same for both trips (80 miles).
time for first trip = 80 ÷ 40 = 2 hours.

time for second trip = 80 ÷ 20 = 4 hours
total distance = 160 miles
total time = 6 hours

average rate = 160 ÷ 6 = $26\frac{2}{3}$ miles per hour

Example: A man travels 200 miles at 40 miles per hour, 100 miles at 50 miles per hour, and 60 miles at 20 miles per hour. What is the average rate for the three trips?

Solution: Time for first trip: 200 ÷ 40 = 5 hours
Time for second trip: 100 ÷ 50 = 2 hours
Time for third trip = 60 ÷ 20 = 3 hours
The total distance is 360 miles
The total time is 10 hours
The average rate is 360 ÷ 10 = 36

Example: If a car travels 200 miles using 8 gallons of gas, what is its gas consumption?

Solution: mph = distance in miles ÷ number of gallons
mph = 200 ÷ 8
mph = 25 mph

5.10.4 Ten Steps for Problem Solving

1. Read the word problem at least twice: first to discover what it is all about, then read it carefully in detail (sentence by sentence or sometimes even phrase by phrase) to make sure you are clear about all the elements of the problem and their relationship, and what you are asked to discover.
2. It may be possible to draw a picture representing the elements of the problem. If it is, do so to clarify the details of the situation.
3. Write down in your own words statements of the facts presented in the problem. One way or another, the problem is likely to say that one part of the problem equals something else. Once you have stated the elements you should be able to write an equation (stating in words, not algebraic symbols) connecting or relating the elements of the problem.
4. When you know what you are asked to find, use an algebraic symbol (variable x, y, or whatever you choose) to represent this element (the unknown) for your developing equation. Clearly state what the symbol represents.
5. See if you can now make algebraic statements of the values of other elements of the problem in terms of the main variable defined in step #4.
6. Now write an equation substituting for step #3 the algebraic expressions (variables) you have worked out in steps #4 and #5.
7. Solve the new algebraic equation for the numerical value of the variable.
8. Use the solution of the equation to determine all answers requested in the problem.
9. Check your answers against the statements and data of the original word problem.
10. Finally, describe with a statement the required answer(s) asked for in the original word problem.

The following sections illustrate special word problems with solutions.

5.10.5 Word Problems Relating Work Rate of Two People

Work problems involve finding the rate at which two or more people working together can do a job. Knowing the rate at which each person works alone, you can find the rate at which they work together.

Steps used to solve work problems are

1. find the fractional part of the job each can do in the time given,
2. multiply each fraction from step 1 by x, and
3. set the sum of the fractions from step 2 equal to the number 1 and solve for x.

The *numerator* represents the time actually spent working. The *denominator* represents the total time needed to do the job alone.

Example: Jane can do housework alone in 3 hours. Bob can do the same job alone in 2 hours. How long will it take the two of them working together to finish the job?

Solution:

1. Express the fraction of the job each can do in 1 hour.
   1/3 = fraction of the job Jane can do in 1 hour. (If she can do the whole job in 3 hours, she can do 1/3 the job in 1 hour.)
   1/2 = fraction of the job Bob can do in 1 hour.

2. Express the fraction of the job each can do in x hours, when x = time it takes to complete the job together.
   1/3 x = fraction of the job Jane can do in x hours.
   1/2 x = fraction of the job Sue can do in x hours.

3. Set the sum of the two fractions equal to 1 and solve for x.

$$\frac{1}{2}x + \frac{1}{3}x = 1$$

$$\frac{5}{6}x = 1$$

$$x = \frac{6}{5}$$

$$x = 1.2 \text{ hours}$$

5.10.6 Word Problems Using Odd and Even Integers

Integers are real numbers. They consist of negative numbers, zero, and positive numbers. The set of integers are (...-4, -3, -2, -1, 0, 1, 2, 3, 4...).

The set of even integers are (...-4, -2, 0, 2, 4...)
The set of odd integers are (...-3, -1, 0, 1, 3...)
All even integers are divisible by 2.

Consecutive integers are integers that are listed in consecutive order. If n is even, three consecutive even integers are n, n + 2, n + 4; e.g., if n = 2, the three consecutive even integers are 2, 4, and 6.

If n is an odd integer, three consecutive odd integers are n, n + 2, n + 4; e.g., if n = 1, then the three consecutive odd integers are 3, 5, and 7.

Example: Find five consecutive odd integers that have a sum equal to 45.

Solution: Let n represent the smallest integer. The other four integers will be expressed in terms of n. Consecutive integers differ by one, therefore consecutive odd integers will differ by 2.

Let n = 1st odd integer
n + 2 = 2nd odd integer
n + 4 = 3rd odd integer
n + 6 = 4th odd integer
n + 8 = 5th odd integer

$$
\begin{aligned}
(n) + (n+2) + (n+4) + (n+6) + (n+8) &= 45 \\
5n + 20 &= 45 \\
5n &= 45 - 20 \\
5n &= 25 \\
n &= 5
\end{aligned}
$$

Answer: 5, 7, 9, 11, 13

Example: Find three consecutive even integers such that the first equals the sum of the second and third.

A. 0, -2, -4
B. -6, -4, -2
C. 4, 6, 8
D. 8, 10, 12
Answer: B

Solution:

$$
\begin{aligned}
\text{Let } n &= \text{first integer} \\
n + 2 &= \text{second integer} \\
n + 4 &= \text{third integer} \\
n &= (n+2) + (n+4) \\
n &= 2n+6 \\
-6 &= n
\end{aligned}
$$

5.10.7 Word Problems Using Coins or Stamps

The best method to solve such problems is to change the value of the money being dealt with to dollars and cents; e.g., the number of nickels should be multiplied by 5 because 1 nickel = $.05. The number of dimes should be multiplied by 10 because 1 dime = $.10. The number of half dollars should be multiplied by 50 because 1 half dollar = $.50, etc.

Example: A cash register contains $30.90 in nickels and quarters. If there are 130 coins in all, how many of each coin are in the cash register?

Let x = number of nickels, then 130-x = number of quarters

number of nickels •	value of nickels	= value in cents
x	5	= 5x

number of quarters • value of quarters = value in cents
130-x   25   = 25 (130-x)

value of nickels + value of quarters = total value in cents

$$5x + 25(130-x) = 3090$$
$$5x - 25x + 3250 = 3090$$
$$-20x = 3090 - 3250$$
$$20x = 160$$
$$x = 8$$

Answer: x = 8 nickels and
130 – x = 130-8 = 122 quarters

Check: 8 (.05) + .25 (122) = .40 + 30.50 = $30.90

Example: A person has 100 stamps with a total value of $18.00. Some stamps are worth 15¢ each and the others are worth 30¢ each. How many stamps of each type does he have?

Solution: Let x = number of 15¢ stamps. 100 – x = number of 30¢ stamps

number of stamps •	values of stamps =	value in cents
x	15	= 15x
100 – x	30	= 30 (100-x)

value of 15¢ stamps + value of 30¢ stamps = total value in cents
15x + 30(100-x) = 1800

$$15x + 30(100-x) = 1800$$
$$15x + 3000 - 30x = 1800$$
$$15x - 30x = 1800 - 3000$$
$$-15x = -1200$$
$$x = 80$$

Answer: x = 80 (15¢) stamps
100x = 100-80 = 20 (30¢) stamps

5.10.8 Word Problems Using Ages of Relatives

Solving age problems is done by comparing ages of relatives at the present, in the future and in the past. If the present age is represented by x, then the future age is found by adding years to x. If the present age is represented by x, then the past age is found by subtracting years from x.

Example: A mother was 36 years old when her daughter was born. How old will the daughter be when her age is 1/4 of the mother's age? What will the mother's age be?

$$
\begin{aligned}
\text{Let } x &= \text{daughter's age} \\
\text{Let } x + 36 &= \text{mother's age} \\
x &= \frac{1}{4}(x + 36) \\
x &= \frac{x}{4} + 9 \\
x - \frac{x}{4} &= 9 \\
4x - x &= 36 \\
3x &= 36 \\
x &= 12
\end{aligned}
$$

Daughter's age = x = 12 years
Mother's age = x + 36 = 48 years

Example: Jack is thrice his son's age. His son Jim is only three years younger than his sister Linda. Linda turned twenty last month and is one-third her mother's age. How old is Jack?

Solution: Let F = father's age, M = mother's age, D = daughter's age and S = son's age.

F = 3S, S = D-3, D = 20, D = 1/3 M

Use symbols that do not overlap or duplicate and which help to convert each problem statement into a mathematical relation. In this situation if D = 20 years then S = 17 years, which makes F = 3(17) = 51 years old. The mother's age is irrelevant in this problem.

5.10.9 Word Problems Using Permutations

Construct a basic diagram showing *all* possible outcomes.

Example: In how many different ways can the letters D, I, G, E, S, T be arranged? How many of these arrangements will start with the letter G?

Solution: D, I, G, E, S, T totals six letters. The first letter, D, can be arranged in any of the six positions shown below:

Position 1	**Position 2**	**Position 3**	**Position 4**	**Position 5**	**Position 6**

6 × 5 × 4 × 3 × 2 × 1

Draw the position diagram, which illustrates that the first letter can go into position 1. There are five letters left to fill the remaining five positions. The second letter can occupy any of the remaining five positions. The second position can be filled in five different ways. The third position can be filled in four different ways (four letters are left), and so on. The total number of *possible* arrangements = $6 \times 5 \times 4 \times 3 \times 2 \times 1 = 720$ for the letters D, I, G, E, S, T. There are six letters, hence $720 \div 6 = 120$, or 120 word arrangements will start with the letter G (e.g., G, S, I, D, E, T, G, I, D, E, S, T; and several others).

5.11 QUANTITATIVE ABILITY SAMPLE TEST

1. If $\frac{1}{3}(x-2) \leq \frac{x+2}{6}$, then

A. $x \geq 6$
B. $x \leq 6$
C. $x \leq 4$
D. $x \geq 3$

2. Simplify: $\frac{-3}{4} + \frac{1}{6} - \frac{5}{8}$

A. $\frac{5}{4}$

B. $1\frac{5}{24}$

C. $\frac{-5}{4}$

D. $-1\frac{5}{24}$

3. $3\frac{1}{3} \times 2\frac{1}{2} = ?$

A. 6

B. 3

C. $6\frac{1}{6}$

D. $8\frac{1}{3}$

4. If $(a^3b^{-2})^{-2}$ is simplified to a form in which exponents are positive, the result is

A. $\frac{b^4}{a^6}$

B. $\frac{1}{a^2b}$

C. $\frac{a^6}{b^4}$

D. a^2b

5. $\frac{\sqrt{12}\sqrt{2}}{\sqrt{18}} = ?$

A. $\frac{2}{5}$

B. $\frac{2\sqrt{5}}{5}$

C. $\frac{\sqrt{3}}{6}$

D. $\frac{2\sqrt{3}}{3}$

6. If $\frac{x-2}{x+2} = \frac{2}{3}$, then x =

A. 12
B. 10
C. no value possible
D. 6

7. A car is run until the gas tank is $\frac{1}{6}$ full. The tank is then filled to capacity by putting in 15 gallons. The capacity of the gas tank of the car is

A. 12 gallons.
B. 15 gallons.
C. 18 gallons.
D. 21 gallons.

8. If John must have a mark of 70% to pass a test of 30 items, the number of items he may miss and still pass the test is

A. 9
B. 8
C. 10
D. 28

9. A man insures 60% of his property and pays a $2\frac{1}{2}$% premium amounting to $348.00. What is the total value of his property?

A. $18,400
B. $19,000
C. $23,200
D. $25,200

10. If the scale of a blue print is $\frac{1}{8}$ inch equals 1 foot, what is to be the actual length of a wall $8\frac{1}{2}$ inches by scale?

A. $5\frac{2}{3}$ feet
B. 8.5 feet
C. 102 feet
D. 68 feet

11. If cards are lettered as follows: T, H, O, M, E, R, R, M, E, E, T, and if you choose one of the cards above without looking, what is the probability that you will choose E?

A. $\frac{2}{9}$
B. $\frac{3}{11}$
C. $\frac{8}{11}$
D. $\frac{3}{8}$

12. Find the perimeter of a roller rink with the following dimensions. Use 3.14 for π.

A. 81.4
B. 101.4
C. 112.8
D. 120

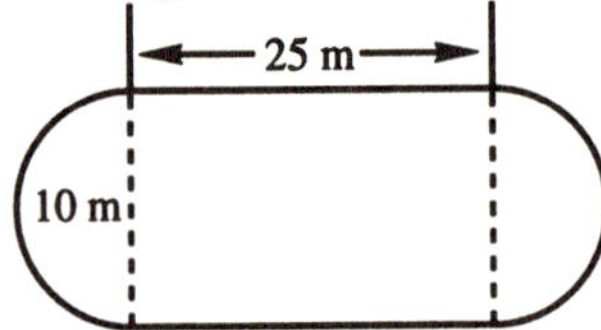

13. Find the area of the following figure. Use 3.14 for π.

A. 150.72 in.^{2}
B. 200.96 in.^{2}
C. 602.88 in.^{2}
D. 25.12 in.^{2}

Radius = 8 in

14. A 25-foot ladder is placed against a building at a point 20 feet from the ground. Find the distance from the base of the building to the base of the ladder.

A. 13 feet
B. 15 feet
C. 25 feet
D. 45 feet

15. Triangles ABC and DEF are similar. Find the area of DEF.

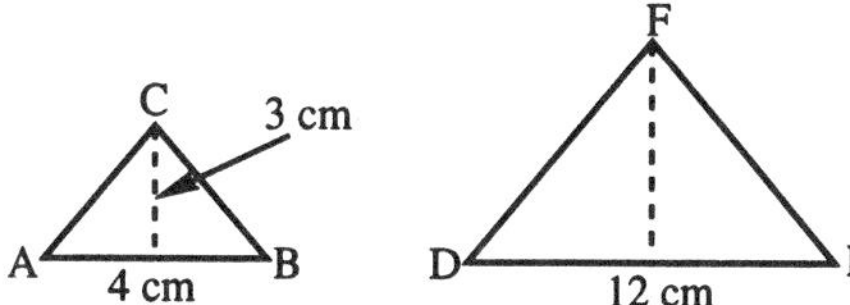

A. 36 cm^2
B. 54 cm^2
C. 48 cm^2
D. 144 cm^2

16. The slope of the line whose equation is $y = -\frac{1}{4}x - 1$

A. $\frac{1}{4}$
B. -1
C. $-\frac{1}{4}$
D. 0

17. How much water must be added to 20 ml of nitric acid to make a 40% nitric acid solution? Assume water temperature is 20°C and pH = 7.0.

A. 50 ml
B. 42 ml
C. 30 ml
D. 8 ml

18. Given $\log p = a^3$, $\log q = a^2$, and $\log t = a^4$, determine: $\frac{\log pq}{\sqrt{\log t}}$

A. $a + 1$
B. a
C. $a - 1$
D. $1/a$

19. If 25% of the inhabitants of a town are foreign born, the ratio of native born to foreign born is

A. 4:1
B. 10:40
C. 300:100
D. 1:3

20. If A finishes the job in 3 hours and B can finish it in 4 hours, how long will it take both if they work together?

A. $3\frac{1}{2}$ hours

B. 7 hours

C. $1\frac{5}{12}$ hours

D. $1\frac{5}{7}$ hours

5.12 ANSWERS TO QUESTIONS IN SECTION 5.11

1. B	2. D	3. D	4. A	5. D	6. B	7. C	8. A	9. C	10. D
11. B	12. A	13. A	14. B	15. B	16. C	17. C	18. A	19. C	20. D

5.13 SOLUTIONS TO QUESTIONS IN SECTION 5.11

Question 1: [B] The answer is found by applying routine steps for solving inequalities. First, clear the fraction by multiplying both sides of the inequality by the GCD, which is 6.

$$
\begin{aligned}
6[\tfrac{1}{3}(x-2)] &\le 6\frac{(x+2)}{6} \\
2(x-2) &\le x+2 \\
2x-4 &\le x+2 \\
2x-x &\le 4+2 \\
x &\le 6
\end{aligned}
$$

Question 2: [D] Find the LCM of 4, 6, 8,

$$
\begin{array}{r|l}
2 & 4,6,8 \\
\hline
1 & 2,3,4 \\
\hline
2 & 1,3,2 \\
\hline
\text{LCM} & 2(2)(3)(2) = 24
\end{array}
$$

$$
\begin{aligned}
4 &= 4, 8, 12, 16, 20, 24 \\
6 &= 6, 12, 18, 24 \\
8 &= 8, 16, 24 \\
\text{LCM} &= 24
\end{aligned}
$$

$$
\begin{aligned}
\frac{-3}{4} + \frac{1}{6} - \frac{5}{8} &= \frac{-18}{24} + \frac{4}{24} - \frac{15}{24} \\
&= \frac{-18+4-15}{24} \\
&= \frac{-29}{24} = -1\frac{5}{24}
\end{aligned}
$$

Question 3: [D] Change $3\frac{1}{3} \times 2\frac{1}{2}$ to an improper fraction.

$$
\begin{aligned}
3\frac{1}{3} &= \frac{9}{3} + \frac{1}{3} = \frac{10}{3} \\
2\frac{1}{2} &= \frac{4}{2} + \frac{1}{2} = \frac{5}{2} \\
\frac{10}{3} \times \frac{5}{2} &= \frac{2 \times 5}{3} \times \frac{5}{2} = \frac{25}{3} = 8\frac{1}{3}
\end{aligned}
$$

Question 4: [A] Use the rule for exponential notation and negative exponent to simplify the algebraic expression.

$$(a^3b^{-2})^{-2} = (a^3)^{-2}(b^{-2})^{-2} = a^{-6}b^4 = \frac{b^4}{a^6}$$

Question 5: [D]

$$\frac{\sqrt{12}\sqrt{2}}{\sqrt{18}}$$

$$= \frac{\sqrt{4 \times 3}\sqrt{2}}{\sqrt{2 \times 9}}$$

$$= \frac{2\sqrt{3}\sqrt{2}}{\sqrt{2}\sqrt{9}}$$

$$= \frac{2\sqrt{3}}{3}$$

Question 6: [B]

$$\begin{aligned}\frac{x-2}{x+2} &= \frac{2}{3}\\ 2(x+2) &= 3(x-2)\\ 2x+4 &= 3x-6\\ 2x-3x &= -6-4\\ -x &= -10\end{aligned}$$

Question 7: [C] If the gas tank is $\frac{1}{6}$ full, then an additional $\frac{5}{6}$ of capacity is left.

$\frac{5}{6}$ of capacity = 15 gallons, therefore

$$\begin{aligned}15 \div \frac{5}{6} &= \frac{15}{1} \times \frac{6}{5}\\ &= \frac{3 \times 5}{1} \times \frac{2 \times 3}{5} = 18\end{aligned}$$

Question 8: [A] Using the formula R/100 = P/B, he must answer 70% of 30 correctly. Therefore, he may miss 30% of 30.

R = 30

P = Unknown

B = 30

$$\begin{aligned}\frac{30}{100} &= \frac{P}{30}\\ 100P &= 30(30)\\ P &= \frac{30(30)}{100}\\ P &= \frac{3(30)}{10}\\ P &= 9\end{aligned}$$

Question 9: [C] Find the solution in two steps. $2\frac{1}{2}$ % of insured value = \$348

1. First find the insured value using the formula $\frac{R}{100} = \frac{P}{B}$

$$R = 2\tfrac{1}{2}\%$$
$$P = \$348$$
$$\frac{2\frac{1}{2}}{100} = \frac{348}{B}$$

Find B, $2\frac{1}{2}B = 348\ (100)$

$$B = \frac{34800}{5/2}$$
$$B = \frac{34800}{1} \times \frac{2}{5} = 13{,}920$$

Therefore the insured value = \$13,920

2. The insured value (\$13,920) is 60% of the total value. Find the total value:

$$R = 60\%$$
$$\frac{60}{100} = \frac{13920}{B}$$
$$P = 13{,}920$$

Find B, $60B = 13{,}920 \times 100$

$$B = \frac{13920 \times (10)\ (10)}{(6)\ (10)}$$
$$B = \frac{139200}{6} = 23{,}200$$

Therefore the total value of the property is \$23,200.

Question 10: [D] Since $\frac{1}{8}$ inch = 1 foot

$$8\tfrac{1}{2} \text{ inches} \div \tfrac{1}{8} \text{ inch} = \frac{17}{2} \times 8 = 68 \text{ feet.}$$

Question 11: [B] Each card has an equally likely chance of being chosen. There are three outcomes that are **E**. There are eleven possible outcomes.

$$\text{Probability of } \mathbf{E} = \frac{\text{number of } \mathbf{E} \text{ outcomes}}{\text{number of possible outcomes}}$$
$$P(M) = \frac{3}{11}.$$

Question 12:[A]
Perimeter = 2(circumference of semicircle) + (perimeter of rectangle) –2(width)

$$P = 2\frac{(\pi d)}{2} + 2(L + W) - 2W$$

$$P = 2\frac{[3.14(10)]}{2} + 2(25 + 10) - 2(10)$$

$$P = 3.14\ (10) + 70 - 20$$

$$P = 31.4 + 50$$

$$P = 81.4 \text{ m}$$

Question 13: [A] To find the area of the figure in this example, use the formula area = πr^2. Notice the figure is $\frac{3}{4}$ of a circle. To find the area of $\frac{3}{4}$ of the circle, take $\frac{3}{4}$ of the area. Therefore,

$$A = \frac{3}{4} \text{ of } \pi r^2$$

$$A = \frac{3}{4} \text{ of } 3.14(8)^2$$

$$A = \frac{3}{4} \times 200.96 = \frac{602.88}{4}$$

$$A = 150.72 \text{ in}^2$$

Question 14: [B] To find the distance from the base of the building to the base of the ladder, draw a figure, then use the pythagorean theorem. The hypotenuse is the length of the ladder (25 feet). One leg is the distance along the building from the ground to the top of the ladder. The distance from the base of the building to the base of the ladder is the unknown leg. Using the pythagorean theorem, $a^2 + b^2 = c^2$, find b.

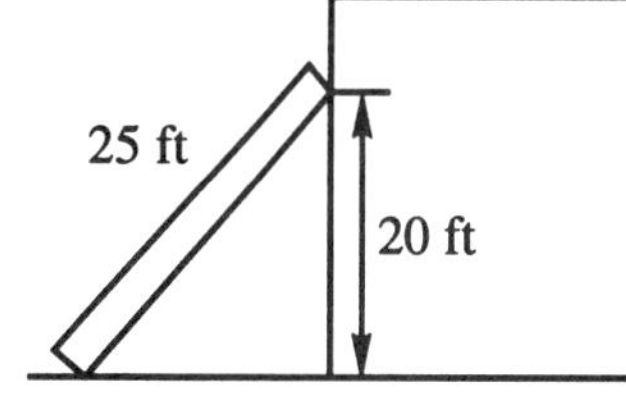

$$a^2 + b^2 = c^2$$

$$(20 \text{ ft})^2 + b^2 = (25 \text{ ft})^2$$

$$400 \text{ ft}^2 + b^2 = 625 \text{ ft}^2$$

$$b^2 = 625 \text{ ft}^2 - 400 \text{ ft}^2$$

$$b^2 = \sqrt{225 \text{ ft}^2}$$

$$b = 15 \text{ ft}$$

The distance from the base of the building to the base of the ladder is 15 feet.

Question 15: [B] To find the area of triangle DEF, (a) solve a proportion to find the height of triangle DFE, and (b) use the formula area = $\frac{1}{2} \times$ base $\times$ height.

$$\frac{AB}{DE} = \frac{\text{height of triangle ABC}}{\text{height of triangle DEF}}$$

$$\frac{4\text{cm}}{12\text{cm}} = \frac{3\text{cm}}{\text{height}}$$

$$4 \times \text{height} = 12 \times 3 \text{ cm}$$

$$4 \times \text{height} = 36 \text{ cm}$$

$$\text{height} = \frac{36 \text{ cm}}{4}$$

$$\text{height} = 9 \text{ cm}$$

$$\text{Area} = \frac{1}{2} \times \text{base} \times \text{height}$$

$$A = \frac{1}{2} BH$$

$$= \frac{1}{2} \times 12 \text{ cm} \times 9 \text{ cm}$$

$$= 54 \text{ cm}^2$$

The area is 54 cm^2.

Question 16: [C] Find two ordered pairs that are solutions of the equation,

$$y = \frac{-1}{4} x - 1$$

$$P_1 = (0, -1)$$

$$P_2 = (1, -1\tfrac{1}{4})$$

Using the slope formula, $M = \dfrac{y_2 - y_1}{x_2 - x_1}$

$$M = \frac{(-1\frac{1}{4}) - (-1)}{1 - 0} = \frac{-1\frac{1}{4} + 1}{1} = \frac{-1}{4}$$

Question 17: [C] 30 ml. Use the given data to construct a block diagram of volumes and percentages of nitric acid and water. This is an example of comparative reasoning.

water +	x ml	=	nitric acid	40%
nitric acid	20 ml		water	60%

Comparing the two block diagrams,

$$\frac{\text{20 ml of nitric acid}}{\text{x ml of water + 20 ml of nitric acid}} = \text{40\% nitric acid solution.}$$

$$\frac{20}{x + 20} = \frac{40}{100} = \frac{2}{5}$$

$$100 = 2x + 40$$

$$2x = 60,$$

$$x = 30 \text{ ml of water}$$

Question 18: [A]

$$\log p = a^3$$
$$\log q = a^2$$
$$\log t = a^4, \text{ because } \sqrt{\log t} = a^2$$
$$\log pq = \log p + \log q = a^3 + a^2 = a^2 (a + 1)$$
$$\frac{\log pq}{\sqrt{\log t}} = \frac{a^2 (a + 1)}{a^2} = a + 1$$

Question 19: [C] If 25% of the inhabitants are foreign born, then 75% are native born. The ratio of native born to foreign born would have to be 3:1, which is equivalent to 300:100.

Question 20: [D] Since multiple choice answers are given, the correct answer is smaller than the shortest time given. No matter how slow a worker is, he does part of the job and therefore it will be completed in less time.

Let $A = \frac{x}{3}$

Let $B = \frac{x}{4}$

The sum of all individual fractions should be 1.

	A		B	
$\frac{\text{Time spent}}{\text{Total time needed to do job}}$	$\frac{x}{3}$	+	$\frac{x}{4}$	= 1

Solve the equation $\frac{x}{3} + \frac{x}{4} = 1$

Find the LCD.

Multiply by 12 to eliminate fraction

$$4x + 3x = 12$$
$$7x = 12$$
$$x = \frac{12}{7}$$
$$x = 1\frac{5}{7} \text{ hours}$$

5.14 REFERENCES

Aufmann, Richard N., and Vernon C. Barker. *Basic College Mathematics: An Applied Approach,* 1st ed. (Boston: Houghton Mifflin, 1985.) Used with permission.

______*Introductory Algebra: An Applied Approach,* 1st ed. (Boston: Houghton Mifflin, 1983.) Used with permission.

Hassan, Aftab, et. al. *A Complete Preparation for the MCAT*, 6th ed. (Rockville, Md.: Betz Publishing Company, 1993.)

Whimbey, Arthur and Jack Lochhead.*Beyond Problem Solving and Comprehension:* (Hillsdale, N.J.: Lawrence Erlbaum Associates, 1984.)

______*Problem Solving & Comprehension,* 5th ed. (Hillsdale, N.J.: Lawrence Erlbaum Associates, 1991.)

Chapter 6: Preparing for PCAT Chemistry

6.0 INTRODUCTION

This section outlines, with brief introductions, the topics in general chemistry required for the PCAT. The material is divided into content groups with a short listing of the topics that should be mastered. Several sample problems are included with explained solutions. Use these questions to gauge your understanding of the general chemistry required on the PCAT and identify specific topics requiring more independent study and review. Consult Betz Publishing's *A Complete Preparation for the MCAT*, Studyware Biology Review (software), and the GRE subject test books, as needed.

6.1 GENERAL CHEMISTRY

6.1.1 General Chemistry Outline

A. Stoichiometry
- **1.** Review of Chemical Compounds
  - **a.** Mole (Definition, Equation, Application)
  - **b.** Equivalent and Gram Equivalent Weight
  - **c.** Percentage Composition
    - **(i)** Structural Formula
    - **(ii)** Molecular Formula
    - **(iii)** Empirical Formula
    - **(iv)** Application to Determine Structural Formula, Molecular Formula, and Empirical Formula
  - **d.** Applications of Mole in Stoichiometry
  - **e.** Use of Mole in Balancing Equations
- **2.** Stoichiometry Problems
  - **a.** Weight/Weight Problems
  - **b.** Weight/Volume Problems
  - **c.** Density Problems

B. Atomic Arrangements in Molecules
- **1.** Definition
  - **a.** Ionic Bond
  - **b.** Covalent Bond
  - **c.** Coordinate Bond
- **2.** Shapes of Molecules
  - **a.** Switching Shapes
  - **b.** Covalent Molecules
    - **(i)** Polar
    - **(ii)** Non-Polar
- **3.** Valence Shell Electron Pair Repulsion Theory
- **4.** Bohr's Atomic Structure

a. Electron Energy States
b. Quantum Theory
(i) Quantum Numbers
(ii) Pauli Exclusion Principle
(iii) Electron Configuration in Orbitals
(iv) Hund's Rule
5. Condensed Phases and Bonds
a. Intermolecular Forces
b. van der Waals Forces
c. Hydrogen Bonding Forces
d. Hydrophobic Bonding Forces
C. Periodic Properties of Elements
1. The Periodic Table
a. Periods
b. Groups
c. Metals
d. Atomic Radius
e. Transition Metals
f. Non-Transition Metals
g. Metalloids
2. Periodic Trends of Elements
a. Ionization Energy
b. Electron Affinity
c. Electronegativity
d. Atomic Radius
e. Oxidation State
f. Diamagnetism
g. Ferromagnetism
h. Paramagnetism
D. Gases
1. Kinetic Molecular Theory of Matter
2. Laws for Gases
a. Boyle's Law
b. Charles's Law
c. Gay-Lussac's Law
d. Dalton's Law of Partial Pressures
e. Avogadro's Law
f. Graham's Law of Gas Diffusion
g. Universal Gas Equation for Ideal Gases
(i) van der Waal's Real Gas Law
(ii) Molar Volume of a Gas
E. Review of Colligative Properties
1. Phase Equilibrium
a. Phase Changes
(i) Boiling Point Elevation
(ii) Freezing Point Depression
(iii) Effects of solutes on BP and FP
b. Definitions
(i) Suspension
(ii) Colloid
(iii) Emulsion

(iv) Foam
(v) Gel
c. Molality

F. Acids, Bases, and Buffers
1. Three Common Definitions of Acids and Bases
a. Arrhenius
b. Brønsted-Lowry
c. Lewis
2. Strength
a. Strong and weak acids
b. Weak and Strong Bases
c. Conjugate Acid and Base
d. pH as a Strength Indicator
e. Molarity
f. Normality
3. Solubility Rules for Acids and Bases
a. Ionization Constant, Percent of Ionization
b. Common Ion Effect
(i) Le Chatelier's Principle
(ii) Buffers (equilibrium constants and pH)

G. Chemical Equilibrium
1. Reversible Reactions
2. Le Chatelier's Principle and Reactants
a. Effect of Concentration
b. Effect of Pressure
c. Effect of Temperature
3. Equilibrium Constant Calculations

H. Thermodynamics and Thermochemistry
1. Energy Changes in Reactions
a. Law of Constant Heat Summation
b. Heat of Formation, Hess's Law
c. Gibbs Free Energy Principle
(i) Free Energy
(ii) Entropy
(iii) Enthalpy
(iv) Spontaneous Reactions
d. Exothermic and Endothermic Reactions

I. Rate Processes in Chemical Reactions/Kinetics
1. Activation Energy Diagram
a. Reversibility of Reaction
b. Reaction Rate
(i) Forward
(ii) Backward
c. Equilibrium Constant

J. Electrochemical Concepts and Calculations
1. Oxidation and Reduction Reactions
a. Oxidation
b. Reduction
c. Anode
d. Cathode
2. Types of Cells

a. Electrolytic
b. Galvanic
c. Concentration
3. Faraday's Laws of Electrolysis
a. Steps to Balance Redox Reactions
b. Problems in Electrolysis

K. Nuclear Structure and Reactions
1. Binding Energy of an Atom
a. Nuclear Binding Energy
b. Fission
c. Fusion
2. Stability of Atoms
3. Nuclear Reactions
a. Radioactive Decay
b. Half life
4. Atomic and Quantum Physics
a. Absorption and Emission Spectra
b. Fluorescent Emission

6.1.2 Basic Concepts and Stoichiometry, With Sample Questions

This section covers concepts related to density, the classification of matter, the law of definite proportions, nomenclature of common polyatomic ions, formula weight of a substance, percent composition, moles, empirical formulas, molecular formulas, the law of conservation of mass, how to balance a chemical equation, the use of a balanced chemical equation, and other information to calculate the quantities of reactants consumed or products produced in a chemical reaction, and how to determine a limiting reactant with percent yield.

1. The chemical compound with the formula of PCl_3 has the name
   A. phosphorus trichlorite.
   B. phosphorus trichloride.
   C. phosphorus trichlorate.
   D. phosphorus trichorine.

2. The chemical compound with the name of barium oxide has the formula of
   A. BaO.
   B. BaO_2.
   C. Ba_2O.
   D. Ba_2O_3.

3. Of the following compounds, which contains the *lowest* % carbon by mass?
   A. CH_4
   B. CH_3CO_2H
   C. $Na_2C_2O_2$
   D. $C_6H_{12}O_6$

4. A compound has the simplest formula CH_2Cl and molecular mass of 196 g mole^{-1}. (Atomic weights: C = 12, H = 1, Cl = 35.5). The molecular formula is
   A. CH_2Cl.
   B. $C_2H_4Cl_2$.
   C. $C_3H_6Cl_3$.
   D. $C_4H_8Cl_4$.

5. Balance the following hypothetical equation using the minimum integral coefficients.

$$CrPO_4 + Bi_2(SiO_4)_3 \rightarrow BiPO_4 + Cr_2(SiO_4)_3$$

   The correct coefficient for $BiPO_4$ is
   A. 1.
   B. 2.
   C. 3.
   D. 4.

6. A chemist, trying to identify the main component in a commercial record cleaner, finds that 25 mL of the substance has a mass of 20 g. Which of these compounds is the most likely choice?
   A. Chloroform, density = 1.5 g/cm^3
   B. Diethyl ether, density = 0.7 g/cm^3
   C. Isopropyl alcohol, density = 0.8 g/cm^3
   D. Toluene, density = 0.9 g/cm^3

7. How many grams of HCl are required to react completely with 1 mole of Zn? (Atomic weights: H = 1, Zn = 65.5, Cl = 35.5)

$$HCl_{(aq)} + Zn_{(s)} \rightarrow ZnCl_{2(aq)} + H_{2(g)}$$

   A. 18 g
   B. 36 g
   C. 54 g
   D. 72 g

6.1.3 Gases, With Sample Questions

Material to be reviewed in this section includes Boyles's Law, Charles's Law, Gay-Lussac's Law, Avogadro's Law, the ideal gas law, and Dalton's Law of Partial Pressures. Other useful topics are gas stoichiometry, STP, kinetic molecular theory, and diffusion.

8. The total pressure of a mixture of gases is
   A. obtained by multiplying the individual pressures by the number of moles and averaging.
   B. the sum of the partial pressures of the components.
   C. dependent only on the pressures of the gas that is present to the greatest extent.
   D. the product of the partial pressures of the components.

9. What volume is occupied by 2.00 moles of methane (CH_4) at 273 K and 2.00 atm?
   A. 22.4 liters
   B. 11.2 liters
   C. 10.00 liters
   D. 44.8 liters

10. Four identical 1.0 L flasks contain the following gases each at 0° C and 1 atm of pressure. Which gas has the lowest density?
    A. He
    B. Cl_2
    C. CH_4
    D. C_3H_6

11. One liter of nitrogen and one liter of carbon dioxide initially at one atmosphere pressure are forced into a single 500 mL vessel. What is the new nitrogen pressure if the temperature remains unchanged?
    A. 1 atm
    B. 2 atm
    C. 3 atm
    D. 4 atm

12. Given the following reaction (not balanced), $N_{2(g)} + Br_{2(g)} \rightarrow NBr_{3(g)}$, how many liters of gaseous bromine are needed to react with 2 liters of nitrogen?
    A. 1 liter
    B. 3 liters
    C. 4 liters
    D. 6 liters

6.1.4 Liquids and Solids, With Sample Questions

This section covers phase changes, intermolecular forces, solutions, colligative properties (freezing point depression, boiling point elevation, and osmotic pressure), hydrogen bonding and hydrophobic bonding forces.

13. You are given the following boiling point data: ethylene glycol bp = 198°, water bp = 100°, formamide = 111°, ethanol bp = 79°, methanol bp = 65°. Which of the compounds has the highest vapor pressure at room temperature?
    A. ethylene glycol
    B. water
    C. ethanol
    D. methanol

Questions 14 and 15 refer to the following phase diagram.

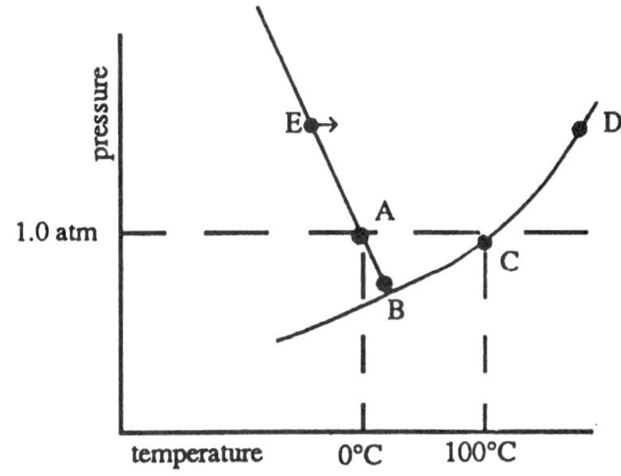

14. The triple point of water is located at the temperature and pressure represented by
A. A.
B. B.
C. C.
D. D.

15. The arrow labeled "E" represents the physical change called
A. sublimation.
B. condensation.
C. melting.
D. deposition.

16. The addition of a nonvolatile solute into a solvent
A. lowers the freezing point and raises the boiling point.
B. raises the freezing point and lowers the boiling point.
C. raises both the freezing and boiling points.
D. lowers both the freezing and boiling points.

17. In any cubic lattice, an atom lying at the corner of a unit cell is shared equally by how many unit cells?
A. 1
B. 2
C. 8
D. 16

6.1.5 Solutions, With Sample Questions

Solution chemistry involves the ideas of concentration, intermolecular forces, and the properties of the solute and solvent.

18. Electrolytes are
A. solutions that contain solvated electrons.
B. solutions that conduct an electric current.
C. solutions that contain soluble salts, strong acids, or strong bases.
D. both B and C.

19. What volume of 2.0 M HCl must be used to prepare 10.0 liters of a 0.50 M HCl solution?
A. 25 L
B. 2.5 L
C. 0.25 L
D. 250 L

20. A factory has 500 L of a 4×10^{-3} M solution of NaOH. How many atoms of sodium are contained in this sample?
A. 6.02×10^{23}
B. 3.01×10^{23}
C. 1.2×10^{24}
D. 4.50×10^{22}

21. Which of the following pairs of liquids would be infinitely miscible?
A. Ethanol and water
B. Benzene and water
C. Ether and water
D. Chloroform and water

22. Which of the following compounds is nonpolar?
A. Ammonia, NH_3
B. Boron trichloride, BCl_3
C. Water, H_2O
D. Carbon monoxide, CO

6.1.6 Acids and Bases, With Sample Questions

Topics reviewed in this section are definitions of acids, conjugate acid/base pairs, neutralization reactions, titrations, buffers, and hydrolysis reactions of salts.

23. What is the conjugate base of NH_3?
A. NH_4^+
B. NH_2^-
C. H_3O^+
D. OH^-

24. When sodium acetate, $NaC_2H_3O_2$, is dissolved in water, the resulting solution is
A. acidic.
B. basic.
C. neutral.
D. colligative.

25. Which of the following systems is a buffer?
A. 10 mL of 0.1 M NH_4Cl and 10 mL of 0.1 M HCl
B. 10 mL of 0.1 M NH_4Cl and 10 mL of 0.1 M NaCl
C. 10 mL of 0.1 M NH_4Cl and 10 mL of 0.1 M NH_3
D. 10 mL of 0.1 M NH_4Cl and 10 mL of 0.1 M NaOH

26. Given the following reaction, $HCl + Ba(OH)_2 \rightarrow BaCl_2 + H_2O$, What volume of 1 N of HCl is required to react completely with 10 mL of 1 N $Ba(OH)_2$?
A. 5 mL
B. 10 mL
C. 15 mL
D. 20 mL

27. Given the following reaction, $BH_3 + N(CH_2CH_3)_3 \rightarrow H_3B{\bullet}N(CH_2CH_3)_3$, the best description of the role of $N(CH_2CH_3)_3$ in this reaction is as
A. Lewis acid.
B. Lewis base.
C. Brønsted-Lowry acid.
D. Brønsted-Lowry base.

6.1.7 Chemical Equilibrium, With Sample Questions

This section reviews how chemical equilibrium can be treated in a quantitative manner. First review the basic principles of chemical equilibrium in the gas phase. Other important equilibria are acid/base and solubility.

28. Consider the equilibrium, $4\ NH_{3(g)} + 3\ O_{2(g)} \leftrightarrow 2\ N_{2(g)} + 6\ H_2O_{(g)}, \Delta H = -803$ kcal, which of the following will cause the equilibrium to shift to the right?
A. Increasing temperature
B. Selectively absorbing the water.
C. Adding a catalyst
D. Selectively absorbing the O_2.

29. Given the reaction, $2\ XY_{(g)} \rightleftharpoons X_{2(g)} + Y_{2(g)}$, $K = 0.9$ at 243 K, 1 mole of XY was injected into a 1 liter container at 243 K. What is the correct equilibrium expression?
A. $0.9 = \frac{(1-2x)^2}{x^2}$
B. $0.9 = \frac{x^2}{(1-2x)^2}$
C. $0.9 = \frac{x^2}{(1-2x)}$
D. $0.9 = \frac{(1-2x)}{x^2}$

30. Which of the following compounds is the most soluble in water?
A. $CaSO_4$, Ksp = 10^{-5}
B. CuI, Ksp = 10^{-12}
C. AgI, Ksp = 10^{-16}
D. CuS, Ksp = 10^{-45}

31. What would be the concentration of silver in a saturated silver iodide solution?
   A. 10^{-16} M
   B. 10^{-32} M
   C. 10^{-4} M
   D. 10^{-8} M

32. The K_{sp} of $Fe(OH)_2$ is 10^{-15}. You are given a system at equilibrium that is a pale green solution, $Fe(OH)_{2(aq)}$, and a brown solid, $Fe(OH)_{2(s)}$. If you add 50 mL of NaOH (assume concentration of NaOH is higher than $Fe(OH)_2$), what will you observe?
   A. Additional solid forms, solution color pales
   B. Some solid dissolves, solution color deepens
   C. A gas is evolved, solution color changes to green
   D. No change would be observed

6.1.8 Thermodynamics, With Sample Questions

Spontaneity of a reaction, the enthalpy change (ΔH), the entropy change (ΔS), and the free energy change (ΔG) are presented with regard to the Second Law of Thermodynamics.

33. The heat of formation of an element in its standard state is
   A. the ΔH of its reaction with hydrogen.
   B. the ΔH of its reaction with oxygen.
   C. zero.
   D. determined by use of the molecular mass.

34. When a sample was burned in a bomb calorimeter containing 1.00 kg of water, the temperature of the water increased 1° C. If the heat capacity of the system was OkJ/K and the specific heat of water is 4.18 J/K g, how much heat was evolved?
   A. 2.09 kJ
   B. 8.36 kJ
   C. 1.00 kJ
   D. 4.18 kJ

35. Calculate the heat of formation of ethanol, C_2H_5OH, using the following information:

$$C_2H_5OH_{(l)} + 3\,O_{2(g)} \rightarrow 2\,CO_{2(g)} + 3\,H_2O_{(l)} \qquad \Delta H = -1300\text{kJ}$$
$$C_{(s)} + O_{2(g)} \rightarrow CO_{2(g)} \qquad \Delta H = -400\text{ kJ}$$
$$H_{2(g)} + 0.5\,O_{2(g)} \rightarrow H_2O_{(l)} \qquad \Delta H = -300\text{ kJ}$$

   A. –2000 kJ
   B. +2000 kJ
   C. –400 kJ
   D. +400 kJ

36. In which case *must* a reaction reach an equilibrium (that is more than 50% complete), independent of T?
   A. $\Delta H = 0, \Delta S > 0$
   B. $\Delta H = 0, \Delta S < 0$
   C. $\Delta S = 0, \Delta H > 0$
   D. $\Delta H < 0, \Delta S > 0$

6.1.9 Kinetics, With Sample Questions

To control the rates of reactions, you must understand the factors that influence the rate. For this section, review the effect of concentration of the reactants, of temperature of the presence of a catalyst, and of activation energy.

37. Which of the following is the rate of a unimolecular reaction?
- **A.** k[A]
- **B.** $k[A]^2$
- **C.** k[A][B]
- **D.** $k[A][B]^2$

38. The rate constant for a certain first order reaction is 0.40 min^{-1}. What is the initial rate in mol L^{-1} min^{-1}, if the initial concentration of the compound is 0.50 M?
- **A.** 0.90
- **B.** 0.10
- **C.** 0.20
- **D.** 0.40

39. Which of the following is necessary for a reaction to occur between two molecules?
- **A.** A particular collision between two molecules has an energy greater than the E_a
- **B.** A particular collision between two molecules has an energy less than the ΔH of the reaction.
- **C.** The activated complex has sufficient vibrational energy to begin bond breaking
- **D.** The activated complex has less potential energy than the reaction products

Questions 40 and 41 refer to the following diagram.

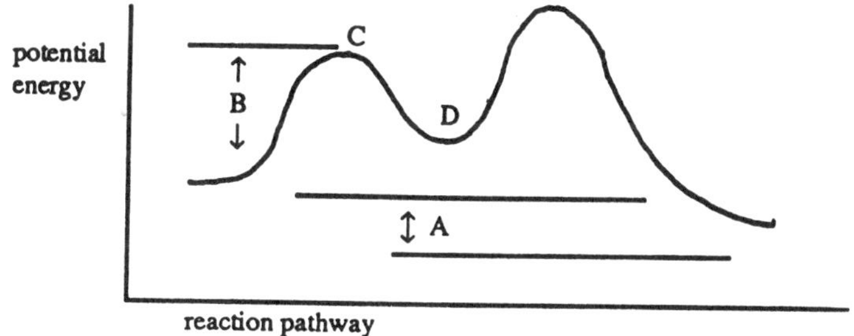

40. What point on the reaction diagram represents a reaction intermediate?
- **A.** A
- **B.** B
- **C.** C
- **D.** D

41. What point on the reaction diagram represents a transition state?
- **A.** A
- **B.** B
- **C.** C
- **D.** D

6.1.10 Redox Reactions, With Sample Questions

This section considers the use of electrical energy to carry out chemical reactions. Important topics include oxidation numbers, the Nernst Equation, and redox chemistry.

Questions 42 and 43 refer to the following information and cell diagram.

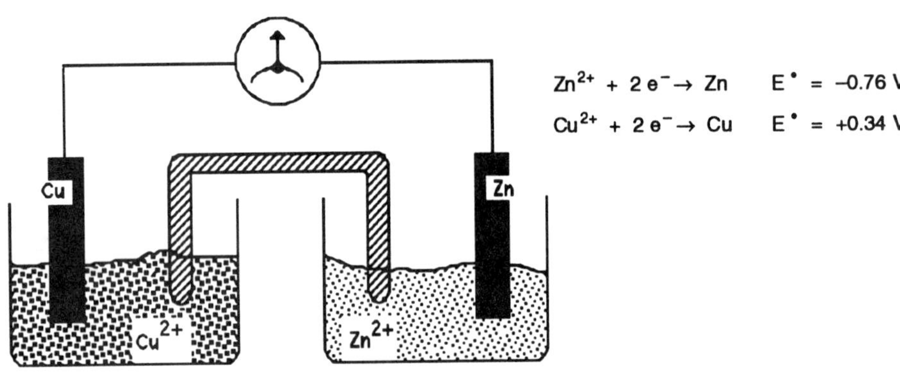

42. Which of the following reactions will give a spontaneous reaction ($\Delta G < 0$) for the above cell?

A. $Cu^{2+} + Zn \rightarrow Cu + Zn^{2+}$

B. $Cu + Zn^{2+} \rightarrow Cu^{2+} + Zn$

C. $Cu^{2+} + Zn^{2+} \rightarrow Cu + Zn + 4\,e^-$

D. $Cu + Zn + 4\,e^- \rightarrow Cu^{2+} + Zn^{2+}$

43. If the above cell contains 1.0 M $CuSO_4$ and 1.0 M $ZnSO_4$, what is the potential, E, of this cell?

A. –1.10 V
B. +1.10 V
C. +2.20 V
D. –2.20 V

44. What is the oxidation state of nitrogen in NO_3^-?

A. -3
B. 0
C. +3
D. +5

45. Based on the following information, which metal is the strongest reducing agent?

(i) $Zn^{2+} + Fe \rightarrow$ no reaction
(ii) $Fe^{2+} + Zn \rightarrow Zn^{2+} + Fe$
(iii) $Mg^{2+} + Zn \rightarrow$ no reaction
(iv) $Zn^{2+} + Mg \rightarrow Mg^{2+} + Zn$
(v) $Cu^{2+} + Zn \rightarrow Cu + Zn^{2+}$

A. Cu
B. Fe
C. Mg
D. Zn

6.1.11 Atomic and Molecular Structure, With Sample Questions

Important topics to review in this section include electron configuration, Hund's Rule, the Pauli Exclusion Principle, the Aufbau Principle, quantum numbers, Lewis Dot structures, and the octet rule.

46. Oxygen has 6 valence electrons. Consider the following electron arrangements. Which represents the ground state for oxygen (O)?

	2s	2p		
A.	↑↓	↑↓	↑↓	
B.	↑↓	↑↓	↑	↑
C.	↑↓	↑↓	↑	↓
D.	↑	↑↓	↑↓	↑

47. Which of the following ions is isoelectronic with Ar?

A. Ca^{+}
B. S^{-}
C. K^{+}
D. P^{2-}

48. Which of the following best describes the bonding in HCN?

A. ionic only
B. 2 sigma bonds and 2 π-bonds
C. 3 sigma bonds and 1 π-bond
D. 4 sigma bonds

49. How many electrons can occupy a shell with n = 3?
A. 2
B. 8
C. 18
D. 42

50. How many electrons can occupy a subshell with $l = 2$?
A. 2
B. 6
C. 10
D. 14

51. Which of the following elements does not have to obey the octet rule?
A. C
B. Ne
C. P
D. Li

52. What element has this electron configuration, [Kr] $4d^5 5s^2$?
A. Mn
B. Tc
C. Re
D. Uns (#107)

6.1.12 Periodic Properties, With Sample Questions

Areas to be reviewed include named groups (halogens, alkali metals, alkaline earth, noble gases, semi-metals, transition metals), and periodic trends (size, ionization potential, electronegativity).

53. Which of the following elements is classified as a semi-metal or metalloid?
A. Carbon
B. Sulfur
C. Arsenic
D. Lead

54. Which of the following elements is a liquid at room temperature?
A. F_2
B. Cl_2
C. Br_2
D. I_2

55. Which of the following lists of elements are known collectively as the noble gases?
A. He, Ne, Ar, Kr, Xe
B. F, Cl, Br, I, At
C. Be, Mg, Ca, Sr, Ba, Ra
D. Li, Na, K, Rb, Cs, Fr

56. How many electrons can be contained in all of the orbitals with $n = 3$?
   A. 2
   B. 8
   C. 18
   D. 32

57. Which of the following orderings of atoms are listed in *increasing* size?
   I Al, Si, P, S
   II S, P, Si, Al
   III I, Br, Cl, F
   IV F, Cl, Br, I

   A. I and III
   B. II and IV
   C. I and IV
   D. II and III

58. What is the value of l for a 3d orbital?
   A. 0
   B. 1
   C. 2
   D. 3

59. Which of the following atoms require the *most* energy to remove a valence electron?
   A. Li
   B. Na
   C. K
   D. Rb

60. Which of the following metals yields an oxide with the formula MO by reaction with oxygen?
   A. Sodium
   B. Potassium
   C. Aluminum
   D. Magnesium

61. Which of the following compounds is caustic soda?
   A. NaOH
   B. Na_2CO_3
   C. NaCl
   D. Na_2SO_4

6.1.13 Nuclear Reactions, With Sample Questions

Several topics should be reviewed, including balancing nuclear equations, decay processes, and particles.

62. Which of the following radioactive decay processes does not involve a change in atomic number?
A. Electron capture
B. Gamma emission
C. Positron emission
D. Beta emission

63. The half-life of Iodine-131 is 8.0 days. How many grams of Iodine-131 remain after 16.0 days in a sample that initially contained 1.00 gram of Iodine-131?
A. 0.50 g
B. 0.25 g
C. 0.13 g
D. 0.05 g

64. What is the missing product of the following reaction? ${}^{43}_{19}K \rightarrow {}^{43}_{20}Ca + ?$

A. ${}^{4}_{2}He$
B. ${}^{0}_{-1}e$
C. ${}^{0}_{1}e$
D. γ

65. What is the missing product of the reaction shown? ${}^{80}_{28}Ni^* \rightarrow {}^{80}_{28}Ni + ?$

A. ${}^{4}_{2}He$
B. ${}^{0}_{-1}e$
C. ${}^{0}_{1}e$
D. γ

6.1.14 Answers and Explanations for General Chemistry Sample Questions

Question 1: [B] Topic: nomenclature. When naming small inorganic compounds, always list the more electropositive element first. The other element is named as an anion. Anion endings are -ide for elemental and -ite and -ate for oxygen-containing polyatomic anions (the ending -ine is the ending used for elements).

Question 2: [A] Topic: nomenclature. Barium is a +2 cation and oxide is a –2 anion. The correct formula would contain 1 barium and 1 oxide.

Question 3: [C] Topic: percent composition. Determine the molecular weight of each species. 1 = 16 g/mole; 2 = 61 g/mole; 3 = 102 g/mole; 4 = 192 g/mole; 5 = 28 g/mole. Next divide the mass of carbon by the molecular weight. 1 = 12/16 = 0.75; 2 = 24/61 = 0.40; 3 = 24/102 = 0.24; 4 = 72/196 = 0.37; 5 = 24/28 = 0.86.

Question 4: [D] Topic: empirical/molecular formula. Determine the mass of empirical formula unit (49 g). Divide into molecular mass (= 4). This means the molecule contains four empirical units.

Question 5: [B] Topic: balancing equations. Start with the most complicated molecule, $Bi_2(SiO_4)_3$. Balance Bi with 2 on product side and $CrPO_4$ with 2.

Question 6: [C] Topic: Density is the ratio of mass to volume. Divide mass of sample by volume.

Question 7: [D] Topic: stoichiometry. First balance the equation by placing 2 with HCl. Mole ratio calculation gives 2 moles of HCl per 1 mole of Zn. Molecular weight of HCl is 36 g/mole.

Question 8: [B] Topic: Dalton's Law of partial pressure. This is the definition of this gas law.

Question 9: [A] Topic: ideal gas law and Avogadro's Gas Law. Remember that at STP one mole of an ideal gas occupies 22.4 L. Avogadro's Law states that the amount of gas present (moles) is directly proportional to the pressure. If the number of moles doubles and the pressure doubles, the volume and temperature are constant.

Question 10: [B] Topic: ideal gas law. Substitute mass/MW for n in the ideal gas law. Solve for density using mass/V. Density is proportional to molecular weight.

Question 11: [B] Topic: Boyle's Law. Boyle's Law states that the pressure of a gas is inversely proportional to its volume. To halve the volume, double the pressure.

Question 12: [D] Topic: law of combining volumes. The law of combining volumes allows us to substitute volumes of gas for moles in stoichiometric calculations in gas-phase reactions.

Question 13: [D] Topic: vapor pressure. The definition of boiling point is when the vapor pressure of the liquid equals the atmospheric pressure. The lower the boiling temperature, the closer the vapor pressure is to the atmospheric pressure.

Question 14: [B] Topic: phase diagrams. **A** = normal freezing point. **C** = normal boiling point. **D**= critical point.

Question 15: [C] Topic: phase changes. The change occurring is from solid to liquid.

Question 16: [A] Topic: colligative properties. The addition of an impurity to a material increases the boiling point according to $\Delta T_b = k_b m$ (ΔT_b is the change in boiling point, k_b is a constant, and m is the molality of the solution). The addition of an impurity lowers the freezing point (why we use salt to melt ice in the winter) according to $\Delta T_f = k_f m$.

Question 17: [C] Topic: cubes. Any atom on the corner of a cube is 1/8 in that cube, so any corner atom is shared by eight atoms. Get 8 shoe boxes and try it.

Question 18: [D] Topic: solutions. Electrolytes are solutions that conduct electrons and are either soluble salts or acids/bases. Any compound that ionizes in solution is an electrolyte.

Question 19: [B] Topic: concentration units. Using the formula $C_1V_1 = C_2V_2$ for this dilution problem, solve for V_1.

Question 20: [C] Topic: concentration units. The definition of molarity is mole per liter. Multiply the concentration by the volume to get moles. Avogadro's number tells us there are 6.02×10^{23} molecules per mole. So there are 2 moles of NaOH and in solution it ionizes to 2 moles of Na^+.

Question 21: [A] Topic: polarity. "Like dissolves like." Water is polar, only another polar compound will be totally miscible.

Question 22: [B] Topic: polarity. You need to draw the molecule in a three-dimensional view and look for a permanent dipole moment.

Question 23: [A] Topic: conjugates. When ammonia ionizes in aqueous solution the reaction is $NH_3 + H_2O \rightleftharpoons NH_4^+ + OH^-$. The definition of a base is a proton acceptor, which makes NH_4^+ the correct response.

Question 24: [B] Topic: salt hydrolysis. Acetate, $C_2H_3O_2^-$, is the conjugate base of a weak acid, acetic acid. The resulting conjugate base of a weak acid is a strong conjugate base that reacts with water.

Question 25: [C] Topic: buffers. The definition of a buffer includes a weak base (acid) and the salt of its conjugate acid (base). See question 23. **A** has a strong acid, **B** has two salts, and **D** has a strong base.

Question 26:[B] Topic: neutralization reaction. Notice the unit of concentration, N (normality). Normality is defined as gram-equivalent weight of a particular substance dissolved in 1 liter of solution. HCl has one reactive H per molecule, giving a gram-equivalent weight equal to the molecular weight. $Ba(OH)_2$ has two reactive hydroxyl ions (each being equivalent to a proton). Therefore, the gram-equivalent weight is one-half the molecular weight. So equal volumes of equal normality solutions are needed for complete reaction.

Question 27: [B] Topic: acid definition. The definition of a Lewis Acid is an electron-pair acceptor. A Lewis Base is an electron pair donor. Brønsted-Lowry Acid is a proton donor. Brønsted-Lowry Base is a proton acceptor. In the course of the reaction no proton is exchanged, ruling out choices **C** and **D**. By knowing the Lewis Dot Structures of the reactants, N possesses a lone pair of electrons [$:N(CH_2CH_3)_3$], making it an electron donor.

Question 28: [B] Topic: equilibrium. The removal of a product will cause the shift to the right, whereas addition of a product shifts to the left; **C** has no effect because catalysts do not cause shifting of equilibrium. Selective absorption of H_2O will cause equilibrium to remain on the right side or shift to the right side as shown in **B**.

Question 29: [B] Topic: equilibrium calculations. To solve any similar problem (gas phase, acid/base, or solubility equilibriums) think of the problem in 3 phases.

$$2\,XY_{(g)} \rightleftharpoons X_{2(g)} + Y_{2(g)} \quad \text{(Phase I)}$$

t_o	1M	0	0	(Phase II)
Δ	$-2x$	$+x$	$+x$	(Phase III)
t_{eq}	1-2x	x	x	

(1) t_o, concentration at the start. (2) Δ, concentration change, and (3) t_{eq}, equilibrium concentration. Place the information into the equilibrium expression for the reaction in question. The general form of an equilibrium expression is [for x A + y B $\leftrightarrow$ aX + bY]

$$K = \frac{\text{concentration of products}}{\text{concentration of reactants}} = \frac{[X]^a\,[Y]^b}{[A]^x\,[B]^y}$$

where a, b, x, and y are the coefficients from the balanced chemical equation.

Question 30: [A] Topic: equilibrium. Since all of the salts in question form the same number of ions in solution, we can compare the K_{sp} values. If the salts formed different numbers of ions in solutions, you would have to calculate the *molar solubility.*

Question 31: [D] Topic: solubility equilibrium. The expression for Ksp for this equilibrium is K_{sp} =
$[Ag^+][I^-]$; substitute x for the concentrations of Ag^+ + I^- and solve for x. The K_{sp} value was given in the previous question.

$$\underset{(s)}{AgI} \rightleftharpoons \underset{\substack{(aq)\\ x}}{Ag^+} + \underset{\substack{(aq)\\ x}}{I^-}$$

Question 32: [A] Topic: common ion effect (Le Chatelier's Principle). The chemical equation describing the equilibrium is $Fe(OH)_{2(s)} \rightleftharpoons Fe^{2+}{}_{(aq)} + 2\,OH^-{}_{(aq)}$. The problem states you have added NaOH, a strong base. Strong bases ionize completely in water, $NaOH_{(aq)} \rightarrow Ag^+ + I^-\ Na^+{}_{(aq)} + OH^-{}_{(aq)}$, notice that both equations have hydroxide as a product. The increased concentration of product of the equilibrium will cause reactants to form.

Question 33: [C] Topic: heat of formation. The heat of formation is the heat needed to form a compound from its component elements. Elements do not need to be formed.

Question 34: [D] Topic: calorimetry. Heat q, evolved in a calorimeter, is q = CΔT (C is heat capacity = specific heat × mass and ΔT is the change in room temperature). C = (4.18 J/Kg)(1.00 kg) = 4.18 kJ/K. q then is equal to (4.18 kJ/K)(1K) = 4.18 kJ.

Question 35: [C] Topic: Hess's Law. Hess's Law states that the energy of a chemical reaction is the same regardless of how you get there. We can use the three given reactions and add them up to the desired reaction. Heat of formation is the formation of the compound from the component elements, in this case $2\,C + 3\,H_2 + 1/2\,O_2 \rightarrow C_2H_5OH$. The first given reaction contains information on ethanol, but as a reactant. To reverse the reaction is equivalent to multiplying by –1. This changes the sign of the heat, ΔH. To remove unwanted species we will use the other reaction to cancel. We need to remove 2 carbon dioxides as reactants. To cancel out you need two carbon dioxides as products. Similar reasoning will remove the water. The problem solved is shown below:

$$-1[C_2H_5OH + 3\,O_2 \rightarrow 2\,CO_2 + 3\,H_2O\ \Delta H = -1300\text{ kJ}] = \cancel{2\,CO_2} + \cancel{3\,H_2O} \rightarrow C_2H_5OH + \cancel{6/2\,O_2} \quad \Delta H = +1300\text{ kJ}$$

$$2[C_{(s)} = O_{2(g)} \rightarrow CO_{2(g)}\ \Delta H = -400\text{ kJ}] = 2C_{(s)} + \cancel{4/2\,O_{2(g)}} \rightarrow \cancel{2\,CO_{2(g)}} \quad \Delta H = -800\text{ kJ}$$

$$3[H_{2(g)} = 1/2\,O_{2(g)} \rightarrow H_2O_{(l)}\ \Delta H = -300\text{ kJ}] = 3H_{2(g)} + (1/2)\cancel{3/2}\,O_{2(g)} \rightarrow \cancel{3\,H_2O_{(l)}} \quad \Delta H = -900\text{ kJ}$$

$$2\,C + 3\,H_2 = 1/2\,O_2 \rightarrow C_2H_5OH,\ \Delta H = -400\text{ kJ}$$

Question 36: [D] Topic: Gibbs free energy. Free energy is the relationship between enthalpy (ΔH, heat that seeks a minimum value) and entropy (ΔS, which seeks a maximum value). The relationship is $\Delta G = \Delta H - T\Delta S$, resulting in

TABLE 5: Gibbs Free Energy Related to Entropy, Enthalpy

ΔH	ΔS	ΔG	Conditions
>0	>0	>0 <0	at low temp (nonspontaneous) at high temp (spontaneous)
>0	<0	>0	at all temperatures (never spontaneous)
<0	>0	<0	at all temperatures (always spontaneous)
<0	<0	>0 <0	at high temp (nonspontaneous) at low temp (spontaneous)

Question 37: [A] Topic: rate laws. Unimolecular refers to one molecule. Bimolecular would refer to two and relates to either **B** or **C** (it doesn't distinguish between two different molecules or two of the same molecules). **D** is trimolecular. The "order" of the reaction is the sum of the coefficients in the rate law and refers to the number of molecules participating in the rate determining step.

Question 38: [C] Topic: reaction rates. See solution for question 37 above and substitute 0.4 for k and 0.5 for the concentration and multiply. A unimolecular reaction is first-order.

Question 39: [A] Topic: activation energies. The criteria for a successful reaction are for the molecules to collide in the correct orientation and with sufficient energy to overcome the activation energy barrier.

Question 40: [D] Topic: reaction diagrams. In a reaction diagram, several concepts are presented. A is the change in enthalpy, ΔH. The energy difference between the reactants and the products, B, is the energy of activation, E_a. The energy required for the reactants to react, C is the transition state (an energy maximum), and D is an intermediate (an energy minimum located between the reactants and products).

Question 41: [C] Topic: reaction diagram.

Question 42: [A] Topic: spontaneity. For the reaction to occur spontaneously, the potential (E°) for the cell must be greater than 0. In thermodynamics, $\Delta G°$ is less than 0 for a spontaneous reaction and $\Delta G° = -nFE°$(n = number of electrons transferred and F is Faraday's constant).

Question 43: [B] Topic: Nernst Equation. Since the concentrations of the ions is equal, log Q = 0, so E = E°.

Question 44: [D] Topic: oxidation states. Since O is –2 and three Os give –6, what positive charge is needed to give a –1? The nitrogen core has a charge of +5.

Question 45: [C] Topic: redox reactions. A reducing agent in a redox reaction is the species that is oxidized. Simply stated for metals, it prefers to be a cation, not the neutral element. By comparing the given reactions, Mg always reacts and Mg^{2+} never does.

Question 46: [B] Topic: electron configurations. The Aufbau principle states that the orbitals of lowest energy must fill first, so this rules out choice **D** (s orbitals are of lower energy than p orbitals). Hund's rule states that the lowest electron configuration has the maximum number of unpaired spins. This means the unpaired spins need to be in the same direction (rules out choices **A** [all electrons are paired], and **C** [unpaired electrons but spins in opposite direction]).

	2s	2p		
A.	↑↓	↑↓	↑↓	
B.	↑↓	↑↓	↑	↑
C.	↑↓	↑↓	↑	↓
D.	↑	↑↓	↑↓	↑

Question 47: [C] Topic: electron configurations. The electron configuration of argon is $[Ne]3s^2 3p^6$. The electron configurations of the choices are

1. $[Ar]3s^1$
2. $[Ne]3s^2 3p^5$
3. [Ar] or $[Ne]3s^2 3p^6$
4. $[Ne]3s^2 3p^5$

Question 48: [B] Topic: bonding. Since ionic bonding usually occurs in compounds consisting of metals and nonmetals and HCN contains only nonmetals, choice **A** is ruled out. To answer this question you need to draw the Lewis Dot structure of HCN. Remember this general rule—H forms 1 bond, N forms 3 and C forms 4, (O will form 2), you will get this result: $H–C \equiv N$. The first bond between atoms will be a sigma bond and if multiple bonds are present, all bonds after the first will be π-bonds. The total number of sigma bonds will be 2, and 2 π-bonds are present.

Question 49: [C] Topic: quantum numbers. For principal quantum number 3, s, p, and d orbitals are allowed. The 3s orbital can contain 2 electrons, the 3 p orbital can contain 6 electrons, and the 3 d orbital can contain 10 electrons, for a total of 18 allowed electrons.

Question 50: [C] Topic: quantum numbers. The azimuthal quantum number refers to the shape of an orbital. $l = 0$ means s, $l = 1$ means p, $l = 2$ means d, and $l = 3$ means f. Since choice A was 2, the question refers to a d orbital that can hold 10 electrons.

Question 51: [C] Topic: octet rule. The elements C, N, O, F, Ne, and H must always obey the octet rule. To violate the octet rule most elements use d orbitals, which for these elements are not allowed by quantum mechanics. Their principal quantum number is 2 (or less), which gives for l allowed values of $0 \rightarrow n-1$, 0 and 1, only s and p orbitals. These orbitals can hold a maximum of 8 electrons.

Question 52: [B] Topic: electron configurations.

Question 53: [C] Topic: metalloids. Most periodic tables have a "red" zig-zag line snaking through the p-block. Elements along this line are metalloids.

Question 54: [C] Topic: halogens. Fluorine and chlorine are gases, bromine is one of two liquid elements (mercury is the other), iodine is a solid. As a general rule, the greater the molecular weight for a series of related elements, the higher the melting and boiling points.

Question 55: [A] Topic: group names. The name groups are (A) noble gases, (B) halogens, (C) alkaline earths, and (D) alkali metals.

Question 56: [C] Topic: electron shells. The electron shells refer to the principal quantum number and increase by +1 for each horizontal row of the periodic table. row 1 ($n = 1$) contains only the s orbital (2 electrons), row 2 ($n = 2$) contains s and p orbitals (8 electrons). Row 3 ($n = 3$) has s, p, and d orbitals available (18 electrons but the d orbitals are not used yet!).

Question 57: [B] Topic: periodic trends. Size increases as you go down the periodic chart and size increases as you go to the *left* across the periodic chart.

Question 58: [C] Topic: quantum numbers. The values of l refer to: $0 \rightarrow s$, $1 \rightarrow p$, $2 \rightarrow d$, and $3 \rightarrow f$.

Question 59: [A] Topic: ionization energy trends. Ionization energies decrease as you go down the periodic chart. Ionization energies increase as you go *right* across the chart.

Question 60: [D] Topic: ionic compounds. O is a –2 anion and needs a +2 cation to form a 1:1 ionic compound.

Question 61: [A] Topic: descriptive chemistry. Sodium hydroxide is known generically as caustic soda, while NaCl is called "salt."

Question 62: [B] Topic: decay process. Gamma radiation is only release of energy. Electron capture and positron emission decrease the atomic number by 1, and beta emission increases the atomic number by 1.

Question 63: [B] Topic: half life. Sixteen days represents two half-life periods, in the first 50% of the sample decayed [1 g$\rightarrow$ 0.5 g], in the second 50% of the sample decayed [0.5 g $\rightarrow$ 0.25g].

Question 64: [B] Topic: nuclear reactions. The atomic mass is unchanged but the atomic number has increased by one (beta emission).

Question 65: [D] Topic: nuclear reactions. The atomic mass and atomic number are unchanged, only energy has been released (gamma emission).

6.2 ORGANIC CHEMISTRY

This section outlines with brief introductions the subject of organic chemistry required for the PCAT. The material is divided into area groups with a short listing of the topics that should be mastered. Specific concepts are covered briefly. Several sample problems are included with explained solutions. Use these questions to gauge your understanding of the organic chemistry required on the PCAT and to identify specific topics requiring further independent study and review. As mentioned in section 5.1, consult *A Complete Preparation for the MCAT* and the GRE subject test books as needed.

6.2.1 Organic Chemistry Outline

A. Chemical Bonding
- **1.** Atomic Orbitals
  - **a.** Aufbau Principle
  - **b.** Pauli's Exclusion Principle
  - **c.** Hund's Rule
- **2.** Molecular Orbitals
  - **a.** Energy and Intermolecular Distance Diagram
  - **b.** Types of Orbitals
    - **(i)** Overlapping Bonding Orbital
    - **(ii)** Overlapping Antibonding Orbital
- **3.** Hybridization
  - **a.** sp^3 hybrids
  - **b.** sp^2 hybrids
  - **c.** sp hybrids
- **4.** Lewis Structures
  - **a.** Lewis Acids
  - **b.** Lewis Bases
  - **c.** Atomic Bonds
    - **(i)** π bonds (pi)
    - **(ii)** σ bonds (sigma)
- **5.** Resonance and Bond Characteristics
  - **a.** Bond Length
    - **(i)** Single Bonds
    - **(ii)** Double Bonds
    - **(iii)** Polar Covalent Bonds
    - **(iv)** Dipole Moment
  - **b.** Bond Angles
    - **(i)** VSEPR Theory
    - **(ii)** Molecule Shapes

B. Mechanism of Reactions
- **1.** Energetics

2. Structure and Stability of Intermediates
   a. S_N1 Reactions
   b. S_N2 Reactions
   c. Elimination Reactions
   d. Addition
3. Free Radical Mechanisms
4. Substitution Mechanisms

C. Properties of Molecules
1. Stability
2. Solubility
3. Polarity
   a. Polar
   b. Non-Polar
4. Inter/Intra Molecular Forces
   a. Separation of Molecules
   b. Purification of Molecules

D. Organic Analysis of Compounds
1. Introduction to Infrared Spectroscopy
2. H-NMR Spectroscopy
3. Simple Chemical Tests

E. Stereochemistry
1. Conformational Analysis
2. Optical Activity
3. Chirality
   a. Chiral Centers
   b. Places of Symmetry
   c. Enantiomers
   d. Diasteriomers
   e. Meso Compounds

F. IUPAC Nomenclature
1. Identification of Functional Groups
2. Naming conventions for Various Functional Groups
3. Reactions of Major Functional Groups
   a. Prediction of Reaction Products
   b. Important Mechanistic Generalities

G. Acid-Base Chemistry
1. Resonance Effects
2. Inductive Effects
3. Prediction of Products
4. Equilibria

H. Chemistry of Aromatic Compounds
1. Concept of Aromaticity
2. Electrophilic Aromatic Substitution
3. Synthesis (Simple Sequence of Reactions)
   a. Identification of the Product
   b. Identification of Reagents

6.2.2 Structure and Stereochemistry, With Sample Questions

Covalent bonds are formed by two atoms sharing a pair of electrons. Covalent bonds generally form between atoms of similar electronegativity (as a rule, the nearer they are to each other in the periodic table the farther apart atoms are located, and the greater the difference in electronegativity the greater likelihood of ionic bonding; for example, NaCl). There are two types of bonds: sigma bonds (orbital overlap in one area in space) and π-bonds (orbital overlap in two areas of space). Topics to be reviewed for this section should include the octet rule, resonance structures, dipoles, optical activity, and assignment of configurations.

1. What is the best description of the bonding in CO_2?
- **A.** One sigma bond and three pi bonds
- **B.** Three sigma bonds and one pi bond
- **C.** No sigma bonds and four pi bonds
- **D.** Two sigma bonds and two pi bonds

2. Which of the following molecules violates the octet rule?
- **A.** BH_3
- **B.** CH_4
- **C.** NH_3
- **D.** H_2O

3. Which of the following molecules represents "molecule 1" in a Fischer projection?

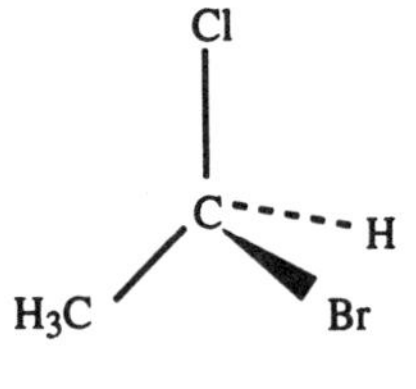

Cl
H₃C — C ··· H
Br

molecule 1

A. 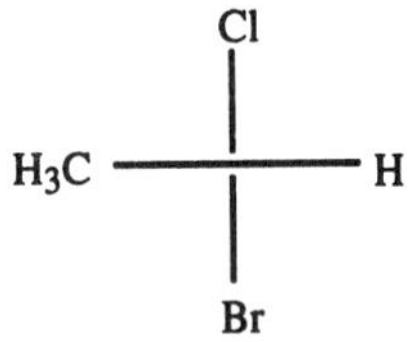 Cl (top), H_3C (left), H (right), Br (bottom)

B. 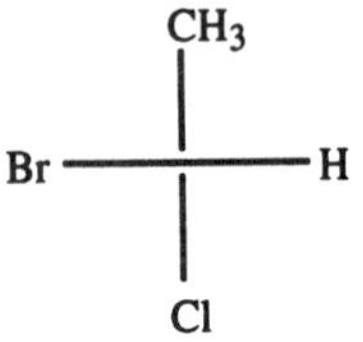 CH_3 (top), Br (left), H (right), Cl (bottom)

C. 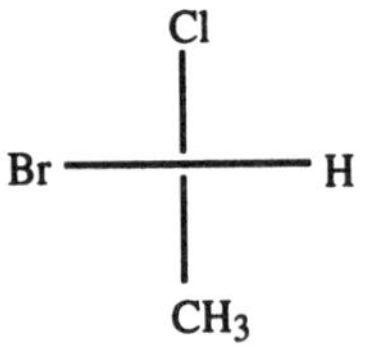 Cl (top), Br (left), H (right), CH_3 (bottom)

D. 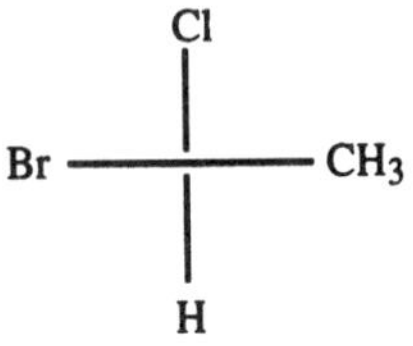 Cl (top), Br (left), CH_3 (right), H (bottom)

4. Which of the following molecules is in the "S" configuration?

A. 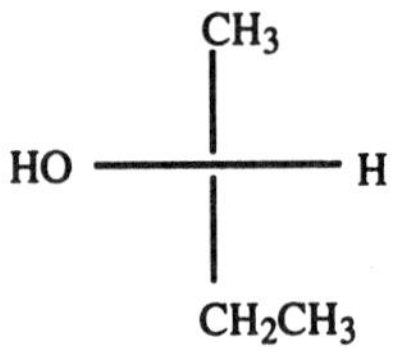 CH_3 (top), HO (left), H (right), CH_2CH_3 (bottom)

B. 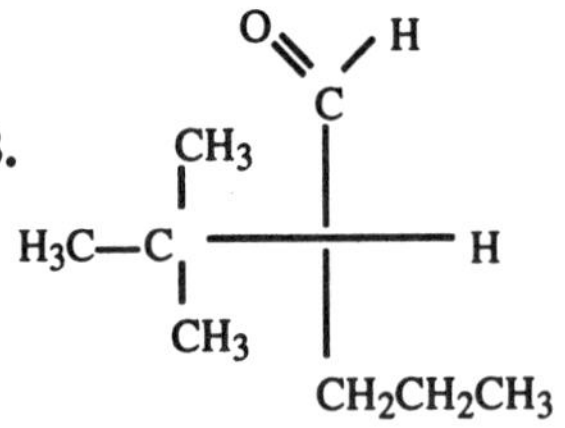 CHO (top; O=C–H), H_3C–C(CH_3)₂ (left), H (right), $CH_2CH_2CH_3$ (bottom)

C. H (top), H_2N (left), CH_3 (right), CH_2CH_3 (bottom)

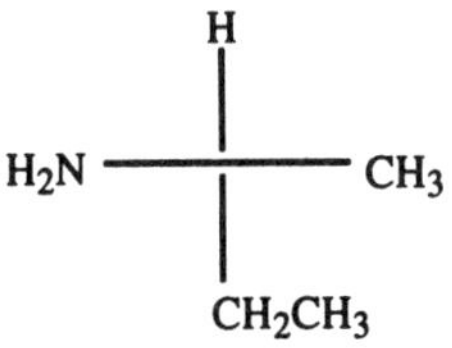

D. 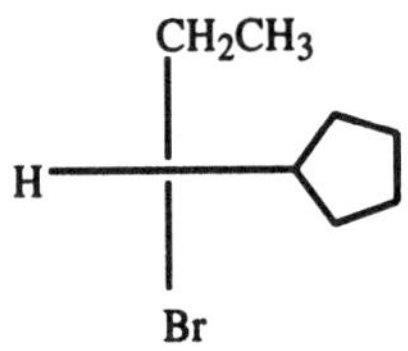 CH_2CH_3 (top), H (left), cyclopentyl (right), Br (bottom)

5. Which of the following molecules is an enantiomer of "molecule 2"?

O=C—H (CHO)
HO—|—H
HO—|—H
H—|—OH
CH_3

molecule 2

A.
O=C—H (CHO)
HO—|—H
HO—|—H
H—|—OH
CH_3

B.
O=C—H (CHO)
H—|—OH
H—|—OH
HO—|—H
CH_3

C.
O=C—H (CHO)
H—|—OH
HO—|—H
H—|—OH
CH_3

D.
O=C—H (CHO)
HO—|—H
HO—|—H
HO—|—H
CH_3

6. How many stereoisomers of "molecule 3" exist?

H I Br Cl H
H—C—C—C—C—C—H
H H H H H

molecule 3

A. 4
B. 8
C. 16
D. 32

Note: For all of the following sections you should review the IUPAC rules for nomenclature of organic compounds relating to the topic. For all sections you should review nomenclature, physical properties, preparation, and reactions.

6.2.3 Alkanes, Alkenes, and Aromatics, With Sample Questions

A few concepts to remember for this section are as follows: Alkanes: the general formula is C_xH_{2x+2}, all names end in -ane, and fragments end in -yl.

Physical properties: (1) the higher the molecular mass the higher the boiling point; (2) branched compounds have lower boiling points than related straight chain compounds; (3) cyclic compounds have higher boiling points than open chains; (4) low densities, and (5) nonpolar.

Unsaturated: the general formula is C_xH_{2x} for one double bond and C_xH_{2x-2} for one triple bond. Alkenes have the ending -ene and alkynes use the ending -yne. Geometric isomers are possible for alkenes, cis, and trans or Z and E.

Aromatics: aromaticity requires a planar ring with all members having sp or sp^2 hybrid orbitals, obeying Hueckel's Rule (number of π-electrons = 4n + 2).

7. Of the labelled carbons in "molecule 4," which represents a tertiary carbon?

```
     1    2     3
     ↓    ↓     ↓
H3 C — CH — CH2 — CH3
          |
         CH2
          |
H3 C — C — CH3
          |  ↖
         CH3   4
```

molecule 4

A. 1
B. 2
C. 3
D. 4

8. Which of the following compounds has the highest boiling point?
A. n-hexane
B. 2-methylpentane
C. 2,3-dimethylbutane
D. Cyclohexane

9. Which of the following Newman projections represents the highest energy conformation?

A. (Newman projection: front H3C, H; H, H; H, CH3)

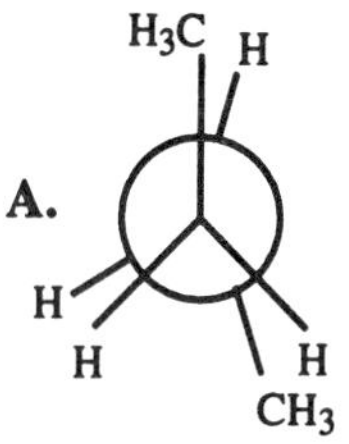

B. (Newman projection: H3C, H, H; H, CH3, H)

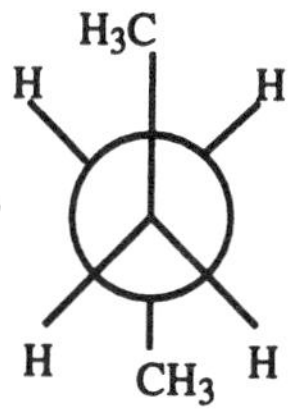

C. (Newman projection: H3C, CH3; H, H; H, H)

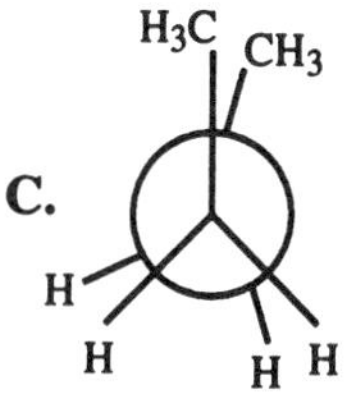

D. (Newman projection: H3C, H, CH3; H, H, H)

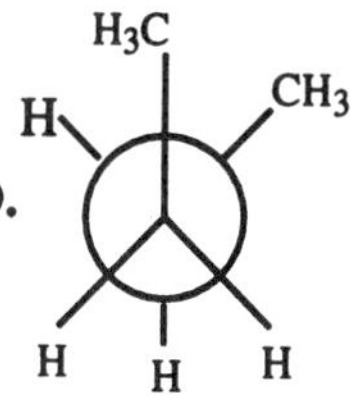

10. What would be the principal organic product of the following reaction?

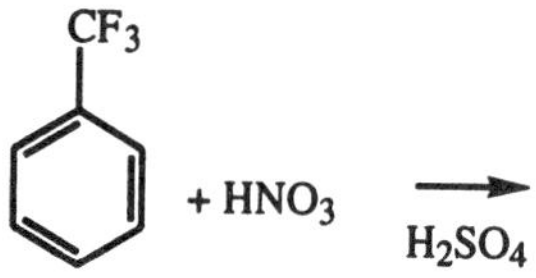

$C_6H_5CF_3 + HNO_3 \xrightarrow{H_2SO_4}$

A. CF_3 / NO_2 (ortho)

B. CF_3 / NO_2 (para)

C. CF_3 / NO_2 (meta)

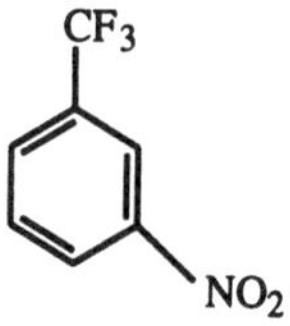

D. NO_2 (nitrobenzene)

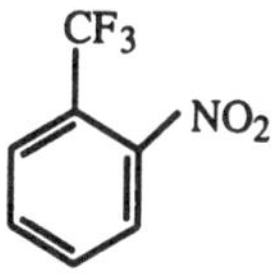

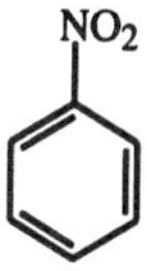

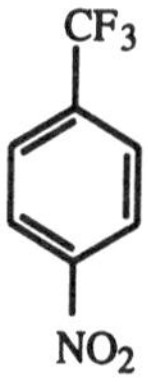

11. Which of the following compounds is not aromatic?

A. 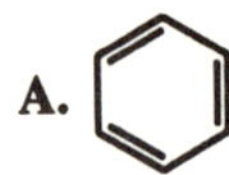

B. 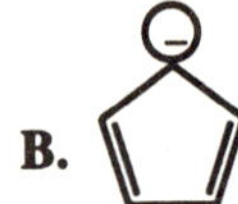

C.

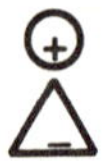

D.

12. What is the principal product of the following reaction?

$H_3CCH{=}CH_2 + HBr \longrightarrow ?$

A. $H_3C\underset{Br}{\underset{|}{C}}H\text{–}\underset{H}{\underset{|}{C}}H_2$

B. $H_3C\underset{H}{\underset{|}{C}}H\text{–}\underset{Br}{\underset{|}{C}}H_2$

C. $H_3CCH{=}C(H)(Br)$

D. $H_3CC(Br){=}CH_2$

6.2.4 Alcohols, Aldehydes and Ketones, Ethers, and Phenols, With Sample Questions

Oxygen-containing groups are as follows:

–OH **Alcohols:** unusually high boiling points, are more soluble in water, polar, named on the basis of the longest carbon chain plus -ol ending.

Ar-OH **Phenols**

$R\text{-}\overset{\overset{O}{\|}}{C}\text{-}H$ **Aldehydes:** name using longest carbon chain with group and ending -al. Carbons are numbered beginning at aldehyde end.

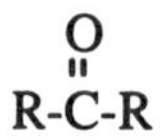

$R\text{-}\overset{O}{\overset{\|}{C}}\text{-}R$ **Ketones:** use the longest chain, numbered to give carbonyl lowest possible number, and use the ending-one.

R-O-R **Ethers:** somewhat polar, named using two alkyl names plus ether or as alkoxyalkanes.

13. The reaction of a secondary alcohol with CrO_3 yields
A. an aldehyde.
B. a carboxylic acid.
C. a ketone.
D. an ether.

14. The Williamson ether synthesis is the reaction of
A. ROH and R'X
B. RCOOH and R'X
C. RONa and R'X
D. ROH and R'Na

15. Which of the following is the correct name for

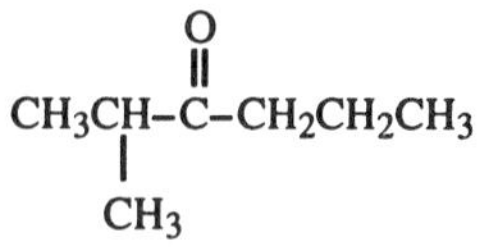

$$CH_3\underset{\underset{CH_3}{|}}{CH}\text{-}\overset{\overset{O}{\|}}{C}\text{-}CH_2CH_2CH_3$$

A. 2-methyl-3-hexanal
B. 1-methyl-3-hexanal
C. 2-methylhexan-3-one
D. 1-methylhexan-3-one

16. Which of the following species represents a ketal?

A. 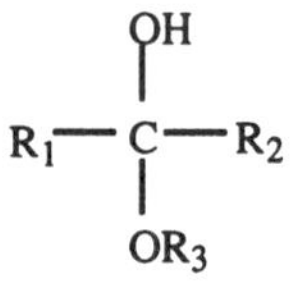 $R_1\text{—}\underset{\underset{OR_3}{|}}{\overset{\overset{OH}{|}}{C}}\text{—}R_2$

B. $R_1\text{—}\underset{\underset{OR_3}{|}}{\overset{\overset{OR_4}{|}}{C}}\text{—}R_2$

C. $R_1\text{—}\overset{\overset{O}{\|}}{C}\text{—}R_2$

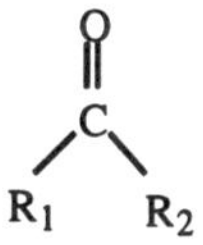

D. 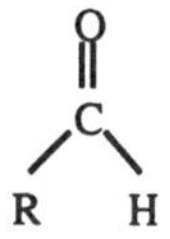 $R\text{—}\overset{\overset{O}{\|}}{C}\text{—}H$

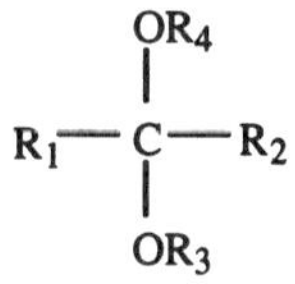

17. Which of the following would be the major product in this reaction?

$$\underset{\text{HO}\quad\text{H}}{CH_3CH_2CH\text{–}CH_2} + H^+ \xrightarrow{\Delta}$$

A. $CH_3CH_2CH{=}CH_2$

B. $CH_3CH{=}CH\text{–}CH_3$

C. $CH_3CH_2\underset{\underset{O}{\|}}{C}CH_3$

D. $CH_3CH_2CH_2CH_3$

18. Alcohols have higher boiling points than the corresponding alkanes (for example, methane boils at –164°C while methanol boils at 65°C). Which of the following accounts for this fact?
A. Higher molecular mass
B. Hydrogen bonding
C. London Dispersion Forces
D. Higher density

6.2.5 Carboxylic Acids and Their Derivatives, With Sample Questions

Carboxylic acids are named using the longest carbon chain and the ending -oic acid.

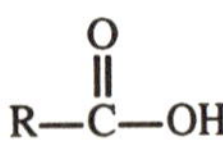

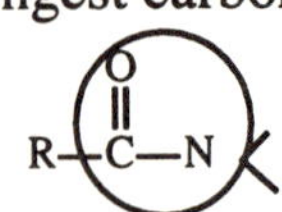

is the amide group.

Anhydrides are formed by the removal of water from two-COOH groups. Anhydrides are more reactive than the corresponding acid.

19. Which of the following carboxylic acids is the strongest acid?

A. H—C(H)(H)COOH

B. H—C(Cl)(H)COOH

C. Cl—C(Cl)(H)COOH

D. Cl—C(Cl)(Cl)COOH

20. The reaction of a carboxylic acid and an alcohol will produce
   A. an anhydride.
   B. an ether.
   C. an ester.
   D. an acid with a longer carbon chain.

21. Which of the following is the correct name for compound shown?

$$CH_3\overset{\overset{\large O}{\|}}{C}{-}OCH_2CH_3$$

   A. Pentanoic acid
   B. Pentanoic anhydride
   C. Ethyl pentanoate
   D. Pentanamide

22. A general reagent for the conversion of an acyl chloride to an ester is
   A. excess ammonia.
   B. an alcohol in the presence of pyridine.
   C. a dialkyl cadium compound.
   D hydrogen in the presence of Pd.

23. Which of the following compounds has the lowest boiling point?
   A. Ethanamide
   B. N-ethylethanamide
   C. N, N-diethylethanamide
   D. Ethene

6.2.6 Amines, With Sample Questions

Amines are weak bases, named either as (organic group) alkylamine or using the longest carbon chain numbered to give the amine-N the lowest possible number.

24. Which of the following compounds is the strongest base in the gas phase?
   A. Trimethylamine
   B. Dimethylamine
   C. Methylamine
   D. Ammonia

25. What is the product of the following reaction after work-up?

$$R\overset{\overset{\large O}{\|}}{C}NH_2 + LiAlH_4 \longrightarrow$$

   A. $R{-}C \equiv N$

   B. RCH_2NH_2

   C. $R\overset{\overset{\large O}{\|}}{C}H$

   D. $R\overset{\overset{\large O}{\|}}{C}NH_3^+$

26. What is the product of the following reaction?

$$CH_2 = CHC \equiv N + H_2/Pt \rightarrow ?$$

A. $CH_3CH_2C \equiv N$
B. $CH_2{=}CHNH_2$
C. $CH_3CH_2CH_2NH_2$
D. $CH_3CH_2CH{=}NH$

27. Which of the following compounds is aniline?

A. 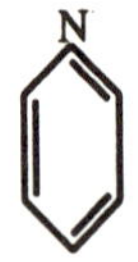 N

B. 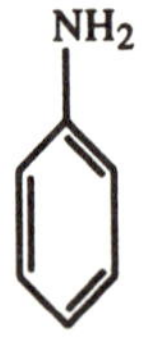 NH_2

C. 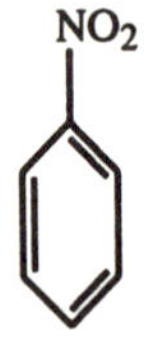 NO_2

D. 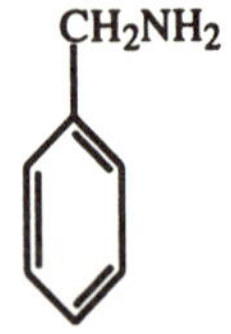 CH_2NH_2

6.2.7 Amino Acids and Proteins, With Sample Questions

Amino acids can act as zwitterions, ions that have both a cation site and anion site in a single molecule, they have high melting points, and are soluble in water.

Proteins are divided into two broad classes, fibrous and globular. These classifications are related to function. The structure of proteins is divided into primary, secondary, tertiary, and quaternary. The primary structure relates the way the atoms of the protein molecule are linked by covalent bonds. The secondary structure yields information on the way the chains are arranged in space (for example: coils or sheets). The tertiary structure involves more details on the intramolecular interactions (hydrogen bonding, van der Waals interactions). The quaternary structure deals with the intermolecular interactions between protein chains.

28. A peptide linkage between two amino acids is best described by
   A. the condensation of two carboxylic acids groups on amino acids.
   B. intramolecular actions between amine and carboxyl groups of amino acids.
   C. a hydrogen bond formed between the –COOH group and $-NH_2$ groups of amino acids.
   D. a new carbon-carbon interaction between amino acids.

29. The isoelectric point of amino acids is defined as
A. occurring when all –COOH sites are protonated.
B. occurring when all $-NH_2$ sites are deprotonated.
C. occurring when the amino acid present as a zwitterion is at a minimum.
D. occurring when the amino acid present as a zwitterion is at a maximum.

30. One useful method for determining the N-terminal amino acid residue is the "Sanger Method." In this reaction, using 2,4-dinitrofluorobenzene, the terminal amino acid contains
A. a nitro group.
B. a fluorophenyl group.
C. a 2,4-dinitrophenyl group.
D. a fluoro group.

31. Which of the following functional groups are not commonly found in amino acids?
A. sulfanyl, –SH
B. nitrosyl, –NO
C. hydroxyl, –OH
D. amino, $-NH_2$

32. How many amino acids occur naturally in proteins?
A. 10
B. 12
C. 18
D. 20

33. What is the product of the reaction of glycine with benzoyl chloride and $NaOH_{(aq)}$?

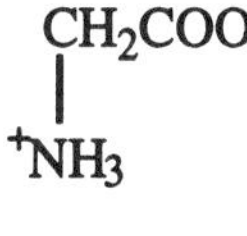

glycine

A. $PhC(=O)NHCH_2COOH$
B. $(Cl^-)(^+H_3NCH_2COOH)$
C. H_2NCH_2COOCl
D. $H_2NCH_2COOCH_2C_6H_5$

34. Which of the following is not characteristic of globular proteins?
A. Insoluble in water
B. Intramolecular hydrogen bonding
C. Folded into compact units
D. Functions usually related to regulation of life processes

35. Stereochemical studies of naturally occurring amino acids have shown they all have the same configurations about the carbon bonded to the alpha-amino group as
A. D-gylceraldehyde.
B. L-glyceraldehyde.
C. D-Tartaric acid.
D. L-Tartaric acid.

6.2.8 Carbohydrates, With Sample Questions

Carbohydrates are polyhydroxy aldehydes, ketones, or related compounds. Monosaccharides cannot be hydrolyzed to simpler compounds, disaccharides can be hydrolyzed to two, and polysaccharides hydrolyzed to many monosaccharides. If it contains an aldehyde group it is an aldose, if it contains a ketone group it is a ketose. For example, a five-carbon monosaccharide containing an aldehyde is classified as an aldepentose.

36. Which of the following labeled carbons is the anomeric carbon?

A. 1
B. 2
C. 3
D. 4

37. Which of the following straight chain aldoses gives the following cyclic structure?

A.
O=C–H
H—|—OH
HO—|—H
H—|—OH
H—|—OH
CH_2OH

B.
O=C–H
H—|—OH
HO—|—H
HO—|—H
H—|—OH
CH_2OH

C.
O=C–H
H—|—OH
H—|—OH
H—|—OH
HO—|—H
CH_2OH

D.
O=C–H
H—|—OH
H—|—OH
HO—|—H
HO—|—H
CH_2OH

38. Which of the following procedures is used in the Kiliani-Fischer synthesis to lengthen the carbon chain of aldoses?
A. Reaction with H_2CO_3 followed by hydrolysis
B. Reaction with $H_2C{=}O$ followed by hydrolysis
C. Reaction with H_3COH followed by hydrolysis
D. Reaction with HCN followed by hydrolysis

39. What is the product of a Ruff degradation starting with

O H
H — OH
H — OH
CH_2OH

$\xrightarrow[H_2O]{Br_2}$ $\xrightarrow{CaCO_3}$ $\xrightarrow[Fe^{3+}]{H_2O_2}$?

A.
O H
H — OH
H — OH
H — OH
CH_2OH

B.
O H
H — OH
CH_2OH

C.
CH_2OH
H — OH
CH_2OH

D.
CH_2OH
H — OH
H — OH
CH_2OH

40. Which of the following reagent tests can be used to differentiate aldoses and ketoses?
A. Fehling's Reagent
B. Tollens' Reagent
C. Bromine water
D. Benedict's Solution

6.2.9 Spectroscopy, With Sample Questions

This section reviews identification of organic compounds using IR and ^1H NMR data. A few important correlations are as follows (ranges given are approximate values):

IR

Functional group	cm^{-1}	Notes
-OH	3640–3610	usually broad peaks
amines	3500–3300	primary amines = doublet, secondary amines = singlet
≡ C-H	3315–3270	
-C-H	3100–3000	aromatics
$=CH_2$	3080	
$-CH_3$, $-CH_2-$	2990–2890	methyl groups have weak intensity, other alkyls are strong
C ≡ N	2300–2200	
C=O	1750–1740	ester
	1740–1720	aldehyde
	1720–1700	ketone

^1H NMR

Group	Chemical shift (∂ in ppm)	Notes
Methyl	0.9	
Methylene	1.3	
Benzylic	2.3–3	Ar-C**H**
Vinyl	4.5–6.0	C = C -**H**
Amino	2.0–2.8	$RC\mathbf{H_2}NH_2$
	1–5	$R\mathbf{NH_2}$
Ketones	2.0–2.7	$RC\mathbf{H_2}C(=O)R$
Alcohols	3.4–4.0	$RC\mathbf{H_2}COH$
	1–5	$RCH_2CO\mathbf{H}$
Ethers	3.3–5.0	$RC\mathbf{H_2}COR$
Esters	3.7–4.1	$RC(=O)OC\mathbf{H_2}R$
	2.0–2.2	$RC\mathbf{H_2}C(=O)OR$
Aromatic	6.0–8.5	Ar-**H**
Aldehydic	9–10	
Carboxylic acids	10–12	

41. High-resolution mass-spectrometric analysis of compound A gave a molecular formula of $C_9H_{10}O_2$. The infrared spectrum showed strong absorption at 1715 cm^{-1} as well as many other medium-intensity bands. The NMR spectrum consisted of three sharp peaks at $\partial = 5.00$ ppm (area 2), $\partial = 1.96$ ppm (area 3), $\partial = 7.22$ ppm (area 5). What is the structure of compound A?

A. $C_6H_5CH_2C(=O)OCH_3$ (phenyl–CH_2COCH_3, C=O on the carbon after CH_2)

B. $C_6H_5CH_2OC(=O)CH_3$ (phenyl–CH_2OCCH_3)

C. $C_6H_5OCH_2C(=O)CH_3$ (phenyl–OCH_2CCH_3)

D. $C_6H_5C(=O)CH_2OCH_3$ (phenyl–CCH_2OCH_3)

42. From a high-resolution mass spectrum of compound B, a molecular formula of $C_6H_{14}O$ could be assigned. In the infrared, the strongest absorption above 1400 cm^{-1} occurred at 2900 cm^{-1}. In the NMR, compound B showed a septet at $\partial = 3.62$ ppm (area 1), J = 7 Hz, and a doublet at $\partial = 1.10$ (area 6), J = 7 Hz. What is the structure of compound B?

A. $(H_3C)_2CH{-}O{-}CH(CH_3)_2$

B. $H_3CH_2C{-}C(=O){-}CH(CH_3)_2$

C. $H_3CH_2CH_2C{-}O{-}CH_2CH_2CH_3$

D. Ring structure: an O atom and four carbons; the two carbons next to O each bear H and CH_3, and the other two ring carbons each bear H and CH_3

6.2.10 Answers and Explanations for Organic Chemistry Sample Questions

Question 1: [D] Topic: covalent bonding. The first step to solve this problem is to draw a Lewis dot structure: O=C=O. In forming covalent bonds, the first bond between atom pairs is a sigma bond and further, multiple bonds are π-bonds.

Question 2: [A] Topic: octet rule. Choices **B–D** have 8 valence electrons. [CH_4 has 4 pairs of bonding electrons, NH_3 has 3 bonding pairs and 1 lone pair, and H_2O has 2 bonding pairs and 2 lone pairs]. BH_3 has 3 bonding pairs but no lone pairs for a total of 6 valence electrons.

Question 3: [C] Topic: stereoview. In a Fischer projection, the horizontal bonds represent bonds pointing out of the page and vertical bonds represent bonds behind (or into the page). Rotating the molecule to the right by about 60° gives the proper orientation.

Question 4: [C] Topic: Cahn-Ingold-Prelog rules. To assign an absolute configuration, (1) assign a rank to the four atoms/groups attached to the chiral carbon by mass. The largest mass is the highest range, #1, and (2) "draw" an arrow from 1 to 2 to 3 to 4. If it is clockwise, assign R for rectus. If it is counterclockwise, assign S for sinister, *unless* the #4 group is in a horizontal position, then reverse the arrow.

Question 5: [B] Topic: enantiomers. An enantiomer is a nonsuperimposable mirror image. Enantiomers have similar chemical and physical properties, except for rotation of light and reactions with chiral reagents. Diastereomers are stereoisomers that are not mirror images. They possess similar chemical properties but different physical properties.

Question 6: [B] Topic: stereoisomers. The number of stereoisomers is 2^n, where N is the number of chiral carbons present.

Question 7: [B] Topic: carbon types. Carbon atoms are typed by the number of carbon-carbon bonds formed. A primary carbon has formed 1 C-C bond, a secondary carbon has formed 2 C-C bonds, a tertiary carbon has formed 3 C-C bonds, and a quaternary carbon has formed 4 C-C bonds.

Question 8: [D] Topic: physical properties of alkanes. Cyclic hydrocarbons have a higher boiling point than straight chain analogs. This is due to London Dispersion Forces.

Question 9: [C] Topic: conformations of alkanes. The highest energy form will have the highest amount of steric interactions. In choice **C** the methyl groups are located in the closest possible arrangement.

Question 10: [C] Topic: directors in aromatic electrophilic substitution reactions. The group $-CF_3$ is a meta director. Some other groups and their influences are:

Activators: ortho & para directors	$-NH_2, -O\overset{O}{\overset{\|}{C}}R, -R, -OH, -NH\overset{O}{\overset{\|}{C}}R, -Ph$
Deactivators: meta directors	$-NO_2, -\overset{O}{\overset{\|}{C}}-R, -\overset{+}{N}H_3, -\overset{O}{\overset{\|}{C}}-OR$
Deactivators: ortho & para directors	Halogens

Question 11: [D] Topic: aromaticity. This compound is not planar and all of the carbons in the ring are not sp^2 or sp hybrids.

Question 12: [A] Topic: addition reactions. This is an addition across a C-C double bond. This class of reaction follows Markovnikov's Rule, which states that the carbon with the most hydrogens gains the added H. If this were a radical reaction, the reverse would be true.

Question 13: [C] Topic: oxidation reactions of alcohols. CrO_3 is an average oxidizing agent and will oxidize primary alcohols to aldehydes. To produce a carboxylic acid you need to use a stronger oxidizing agent, like $KMnO_4$. Oxidizing agents will react with secondary alcohols to form ketones and will not react with tertiary alcohols. For a reaction to occur, the alcohol carbon must possess an H.

Question 14: [C] Topic: name reactions. The Williamson Ether Synthesis is the reaction of an alkoxide and alkyl halide.

Question 15: [C] Topic: nomenclature. The compound is a ketone so the ending is -one. The longest carbon chain is 6 (hexane). Finally, use the lowest number combination from an end.

Question 16: [B] Topic: reaction products. A ketal is produced in the reaction of a ketone with two alcohols under acidic conditions. Choice **A** is the hemiketal, which is produced by reaction with one alcohol. Further reaction will produce the ketal. If your starting material is an aldehyde, you will produce an acetal.

Question 17: [B] Topic: reaction products. The reaction in question is a dehydration, which results in a C=C. The major product is the most substituted double bond, due to a rearrangement. Choice **A** would be a minor product.

Question 18: [B] Topic: physical properties. Alcohols meet the criteria for hydrogen bonding (electronegative element, N, O, or F, with an H attached and a lone pair of electrons). This is the strongest intermolecular force and gives the higher boiling points.

Question 19: [D] Topic: acid strength. Cl is an electron withdrawing group. The inductive effect results in a withdrawing of electrons from the O-H bond, weakening the bond, and resulting in a stronger acid. The higher the degree of substitution, the larger the effect.

Question 20: [C] Topic: reaction products. Anhydrides are formed by the removal of water from two carboxylic groups and ethers would form from alcohols in the Williamson ether synthesis.

Question 21: [C] Topic: nomenclature. The compound in question is an ester, named by changing the acid ending with -ioc to -ate, and naming the organic group attached to the oxygen. The others would be

A. CH_3COOH (common name = acetic acid) **B.** $CH_3\overset{O}{\overset{\|}{C}}O\overset{O}{\overset{\|}{C}}CH_3$ **D.** $CH_3\overset{O}{\overset{\|}{C}}NH_2$ **E.** $CH_3\overset{O}{\overset{\|}{C}}CH_2CH_3$

Question 22: [B] Topic: reaction reagents. Acyl chlorides, RC(=O)Cl show these general reactions (to name a few):

1. with excess ammonia to form amides
2. with an alcohol to form esters
3. with a dialkyl cadium compound, R_2Cd, to form ketones
4. with H_2/Pd to form aldehydes

Question 23: [C] Topic: Physical properties. The trisubstituted N does not possess a bond for use in hydrogen bonding. This would result in a lower melting point. Both choices **A** and **B** can form strong hydrogen bonds resulting in higher melting and boiling points. Choice D is a salt.

Question 24: [A] Topic: physical properties. In the gas phase, the inductive effect of the donor group, Me, results in increasing the electron density on the central N. The higher the degree of substitution, the larger the effect. This is similar to question 19.

Question 25: [B] Topic: reaction products. $LiAlH_4$ is a reducing agent. This example reduces a C=O group to a CH_2 group. This is a typical reaction result with $LiAlH_4$.

Question 26: [C] Topic: reaction products. H_2/M is also a reducing agent. The product will generally contain hydrogens at the site of the original unit of unsaturation. In this example there are two units of unsaturation, C=C and C≡N. Both units are reduced by this strong reducing agent.

Question 27: [B] Topic: nomenclature. The correct names are

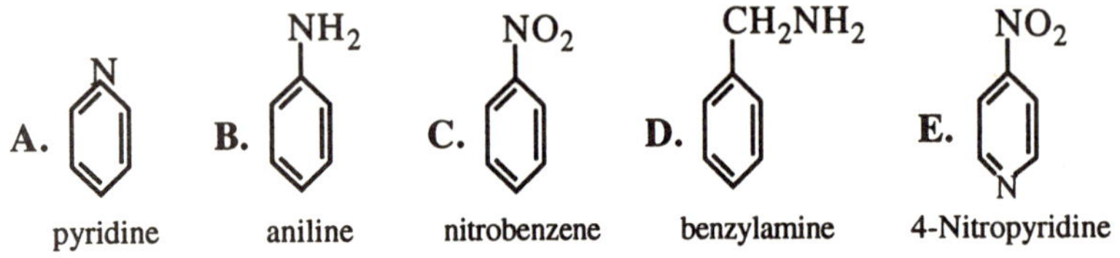

A. pyridine
B. aniline (NH_2)
C. nitrobenzene (NO_2)
D. benzylamine (CH_2NH_2)
E. 4-Nitropyridine (NO_2)

Question 28: [B] Topic: peptides. A peptide linkage is formed by loss of water from the -COOH and NH_2 groups on amino acids. The formation is shown and the correct way to draw the peptide. For example:

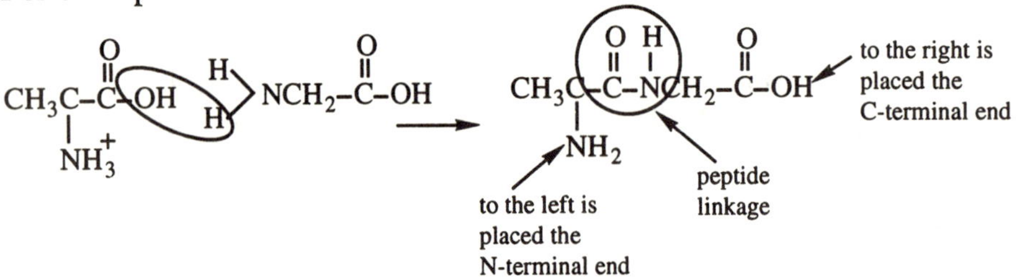

$$CH_3C(NH_3^+)-C(=O)-OH + H-NH-CH_2-C(=O)-OH \longrightarrow CH_3C(NH_2)-C(=O)-NH-CH_2-C(=O)-OH$$

to the right is placed the C-terminal end

peptide linkage

to the left is placed the N-terminal end

Question 29: [D] Topic: properties. The isoelectric point is when the rate of reaction 1 is equal to the rate of reaction 2, and the concentration of the zwitterion is maximized.

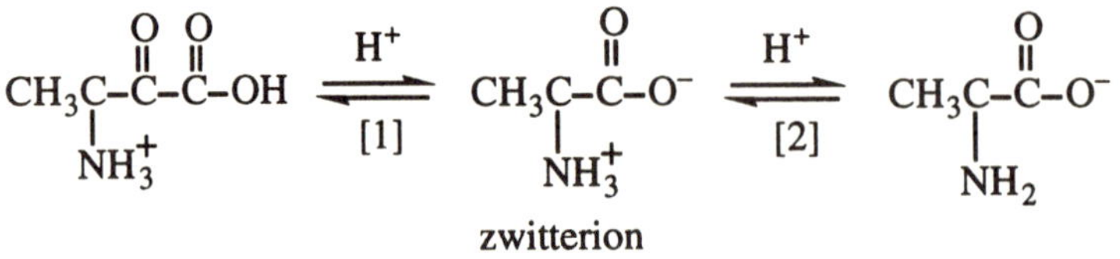

$$CH_3C(NH_3^+)-C(=O)-C(=O)-OH \underset{[1]}{\overset{H^+}{\rightleftharpoons}} CH_3C(NH_3^+)-C(=O)-O^- \underset{[2]}{\overset{H^+}{\rightleftharpoons}} CH_3C(NH_2)-C(=O)-O^-$$

zwitterion

Question 30: [C] Topic: reaction types. The Sanger method labels the N-terminal end with 2,4-dinitrophenyl group. The DNFB will react with any free amino group, but only an α-amino group is at the N-terminal end.

Question 31: [B] Topic: amino acids. Nitroso groups are normally found bonded to transition metals as in nitrosamines.

Question 32: [D] Topic: amino acids. There are 20 naturally occurring amino acids.

Question 33: [A] Topic: reactions. Amino acids exhibit the reactions the functional groups possess. Amines react with acid chlorides, and -Cl is replaced by the -NHR group yielding the observed product.

Question 34: [A] Topic: globular proteins. Hemoglobin and lysozome are globular proteins that are soluble in water. Globular proteins have low molecular weights, e.g., lysozome is an enzyme with a molecular weight of 14,600.

Question 35: [B] Topic: configuration of amino acids. All naturally occurring amino acids have the same configuration as L-glyceraldehyde.

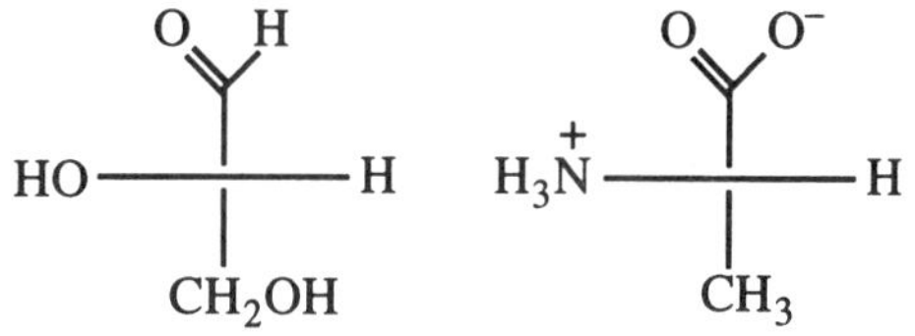

L-Glyceraldehyde L-Alanine

Question 36: [A] Topic: diastereomeric forms. The "1" carbon in a cyclic representation of the structure is called the anomeric carbon. The forms are designated as the α-anomer or the β-anomer, depending on the orientation of the OH group. The α-anomer refers to the -OH in the down orientation and β-anomer has the -OH in the up orientation. Which is this one?

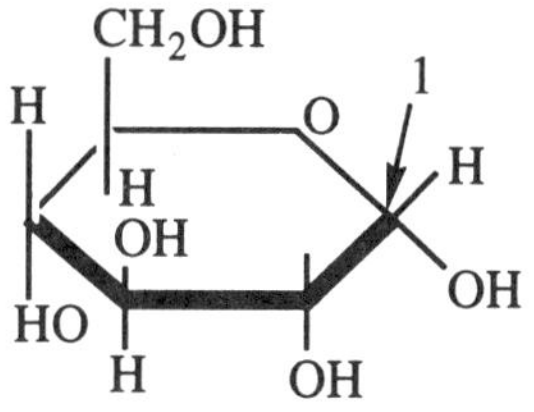

Question 37: [A] Topic: sugar structures. To relate a linear structure to a cyclic structure, follow this procedure:

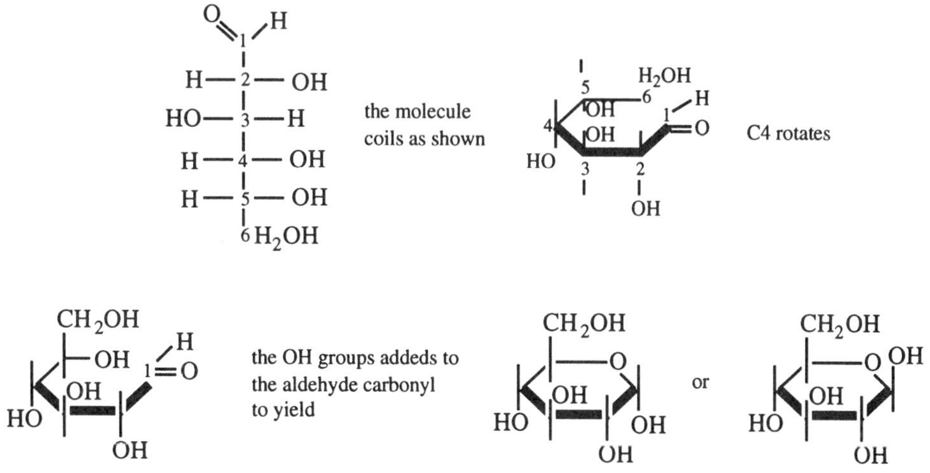

the molecule coils as shown

C4 rotates

the OH groups addeds to the aldehyde carbonyl to yield

or

Question 38: [D] Topic: name reactions. The Kiliani-Fischer synthesis uses HCN followed by hydrolysis to lengthen the carbon chain by one unit. In this process, the product would be the carboxylic acid, reduction of the nitrile is required for obtaining an aldose.

Question 39: [B] Topic: name reactions. The Ruff degradation shortens the carbon chain by one H-C-OH unit. It is the reverse reaction of the Kiliani-Fischer synthesis.

Question 40: [C] Topic: chemical tests. Fehling's Reagent, Tollens' Reagent, and Benedict's Solution are all tests for sugars. They do not differentiate between aldoses and ketoses. Bromine water will only react with aldoses. It converts aldoses to an aldonic acid.

$$\mathrm{O{=}C(H)-(H-C-OH)_n-CH_2OH \xrightarrow[H_2O]{Br_2} O{=}C(OH)-(H-C-OH)_n-CH_2OH}$$

Question 41: [C] Topic: spectroscopy. The IR signal at 1715 cm^{-1} indicates a ketone (this rules out choices **A** and **B**). The NMR signal at 7.22 indicates C_6H_5, the other signals are not coupled. A peak of area 2 suggests CH_2 and a peak of area 3 suggests CH_3. A group neighboring an O is in the range of 3–5 and this suggests choice **C**.

Question 42: [A] Topic: spectroscopy. The IR information suggests there is no carbonyl, C=O, in this molecule (rules out choice **B**). The formula tells you that there is only 6 carbons (rules out choice **C**). The NMR data of a doublet at 1.10 ppm suggests a group next to a carbon with one hydrogen, and the septet suggests a group next to carbon(s) with six hydrogens. This is choice **A**.

6.3 REFERENCES

Burkett, A., and J. Sedenair. *Test Bank for Chemistry,* 2nd ed. (Allen and Baker, 1989).

Jacob, Stanley W., M.D., and Clarice A. Francone. *Structure and Function of Man*, 3rd ed. (W. B. Saunders Company, 1974).

Masterton, W., and C. Hurley. *Test Bank for Chemistry* (Saunders College Pub., 1989).

PART III

TEST-TAKING SKILLS AND SAMPLE PCAT

Chapter 7: **Test-Taking Skills**

7.0 INTRODUCTION TO TEST-TAKING SKILLS

The PCAT requires half a day for administration; the exam takes approximately four to five hours total. The PCAT is given twice every year, in April and October. Candidates report at 8:00 a.m. and the exam will usually begin at 8:45 a.m. and end at 1:50 p.m. There is a fifteen-minute break, but no lunch break. Any other breaks are decided upon by the proctor and vary from test center to test center.

There are 270 test items on the exam, but the time allowed per item for each section may vary slightly depending on the length and difficulty of the questions in that section. Writing in the test booklet is allowed, including marking with highlighter pens. Calculators and electronic watches are not allowed. When the PCAT is given, the order of the sections is sometimes randomized. For example, Reading Comprehension may come first in California, whereas Verbal Ability may come first in Alabama. This information is based on previous data and it may or may not happen at your test center.

7.1 SELF-ASSESSMENT

This chapter trains you to be test-wise. By now you are familiar with the PCAT test item format. You have developed your skills for accuracy, even if you are not yet working at PCAT speed; you have reviewed the natural science sections, concentrating to master weak areas while maintaining your mastery of strong areas. You have also practiced Reading Comprehension, Quantitative Ability, and Verbal Ability skills through test-item practice. Can you concentrate for two-hour segments, including short, structured breaks?

Now is the moment for honesty. If you have procrastinated, you may consider postponing your application until the next test date. Doing poorly on the test is personally demoralizing and does not enhance your standing with application committees. On the other hand, you may have prepared wisely for the PCAT and with discipline, and you are now ready to develop your test-taking strategies.

7.2 PCAT TEST-TAKING SPEED

If your accuracy level (without time considerations) is high on all sections of the PCAT, you should now add speed as a variable. The actual PCAT takes approximately four hours. The following chart provides information on the timing requirements of each subtest.

TABLE 6: PCAT Test Day Schedule

Examination Section	Number of Questions	Maximum Time (Minutes)	Average (Seconds / item)
Verbal Ability - Antonyms (25) - Analogies (25)	50	30	(36 secs/item)
Biology	50	30	(36 secs/item)
Reading Comprehension	45	45	(60 secs/item)
——— *Break* ———	—	30	—
Quantitative Ability	65	45	(42 secs/item)
Chemistry	60	30	(30 secs/item)
Reading Comprehension (not graded)	45	45	(60 secs/item)

Managing your time well on the PCAT is a major ingredient of test-wiseness. First, you must keep in mind that there are no extra points for finishing a subtest. You need to develop your speed, but speed is always a trade-off with accuracy, so you will need to gauge for yourself what is the best speed/accuracy ratio to achieve the highest possible score on the exam. Second, it is clear from the chart that your speed will have to vary from section to section. On average, you have approximately twice as much time for the reading comprehension items as for the verbal ability items. But additionally, within each subtest, some questions are designed to take longer than others. This means that the test-wise student will not spend an equal amount of time on each item within a given subtest, but rather will take less time on those that are simpler and save time for the more difficult items.

A good test-taking strategy is to work the relatively easy questions quickly, thereby earning the more certain points and saving time for the harder questions. Keep in mind that there are no extra points for answering the single hardest question. A better strategy is to take the same time you might spend on the single hardest question to answer three easier questions.

Separate subscores are given for each topic. It is natural to spend more time on the science topics you like, avoiding those areas you don't like. If you have studied in accord with the suggestions in this manual, you should be fairly disciplined in your approach, and no longer tempted to dawdle over biology, simply because you are in no hurry to get to organic chemistry. On the other hand, the pressure of real testing situations has a tendency to make everyone revert to past behaviors. Don't let the test take you!

7.2.1 How to Work on Speed

Serious work on increasing your speed should begin approximately six weeks before the exam.

Work with a clock in front of you. Take approximately ten items at a time, work first for accuracy and note how much time it takes you to achieve the accuracy level you require for a good score. On the next set of practice items, push yourself to work still faster. If your accuracy level stays the same, work just a little bit faster on the next practice set. At the point where your accuracy level begins to suffer, work at that speed to bring the accuracy level back up. Increase your speed only when the accuracy level is high. Work in this way on all the subtests.

As you build your test-taking speed, look for "short-cuts." Would a quick estimate have allowed you to eliminate several answer possibilities quickly? Were there other ways to answer a question that would have been faster? Did you stubbornly work at answering a question that simply ate up too much time? (Note: this may be a virtue when you are a practicing pharmacist, but not when you are taking the PCAT!)

7.3 THREE WEEKS BEFORE THE TEST

1. Plan to take a full simulated mock PCAT about three or four Saturdays before the actual test. The PCAT practice test in Chapter 8 could be used for this purpose. From the results you should be able to determine both whether you are ready to take the PCAT and how you might spend your last few weeks of study most profitably. The practice test provided in this manual will also help you understand your weaknesses.

If you can get others to participate in the simulation with you, so much the better. But remember, even if you do it on your own, the closer you simulate the real thing, the more benefit you can derive from the experience. For example, if you take the test at home, do not play the radio or take phone calls while you are testing. Carefully follow the time limits in the PCAT test booklet.

2. Part of the benefit, of course, will be a careful analysis of the results. Score one point for each correct answer. There is no penalty for incorrect or unanswered items. Now make a percentage to discover your raw score. For example, if there are fifty questions and you answered thirty-five correctly, your raw score is 70 percent. You will now be able to tabulate your converted or scaled score exactly the way the PCAT does. It varies from test to test, depending on test difficulty, item analysis, and other variables.

There is no advantage in taking the test just to learn that you were not yet ready. You can take the PCAT as many times as you want, but all your scores will be forwarded to the schools where you apply.

3. Insofar as it is possible, maintain a daily schedule that corresponds to the PCAT test day. This includes the time you wake up, what you do when you get up, food intake (do not forget to eat a nourishing breakfast), and the time you go to sleep. You cannot be at your best on a morning test if you have maintained a night-study schedule up until the test day.

7.4 THE LAST WEEK BEFORE THE TEST

1. If possible, on the Saturday before the actual PCAT, drive to the testing location at the same time as you will on the day the PCAT is given. Pay attention to route, traffic, parking, and so forth. Locate the testing room, bathroom, snack bar. Over-preparation is a good antidote to anxiety.

2. Schedule review sessions that emphasize short-term memory tasks. The rest of your PCAT study time should be spent working item sets from each section under timed conditions. During these final sessions, simulate real test situations as closely as possible. For example, do not allow yourself to spend too much time solving one problem. In a good simulation, the adrenaline should be flowing just enough so you feel the stress, but not enough to make you anxious.

3. In these final practice sessions, stay with the strategies you have developed and practiced. Be deliberate. Mark the answer clues in the questions. Cross out wrong answers. Work with the watch that you intend to bring to the real PCAT. It should have a large, clear face and a minute hand. Remember, no calculators are allowed. Accuracy and speed are a trade-off. You should know beforehand what speed on each subtest gives you the highest level of accuracy.

4. Put yourself on the PCAT schedule, doing each morning what you intend to do on the test day itself. Working with your plan of "things to do today" should now be a habit.

7.5 THE TEST DAY ITSELF

1. Prepare in advance what you will take with you. This may include your watch, three or four well-sharpened pencils with erasers, juice or water, and small boxes of raisins. (Raisins are a better source of quick energy than a candy bar. They are metabolized fast and you do not risk the same "sugar low" that you can get from candy. As an added bonus, opening the little box makes no noise!)

2. The night before the test eat a high-carbohydrate dinner. Called "carbohydrate loading," athletes do this the night before a game because the carbohydrates convert to energy by morning.

3. In the morning of the test, eat a high-protein breakfast. Research at Johns Hopkins shows that protein at breakfast is particularly important for problem-solving activities. Get up in time to have your breakfast calmly.

4. Get to the testing room in plenty of time to settle in.

5. Once the test starts, you may want to note down certain short-term memory items.

6. Remember to stick to your strategies throughout the test. Do not be distracted by what others are doing around you. Periodically make sure your mark on the answer sheet corresponds to the number of the question you are answering.

7. If you go blank reading the first item, go on to the next. Continue searching until you find one you can answer. Then go back. Once started, keeping to the pace that you know from the practice sessions gives you the highest level of accuracy.

8. Do not omit any items. For those you don't know, simply fill in your predetermined "guess answer." There is no penalty for wrong answers.

9. During breaks, do not talk to other test takers. Keep your energies focused on the test.

10. Stay in control of your time and energy. Remember, you are taking the test. Do not let the test take you.

7.6 AFTER THE TEST

1. If you feel sick during the exam or you realize that you are not adequately prepared, you can void your test. If you do this, you will not receive scores (the proctor will void the test in front of you), and unsatisfactory scores will not be recorded against your name.

2. After the test is over, do not compare what you remember answering with what someone else remembers answering. It is unreliable at best and often depressing. Be good to yourself!

3. If you have not performed as well as you needed to, you can take the test again. Do not waste much time in depression; rather, analyze your weaknesses and figure out the best ways to correct them.

7.7 REFERENCES

PCAT Candidate Information Booklet (obtain latest edition from The Psychological Corporation, based on information in Chapter 1)

Chapter 8

Pharmacy College Admission Test: Model Examination

8.0 INTRODUCTION

This sample test consists of five separate examinations, one each in Verbal Ability, Biology, Chemistry, Reading Comprehension, and Quantitative Ability. The sample (model) test is designed in accordance with the Psychological Corporation's Pharmacy College Admission Testing Program in conformity with sample items and proper course outlines. We emphasize that this examination is not a copy of the actual exam, which is guarded closely and may not be duplicated. The actual exam you'll take may have more difficult questions in some areas than you will encounter on this model test, or some questions may be easier.

The time allotted for each subtest in the sample model test is based on a careful analysis of the Psychological Corporation test schedule. The time we allot for each test, therefore, merely suggests how much time you should spend on each subject when you take the actual exam. We have not, in every case, provided precisely the number of questions you will see on the examination. It might be a good idea to jot down your "running" time for each test and make comparisons later on. If you find that you're working faster, you may assume you are making progress. Remember, we have timed each section uniformly. If you follow all our directions, your scores will all be comparable.

The actual PCAT is given with a different schedule than the one in this book. The chart below shows the schedule for the actual PCAT:

Actual Test Schedule	Time Allowed
Verbal Ability	30 minutes
Biology	30 minutes
Reading Comprehension (Set 1)	45 minutes
Quantitative Ability	45 minutes
Chemistry	30 minutes
Reading Comprehension (Set 2)	45 minutes

8.1 BIOLOGY

DIRECTIONS: For each question, read all the choices carefully. Then select the answer that you consider correct or most nearly correct. Blacken the answer space corresponding to your best choice just as you would do on the actual examination. **This examination is comprised of 53 items.**

Time limit: 30 minutes

1. Which of the following organelles is incorrectly matched with a function?
- **A.** Mitochondria – fermentation
- **B.** Chloroplast – fixation of CO_2
- **C.** Lysosome – storage of hydrolytic enzymes
- **D.** Golgi Apparatus – packaging and secretion of glycoprotein

2. The corpus luteum secretes:
- **A.** LH.
- **B.** progesterone.
- **C.** FSH.
- **D.** hCG.

3. When members of two species both benefit from living together in close association, the relationship is called
- **A.** mutualism.
- **B.** commensalism.
- **C.** parasitism.
- **D.** predation.

4. Which substance has the highest energy content per gram?
- **A.** Proteins
- **B.** Fats
- **C.** Carbohydrates
- **D.** Phospholipids

5. Cyanide blocks cellular production of energy at which stage?
- **A.** Glycolysis
- **B.** Citric acid cycle
- **C.** Electron transport system
- **D.** Oxidative phosphorylation

6. Lysosomes
- **A.** are a site of protein synthesis.
- **B.** form the rough endoplasmic reticulum.
- **C.** contain digestive enzymes.
- **D.** contain the enzymes for oxidative phosphorylation.

7. Which of the following conditions will cause a gene frequency to depart from the equilibrium expected from the Hardy-Weinberg law?
- **A.** Random assortment
- **B.** Nonrandom mating
- **C.** Large population
- **D.** No mutation

8. Which of the following substances is NOT secreted into the human digestive tract?
- **A.** Bile
- **B.** Insulin
- **C.** Ptyalin
- **D.** Pepsinogen

9. Which of the following is a characteristic of both eukaryotic animal cells and animal viruses?
- **A.** The ability to undergo mutation.
- **B.** The ability to reproduce through mitosis.
- **C.** The ability to produce proteins.
- **D.** The ability to enter other cells and cause lysis.

10. One of the major differences between fungi and bacteria is that only fungi
A. are photosynthetic.
B. can produce spores.
C. are always diploid.
D. can undergo meiosis and mitosis.

11. Blood that is pumped from the left ventricle of the heart
A. is highly oxygenated.
B. flows into the aorta.
C. is under high pressure.
D. all of the above.

12. Muscles are bound to joints by
A. cartilage.
B. tendons.
C. ligaments.
D. myosin fibers.

13. The development of the ovarian follicle is initiated by
A. FSH.
B. LH.
C. estrogen.
D. progesterone.

14. In the immune system, B cells
A. are lymphocytes that eventually release antibodies.
B. are special phagocytic neutrophils.
C. are transformed into macrophages at the site of inflammation.
D. are lymphocytes that destroy foreign cells.

15. When one species benefits and the other is exploited, the relationship is called
A. mutualism.
B. socialism.
C. commensalism.
D. parasitism.

16. Translation of the genetic code does not directly require
A. activated tRNA - AA.
B. mesosomes.
C. mRNA.
D. DNA.

17. What is the correct hierarchy (from the highest to lowest) of given levels of taxonomy?
A. Class, order, family, genus
B. Order, family, genus, class
C. Family, genus, class, order
D. Family, class, order, genus

18. "Under certain conditions gene frequencies and genotypic frequencies remain constant from generation to generation in sexually reproducing populations" was put forth by
A. Dalton.
B. Hardy-Weinberg.
C. Mendel.
D. Mendeleev.

19. Given the following representative pedigree, what is the most likely pattern of inheritance (blackened symbol means trait is present)?

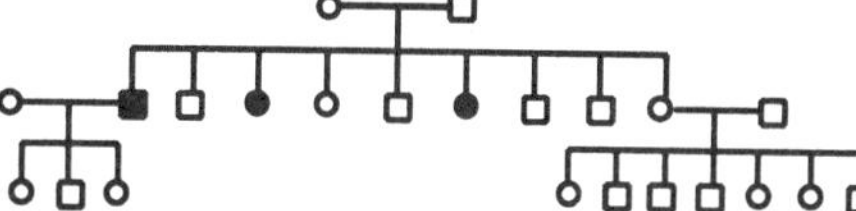

A. Autosomal dominant
B. Autosomal recessive
C. Sex-influenced
D. Heterozygous

20. Which of the following substances is NOT generally absorbed into the blood capillaries of the intestinal villi?
A. Water
B. Glucose
C. Amino acids
D. Triglycerides

21. Which of the following is required for the conversion of fructose-6-phosphate to fructose 1, 6- diphosphate during glycolysis?
A. Oxygen
B. An excess of fructose-6-phosphate
C. A kinase enzyme, specific for fructose-6-phosphate.
D. Any of the enzymes that catalyze the reactions of glycolysis

22. A membrane may be found on all of the following structures except
A. lysosomes.
B. endoplasmic reticulum.
C. mitochondria.
D. centrioles.

23. During facilitated diffusion
A. carrier substances carry molecules across the membrane.
B. molecules can go against the concentration gradient.
C. molecules require energy.
D. saturation kinetics is not observed.

24. If red blood cells are put in a hypertonic solution, they will
A. remain the same.
B. hemolyze.
C. crenate.
D. swell up.

25. What anatomical structure(s) is (are) used to prevent the bronchi from collapsing?
A. Cartilage rings
B. Alveolus
C. Bony rings
D. Epiglottis

26. The greatest resistance to blood flow is in the
A. capillaries.
B. veins.
C. arteries.
D. arterioles.

27. Bacteriophages
A. cause disease in humans.
B. contain both DNA and RNA.
C. are viruses.
D. are bacteria.

28. Which structure may protect a bacteria from phagocytosis by white blood cells?
A. Mesosome
B. Cilia
C. Capsule
D. Nucleoid

29. The chromosomes become coiled and visible and the nuclear membrane disintegrates. This is what phase of mitosis?
A. Anaphase
B. Telophase
C. Prophase
D. Metaphase

30. The genetic code is composed of sequences of
A. three nucleotides.
B. three nucleosides.
C. three amino acids.
D. two amino acids.

31. The following is one strand of a double helix of DNA (showing only nitrogen bases). What is the structure of its complementary DNA strand? (A = adenine, G = guanine, T = thymine, C = cytosine, U = uracil)

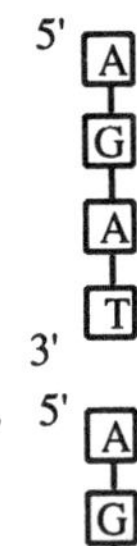

A. 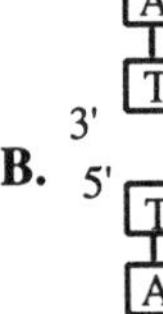

B. 5' T A G A 3'

C. 3' T C T A 5'

D. 3' T A G A 5'

32. Which of the following is least involved in immune reaction and most in coagulation?
A. Neutrophils
B. Platelets
C. Lymphocytes
D. Basophils

33. All are part of the kidney except
A. glomerulus.
B. loop of Henle.
C. Bowman's capsule.
D. Malpighian tubules.

34. Reabsorption of most of the water, glucose, amino acids, sodium, and other nutrients occurs in the
A. calyx.
B. collecting duct.
C. distal convoluted tubules.
D. proximal convoluted tubules.

35. Control of body temperature is localized in the
A. skin.
B. heart.
C. cerebrum.
D. hypothalamus.

36. Which of the following is not a feature of the unit membrane model of the cell membrane?
A. Continuous lipid bilayer present
B. Globular proteins floating in lipids
C. Hydrophobic ends of lipids in contact with water
D. Continuous protein bilayers outside lipid layer

37. If a cell is placed in a solution that causes it to shrink because of water loss, that solution is said to be
A. hypotonic.
B. isotonic.
C. hypertonic.
D. homeostatic.

38. The term glycolysis, which is the first series of reactions in the breakdown of glucose, is sometimes used as a synonym for the
A. Kreb's cycle.
B. Calvin cycle.
C. Embden-Meyerhof Pathway.
D. electron transport system.

39. Fertilization of an ovum by sperm normally occurs in the
A. uterus.
B. vagina.
C. seminal vesicle.
D. fallopian tube.

40. Which of the following is not a function of the liver?
A. Synthesis of insulin
B. Synthesis of carbohydrates, proteins, and fats
C. Detoxification of drugs
D. Synthesis of bile

41. Which of the following is correct for gene mapping?
A. Only three-factor crosses may be used to sequence gene loci.
B. The recombination frequencies are always representative of the recombination rates of the gene loci.
C. The recombination frequency is equal to the map units.
D. Viral DNAs are used for gene mapping.

42. Cytoplasmic inheritance:
A. does not follow Mendelian Laws.
B. the maternal cytoplasm plays the dominant role.
C. replication of mitochondria is an example.
D. all of the above.

43. Homozygous refers to
   A. similar types of chromosomes.
   B. having similar functions on an evolutionary basis.
   C. particles in a solution not being separable microscopically.
   D. identical alleles for a given trait.

44. Which statement is *incorrect* concerning X and Y chromosomes?
   A. X is larger than Y.
   B. They are not homologous.
   C. XY is a genotypic male.
   D. Traits due to X but not Y are called sex-linked traits.

45. Select the *incorrect* statement:
   A. Genotype is the alleles for a given trait in an individual.
   B. Phenotype is the expression of the genotype.
   C. A given genotype may express different phenotypes.
   D. Different genotypes may express to the same phenotype.

46. Blights, wilts, and galls are caused by
   A. fungi.
   B. viroids.
   C. rickettsia.
   D. bacteria.

47. Which of the following is a fungal disease?
   A. Influenza
   B. Pneumonia
   C. Typhus
   D. Ringworm

48. All of the following are families in Suborder Eubacteriineae, except
   A. rhizobiaceae.
   B. chlamydobacteriales.
   C. achromobacteriaceae.
   D. parvobacteriaceae.

49. A vaccine usually stimulates:
   A. passive immunity.
   B. active immunity.
   C. production of antibodies.
   D. both B and C.

50. Which of the following is a viral disease?
   A. Anthrax
   B. Syphilis
   C. Poliomyelitis
   D. Tuberculosis

51. All of the following are infections except
   A. typhoid.
   B. botulism.
   C. influenza
   D. strep throat.

52. All of the following are types of bacteria except
   A. metatrophic.
   B. parasitic.
   C. autotrophic.
   D. eucalyptus.

53. Infectious diseases are always caused by:
   A. inherited genes.
   B. pathogens.
   C. rickettsias.
   D. bacterial respiration.

8.2 CHEMISTRY

DIRECTIONS: For each question, read all the choices carefully. Then select the answer that you consider correct or most nearly correct. Blacken the answer space corresponding to your best choice just as you would do on the actual examination. **This examination is comprised of 60 items: General Chemistry (1–30), and Organic Chemistry (31–60).**

Time limit: 30 minutes

1. A neutral atom that has 53 electrons and an atomic mass of 111 has
   A. no other isotopes.
   B. an atomic number of 58.
   C. a nucleus containing 58 neutrons.
   D. a nucleus containing 53 neutrons.

2. Which of the following measurements or techniques can be used to find the atomic weight, or molecular weight of a substance?
   A. Heat of combustion
   B. Boiling point elevation
   C. Boiling point of the pure substance
   D. Electrical conductivity

3. How many grams of HCl are required to react completely with 32.5 grams of Zn (producing zinc chloride and hydrogen)?
   A. 9 g
   B. 18 g
   C. 36 g
   D. 72 g

4. What is the sum of the coefficients of all species in the balanced equation

$$Pb(NO_3)_2 \rightarrow NO_2 + PbO + O_2$$

   A. 18
   B. 15
   C. 12
   D. 9

5. Estimate the boiling point of a low concentration solution of a non-electrolyte in acetic acid. The boiling point of acetic acid is 118°C.
   A. 115°
   B. 118°
   C. 120°
   D. 100°

6. Given that the standard heats of formation of SO_2 and SO_3 are –70 and –95 kcal/mole respectively, find the heat of reaction for

$$SO_2 + 1/2\ O_2 \rightarrow SO_3$$

   A. –25 kcal
   B. –165 kcal
   C. 25 kcal
   D. 165 kcal

7. If 50 mL of 2.0 M NaOH is mixed with 50 mL of 4.0 M nitric acid, what is the pH of the final solution?
   A. 1.00
   B. 7.00
   C. 14.00
   D. 10.00

8. What is the volume occupied by 0.50 moles of an ideal gas at 760 torr and 0°C?
   A. 2.24 L
   B. 11.2 L
   C. 22.4 L
   D. 44.8 L

9. What volume of HBr can be made if 14.2 L of hydrogen and 23.5 L of bromine react at STP?

$$H_2 + Br_2 \rightarrow 2\ HBr$$

   A. 14.2 L
   B. 23.5 L
   C. 28.4 L
   D. 47.0 L

10. A gas mixture contains equal numbers of CO molecules and CO_2 molecules, and no others. Assuming ideal gas behavior, which of the following statements is true?
   A. The total mass of CO_2 and CO is the same.
   B. The partial pressure of CO_2 and CO is the same.
   C. Since carbon dioxide molecules have more mass, they have more inertia and contribute more to the total pressure.
   D. The density of CO_2 and CO is the same.

11. Which of the following compounds is incorrectly named?
   A. V $(ClO_3)_3$; vanadium (III) chlorate
   B. $Na_2C_2O_4$; sodium oxalate
   C. $AlPO_4$; aluminum phosphate
   D. $KHSO_4$; krypton bisulfate

12. Fe metal adopts a body-center cube structure. How many Fe atoms are present in the unit cell?
   A. 1
   B. 2
   C. 4
   D. 6

13. Which of the following combinations of quantum numbers DO NOT represent permissible solutions of the Schroedinger wave equation for the hydrogen atom?

	n	l	m	s
(i)	9	0	0	–5/2
(ii)	2	1	0	–1/2
(iii)	1	3	3	1/2

   A. (i)
   B. (iii)
   C. (i) and (ii)
   D. (i) and (iii)

14. Atom A has 3 valence electrons and atom B has 7 valence electrons. The formula expected for an ionic compound of A and B is
   A. AB.
   B. AB_3.
   C. AB_2.
   D. A_2B.

15. Which of the following trends in first ionization potential is NOT correct?
   A. Rb<Sb<Cl<Ne
   B. Na<Mg<P<Cl
   C. Be<Sb<P<N
   D. F<N<B<Li

16. In which of the following molecules is the octet rule violated?
   A. $SnCl_2$
   B. $PbCl_4$
   C. F_2
   D. All of the above.

17. Which of the following oxidations states would not be expected?
   A. Ar(0)
   B. Pb(IV)
   C. Nb(V)
   D. N(VI)

18. Which of the following molecules are polar?

   1. NO 2. SO_3 3. HF 4. $COCl_2$

   A. 1
   B. 2 and 4
   C. 1, 3, and 4
   D. 1, 2, and 3

19. What is the pH of a 0.0100 molar HNO_3 aqueous solution?
   A. 7.00
   B. 12.00
   C. 2.00
   D. 2.76

20. Given the following hypothetical half-reactions,

$$M^2 + e^- \rightarrow M^+ \ , E° = -0.579 \text{ V}$$
$$M^3 + e^- \rightarrow M^2 \ , E° = 0.735 \text{ V}$$

Which of the following is true?
- **A.** M^{2+} is reduced.
- **B.** M^{3+} is reduced.
- **C.** This reaction is never spontaneous.
- **D.** More information is needed.

21. If 75% of a radioactive isotope decays in 300 days, what is its half-life?
- **A.** 100 days
- **B.** 150 days
- **C.** 200 days
- **D.** 300 days

22. Which of the following arrangements of atoms is most likely?
- **A.** $O{=}C{=}\overset{+}{O}{-}\overset{-}{O}$
- **B.** (ring of two O atoms and C, with C=O)
- **C.** $O{=}C(O\cdot)(O\cdot)$
- **D.** $\overset{-}{C}{=}\overset{+}{O}$, ring with O—O

23. A compound was found to have an empirical formula of NO and a molecular mass of 90g/mole. What is the molecular formula?
- **A.** NO
- **B.** N_2O_2
- **C.** N_3O_3
- **D.** N_4O_4

24. An element with this electron configuration, $1s^2 2s^2 2p^4$, will form which of the following ions?
- **A.** +2
- **B.** +4
- **C.** −2
- **D.** −4

25. Element A exists in three isotopic forms with masses of 21.0, 25.0, and 26.0 amu, respectively. Element B also exists in three isotopic forms with masses of 22.0, 24.0, and 26.0 amu respectively. It is true that
- **A.** element A has a higher atomic mass than B.
- **B.** element B has a higher atomic mass than A.
- **C.** A and B have identical atomic masses since the sum of their isotopic masses are equal.
- **D.** you cannot predict which atomic mass is greater from the data given.

26. Which of the following oxidation states would not be expected?
- **A.** Ar(0)
- **B.** Ag(I)
- **C.** S (VII)
- **D.** Na(III)

27. Which one of the following gives the correct hybridization for the central atom in the molecule?

$AlCl_3$ N_3^- CS_2

- **A.** sp^3 sp^2 sp^2
- **B.** sp^3 sp sp^2
- **C.** sp sp^3 sp^2
- **D.** sp^2 sp sp^2

28. The biological affect of radiation is measured in units of
- **A.** geigers.
- **B.** electron volts.
- **C.** curies.
- **D.** rems.

29. When sulfuric acid is added to sodium chloride, the gas given off has the formula
- **A.** Cl_2.
- **B.** HCl.
- **C.** H_2S.
- **D.** SO_3.

30. Which species cannot behave as a reducing agent?

A. ClO^-

B. ClO_2^-

C. ClO_3^-

D. ClO_4^-

31. Which of the following carbon backbones forms the structure of 2,3,6-trimethyloctane?

```
     C   C C
     |   | |
A. C-C-C-C-C-C-C
```

```
             C
             |
     C   C   C
     |   |   |
B. C-C-C-C-C-C-C
```

```
     C
     |
C. C-C-C-C-C-C-C
         | |
         C C
```

```
       C
       |
D. C-C-C-C-C-C-C
         |   |
         C   C
```

32. Which of the following compounds has the highest dipole moment?

A. H_3C–CH=CH–CH_3 (cis)

B. H_3C–CH=CH–CH_3 (trans)

C. $H_3C-\equiv-CH_3$

D. H_3C–CH_2–CH_2–CH_3

33. What is the product of the reaction between 1,1,1-tribromo-2-butene and HBr?

A. Br_3C–CH=C(Br)–CH_3

B. Br_3C–CH(Br)–CH_2–CH_3

C. $Br_3C-\equiv-CH_3$

D. Br_3C–CH_2–CH(Br)–CH_3

34. What is the product of the reaction between Br^+ and anisole?

A. benzene ring with OCH_3 and Br (meta)

B. benzene ring with OCH_3 and Br (para)

C. benzene ring with OCH_2Br

D. benzene ring with Br

35. Which of the following is the strongest acid?

A. Isopropanol

B. Sec-butanol

C. Tert-butanol

D. Propanol

36. Which of the following is the least soluble in water?

A. Ethanol

B. Propanol

C. Butanol

D. Pentanol

37. Which of the following alcohols is most likely to undergo S_N2 substitutions?

A. CH_3OH

B. CH_3CH_3OH

C. $(CH_3)_2CHOH$

D. $(CH_3)_3COH$

38. What is the relationship between these straight-chain aldoses?

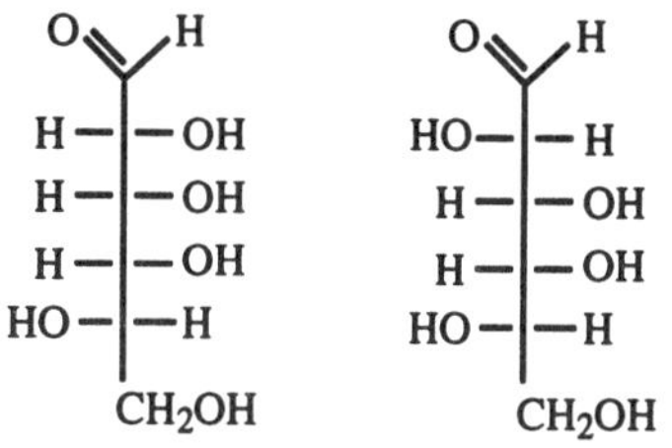

```
  O  H            O  H
   \/              \/
H-|-OH          HO-|-H
H-|-OH           H-|-OH
H-|-OH           H-|-OH
HO-|-H          HO-|-H
  CH2OH            CH2OH
```

A. Anomers
B. Enantiomers
C. Epimers
D. Racemers

39. Which of the following is not a product of this reaction?

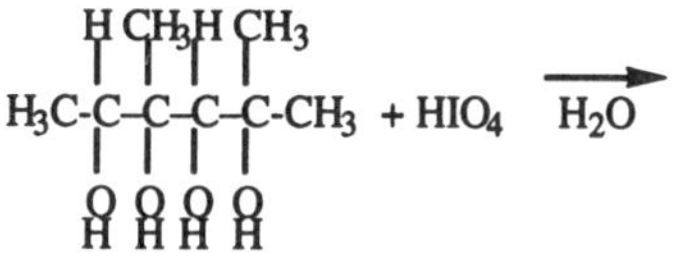

```
   H CH3 H CH3
   |  |  |  |
H3C-C--C--C--C-CH3 + HIO4 --H2O-->
   |  |  |  |
   O  O  O  O
   H  H  H  H
```

A. H_3CCH (with C=O)

B. $H_2C{=}O$

C. $(CH_3)_2C{=}O$

D. $(CH_3)_3COH$

40. Name the following compound.

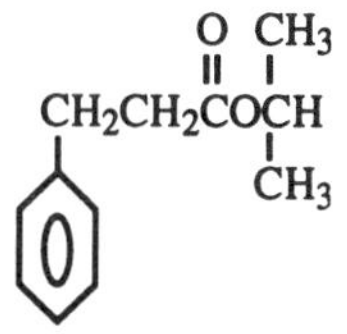

```
           O  CH3
           ‖  |
CH2CH2COCH
|          |
C6H5       CH3
```

A. Isopropyl benzoate
B. Benzyl isopropyl ester
C. Isopropyl-3-phenylproponate
D. Isoalkyl chloride

41. What is the product of the following reaction?

$(CH_3)_3CCH_2CH_2OH + KMnO_4 \rightarrow$

A. $(CH_3)_3CCH_2\overset{O}{\overset{\|}{C}}H$
B. $(CH_3)_3CCH{=}CH_2$
C. $(CH_3)_3C\overset{O}{\overset{\|}{C}}CH_3$
D. CH_3COOH

42. Which of the following is not a property of phenols?
A. They are more acidic than alcohols, but less acidic than carboxylic acids.
B. Most reactions involve breaking the O–H bond.
C. They can be esterified with acid chlorides.
D. They are easily oxidized to ketones.

43. Which of the following reagents is used in a Fridel-Crafts acylation?
A. CuX
B. RX and $AlCl_3$
C. $KMnO_4$
D. RC(=O)X and $AlCl_3$

44. Which of the following sugars is a furanose?

A. 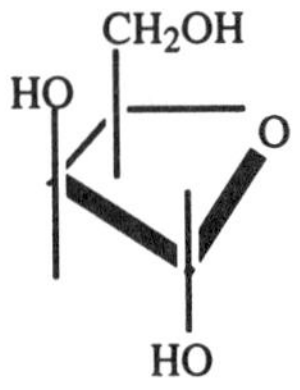
CH_2OH
HO
O
HO

B. 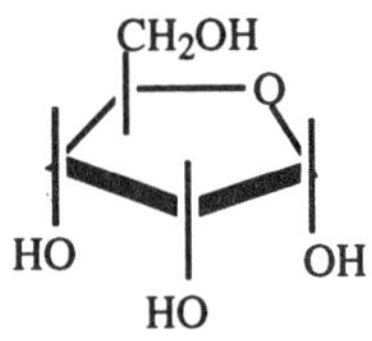
CH_2OH
O
HO OH
HO

C. 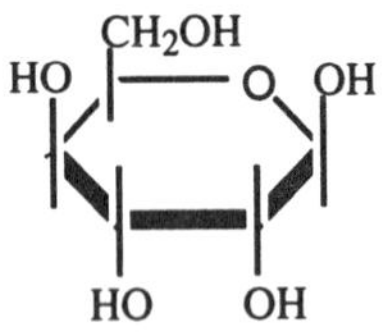
CH_2OH
HO O OH
HO OH

D. 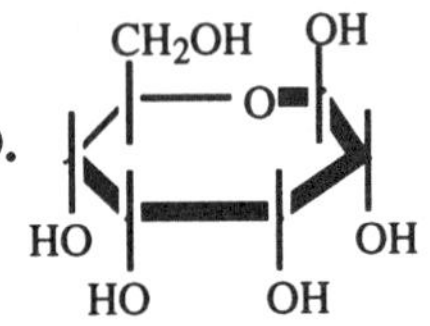
CH_2OH OH
O
HO OH
HO OH

45. Which of the following structures is consistent with this IR and ^{1}H NMR data?

IR: 3620 cm^{-1} broad peak
2980 cm^{-1} strong peak
no other strong peaks

NMR: 1.1 doublet, area 6
2.6 broad, area 1
3.9 septet, area 1

Mass Spec: C_3H_8O

A. 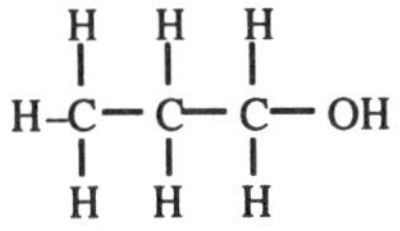 H–C–C–C–OH (each C bearing two H)

B. H–C–C–C–H (central C bearing OH and H; outer C each bearing two H)

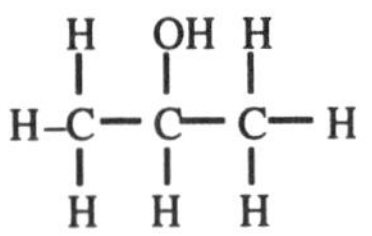

C. H–C–C–C–H (central C=O; outer C each bearing two H)

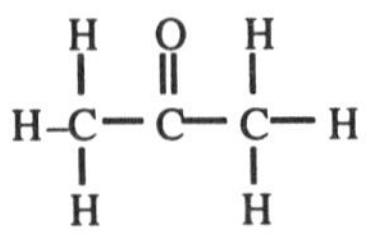

D. 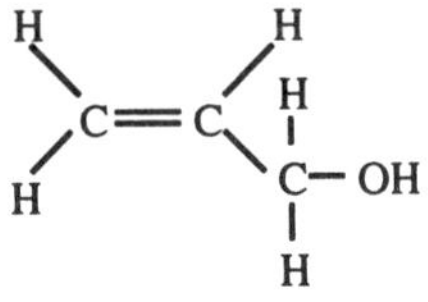 $H_2C{=}CH–CH_2–OH$ (H, H on first C; H on second C; H, H on C–OH)

46. Aldehydes and ketones react with secondary amines to form compounds called

A. amides.
B. enamines.
C. lipids.
D. barbiturates.

47. Which of the following best describes a *transesterification* reaction?

A. High boiling ester + high-boiling alcohol → higher-boiling ester + low-boiling alcohol.
B. High boiling ester + low-boiling alcohol → higher-boiling ester + high-boiling alcohol.
C. Low boiling ester + high-boiling alcohol → high-boiling ester + low-boiling alcohol.
D. Low-boiling ester + low-boiling alcohol → high-boiling ester + high-boiling alcohol.

48. What is the product of the following reaction?

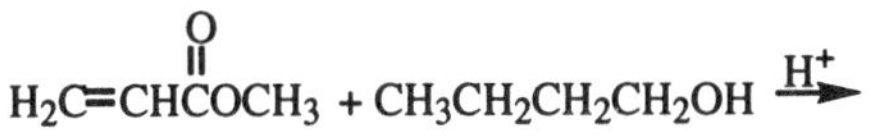

$$H_2C{=}CH\overset{O}{\overset{\|}{C}}OCH_3 + CH_3CH_2CH_2CH_2OH \xrightarrow{H^+}$$

A. $H_2C{=}CH\overset{O}{\overset{\|}{C}}OCH_2(CH_2)_2CH_3$

B.
CH_2 CH_3
CH_2 CH
O O
H_2C–$CHCOCH_3$
H

C. $CH_3(CH_2)_2CH_2O$
$H_2C{=}CHCOCH_3$
H

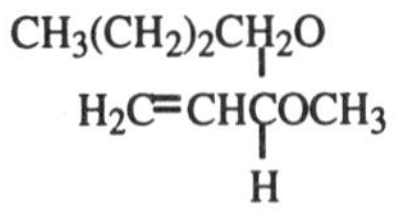

D. 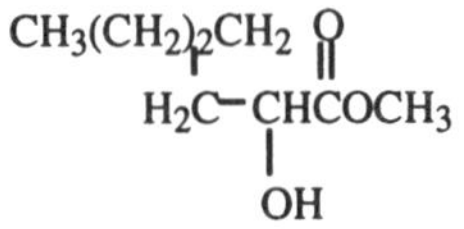 $CH_3(CH_2)_2CH_2$ O
H_2C–$CH\overset{\|}{C}OCH_3$
OH

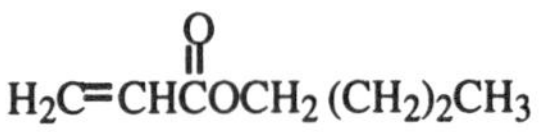

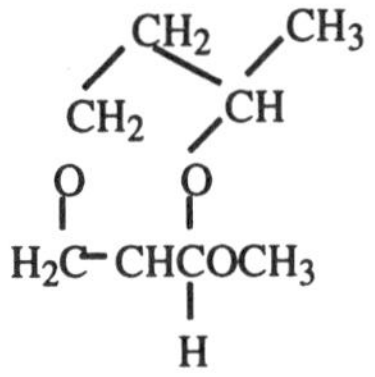

49. Which of the following steps is not a chain-propagating step for a radical reaction?
A. $(C_6H_5)_3C\bullet + O_2 \rightarrow (C_6H_5)_3C\text{-}O\text{-}O\bullet$
B. $(C_6H_5)_3C\text{-}O\text{-}O\bullet + (C_6H_5)_3CH \rightarrow$
$(C_6H_5)_3C\bullet + (C_6H_5)_3C\text{-}O\text{-}OH$
C. $(C_6H_5)_3C\bullet + (C_6H_5)_3C\text{-}O\text{-}OH \rightarrow$
$(C_6H_5)_3C\text{-}O\text{-}O\bullet + (C_6H_5)_3CH$
D. $(C_6H_5)_3C\bullet + (C_6H_5)_3C\bullet \rightarrow$
$(C_6H_5)_3C\text{-}C(C_6H_5)_3$

50. Reduction of an organic compound usually entails
A. a decrease in its oxygen content.
B. an increase in its oxygen content.
C. a decrease in the length of the longest carbon chain.
D. an increase in the length of the longest carbon chain.

51. A compound with an empirical formula of $C_5H_{10}O$ showed the following spectral characteristics: IR: strong peak near 1710 cm^{-1}, NMR: doublet at 1.10 ppm (6H), singlet at 2.10 ppm (3H), and a septet and 2.50 ppm (1H). Which of the following compounds agrees best with this data?

A. 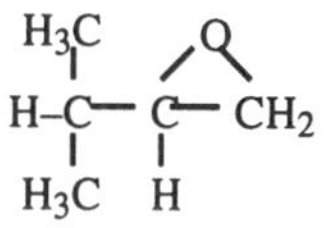 $(H_3C)_2CH\text{-}CH(O)CH_2$ (H–C(H₃C)(H₃C)–CH–CH₂ epoxide)

B. $(H_3C)_2CH\text{-}C(=O)\text{-}CH_2$

C. $(H_3C)_2C{=}CH\text{-}CH_2OH$

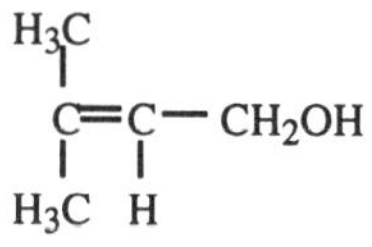

D. 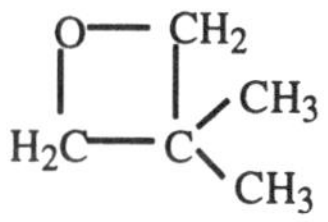 4-membered ring O–CH₂–C(CH₃)₂–CH₂ (H_2C, O, CH_2, $C(CH_3)_2$)

52. Which of the following is the major product for the reaction

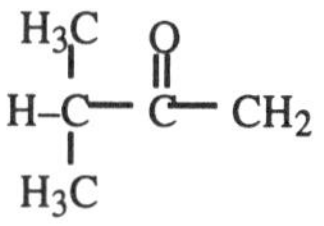

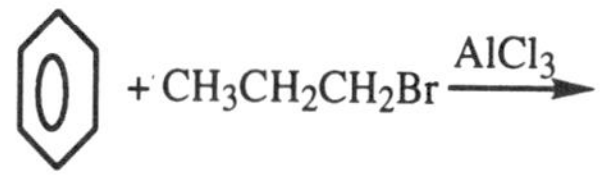

benzene + $CH_3CH_2CH_2Br \xrightarrow{AlCl_3}$

A. 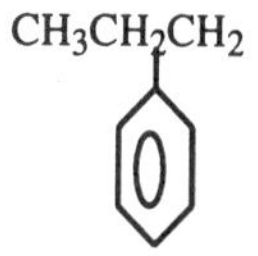 benzene with $CH_3CH_2CH_2$

B. 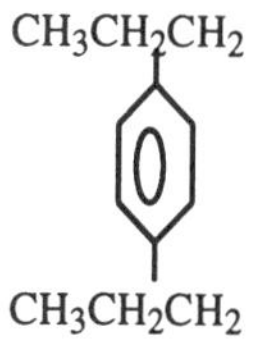 benzene with $CH_3CH_2CH_2$ (para) and $CH_3CH_2CH_2$

C. 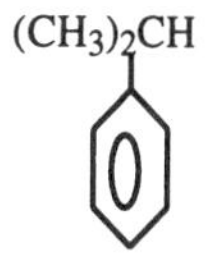 benzene with $(CH_3)_2CH$

D. 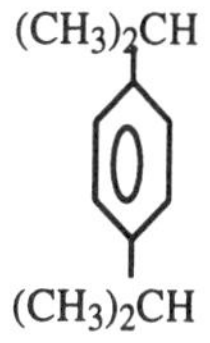 benzene with $(CH_3)_2CH$ (para) and $(CH_3)_2CH$

53. Which of the following substituent groups functions as a meta-director on electrophilic aromatic substitution reactions?
A. $-NH_2$
B. $-CH_3$
C. $-CF_3$
D. $-F$

54. Cyclooctatetrene reacts with 2 equivalents of potassium to yield the very stable compound, $K_2C_8H_8$. The NMR spectrum of this compound indicates all of the hydrogens are equivalent. Which of the following statements accounts for these observations?
A. The compound is covalent.
B. The compound is cyclic.
C. The compound is planar.
D. The compound is aromatic.

55. Which of the following sets of reactants would produce

H, $\overset{O}{\parallel}$COCH$_3$, $\overset{O}{\parallel}$COCH$_3$, H

A. [diene] + H, $\overset{O}{\parallel}$COCH$_3$, $H_3CO\overset{O}{\parallel}C$, H

B. [diene] + H, $\overset{O}{\parallel}$COCH$_3$, H, $\overset{O}{\parallel}$COCH$_3$

C. [diene] + H, $\overset{O}{\parallel}$COCH$_3$, $H_3CO\overset{O}{\parallel}C$, H

D. [diene] + $\overset{O}{\parallel}$COCH$_3$, H, $\overset{O}{\parallel}$COCH$_3$

56. Which of the following is the strongest carbon acid?
A. Acetylene
B. Ethene
C. Ethane
D. Methane

57. Which of the following compounds is drawn as a "trans" isomer?

A. F, Cl / Br, H

B. H_3C, CH_3 / H, H

C. H_3C, CH_3 / H, Br

D. H, CH_3 / H_3C, H

58. In the following reaction

$$(-)CH_3\underset{OH}{\underset{|}{C}}HCHO + Br_2 \xrightarrow{H_2O} CH_3\underset{OH}{\underset{|}{C}}HCOOH$$

What occurs to the configuration of the chiral carbon?
A. Retention
B. Inversion
C. Racemization
D. Chirality is lost

59. Which of the following are cis-isomers?

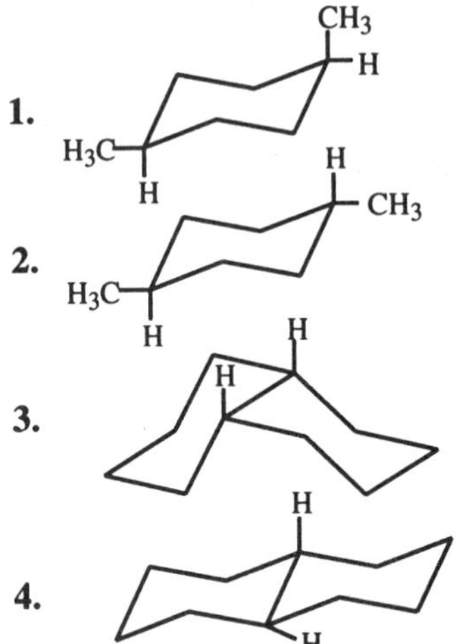

A. 1 and 2
B. 1 and 3
C. 1 and 4
D. 2 and 3

60. A Grignard reagent reacts with esters to form
A. primary alcohols.
B. secondary alcohols.
C. tertiary alcohols.
D. ketones.

8.3 READING COMPREHENSION TEST

Read each passage to get the general idea. Then reread the passage more carefully to answer the questions based on the passage. For each question read all choices carefully. Then select the answer you consider correct or most nearly correct. Blacken the answer space corresponding to your best choice, just as you would do on the actual examination.

Time limit: 45 minutes

Passage 1:
Taken from "Achieving Electronic Privacy"
David Chaum
Scientific American, August, 1992 p. 101

Computerized transactions of all kinds are becoming ever more pervasive. More than half a dozen countries have developed or are testing chip cards that would replace cash. In Denmark, a consortium of banking, utility and transport companies has announced a card that would replace coins and small bills; in France, the telecommunications authorities have proposed general use of the smart cards now used at pay telephones. The government of Singapore has requested bids for a system that would communicate with cars and charge their smart cards as they pass various points on a road (as opposed to the simple vehicle identification systems already in use in the U.S. elsewhere). And cable and satellite broadcasters are experimenting with smart cards for delivering pay-per-view television. All these systems, however, are based on cards that identify themselves during every transaction.

If the trend toward identifier-based smart cards continues, personal privacy will be increasingly eroded. But in this conflict between organizational security and individual liberty, neither side emerges as a clear winner. Each round of improved identification techniques, sophisticated data analysis or extended linking can be frustrated by widespread noncompliance or even legislated limits, which in turn may engender attempts at further control.

Meanwhile, in a system based on representatives and observers, organizations stand to gain competitive and political advantages from increased public confidence (in addition to the lower costs of pseudonymous record-keeping). And individuals, by maintaining their own cryptographically guaranteed records and making only necessary disclosures, will be able to protect their privacy without infringing on the legitimate needs of those with whom they do business.

1. The passage suggests that chip cards are being developed because
   A. they are easier to handle than cash.
   B. they provide greater privacy.
   C. they generate sophisticated data to analyze.
   D. the technology exists and should be used.

2. How does the author characterize the trend toward identifier-based smart cards?
   A. As a technological advance
   B. As a potential threat to personal privacy
   C. Providing a competitive edge for innovative corporations
   D. Offering greater choices to consumers

3. It can be inferred from the passage that the key technological innovation that made smart cards possible was
   A. sophisticated data analysis.
   B. miniaturization of computer components.
   C. sophisticated security systems.
   D. advances in telecommunications.

4. According to the passage all of the following are advantages of a system based on representatives EXCEPT
   A. competitive advantages for organizations.
   B. protection of individual privacy.
   C. increased public confidence.
   D. improved identification systems.

5. All of the following could potentially gather data generated by identifier-based smart cards EXCEPT
   A. businesses.
   B. governments.
   C. individuals.
   D. organizations.

6. In the context of the passage what does cryptographically mean?
   A. Simple
   B. Complex
   C. Coded
   D. Anonymous

7. What does the author suggest is the difference between identifier-based systems and systems based on representatives and observers?
   A. Identifier-based systems are more economical.
   B. Systems based on representatives and observers threaten organizational security.
   C. Systems based on representatives and observers can better protect individuals.
   D. Identifier-based systems can deliver a larger range of services.

Passage 2:
Taken from "Carbohydrates in Cell Recognition"
Nathan Sharon and Halina Lis
Scientific American, January, 1993.
pp 82–83

Biologists generally accept that cells recognize one another through pairs of complementary structure on their surfaces: a structure on one cell carries encoded biological information that the structure of the other of the other cell can decipher. That idea represents an extension of the lock-and-key hypothesis formulated in 1897 by Emil Fisher, the noted German chemist. He used it to explain the specificity of interactions between enzymes and their substrates. Pioneering immunologist Paul Ehrlich extended it in 1900 to account for the highly specific reactions of the immune system, and in 1914 Frank Rattray Lillie of the University of Chicago invoked it to describe recognition between sperm and eggs.

By the 1920s the lock-and-key hypothesis had become one of the central theoretical assumptions of cellular biology. Yet for many years thereafter, the nature and identity of the molecules involved in cellular recognition remained a complete mystery.

To most biologists, the idea that the molecules might be carbohydrates seemed farfetched. That large class of compounds consists of monosaccharides (simple sugars such as glucose and fructose) and of oligosaccharides and polysaccharides, which are composed of linked monosaccharides. Until the late 1960s, carbohydrates were thought to serve only as energy sources (in the forms of monosaccharides and storage molecules such as the polysaccharide starch) and as structural materials (the polysaccharides cellulose in plants and chitin in the exoskeletons of insects). The two other major classes of biological materials—nucleic acids, which carry genetic information, and proteins—were obviously far more versatile. By comparison, carbohydrates looked like dull, second-class citizens.

Interest in carbohydrates was further discourage by the extraordinary complexity of their structures. In contrast to the nucleotides in nucleic acids and the amino acids in proteins, which can interconnect in only one way, the monosaccharide units in oligosaccharides and polysaccharides can attach to one another at multiple points. Two identical monosaccharides can bond to form 11 different disaccharides, whereas two amino acids can make only one dipeptide. Even a small number of monosaccharides can create a staggering diversity of compounds, including many with branching structures. Four different nucleotides can make only 24 distinct tetranucleotides, but four different monosaccharides can make 35,560 unique tetrasaccharides.

This potential for structural diversity is the bane of the carbohydrate chemist, but it is a boon to cells: it makes sugar polymers superbly effective carriers of information. Carbohydrates can carry much more information per unit weight than do either nucleic acids or proteins. Monosaccharides can therefore serve as letters in a vocabulary of biological specificity; the carbohydrate words are spelled out by variations in the monosaccharides, differences in the links between them and the presence or absence of branches.

Scattered reports that carbohydrates could define specificity began to appear quite early in the scientific literature, although they often went unnoticed. By the 1950s, for example, it was well established that injected polysaccharides could stimulate the production of antibodies in animals. Researchers also knew that the major ABO blood types are determined by sugars on blood cells and that the influenza virus binds to a red blood cell through a sugar, sialic acid. Yet not until the 1960s did sugars come into their own.

Two major developments prompted that change. The first was the realization that all cells carry a sugar coat. This coat consists for the most part of glycoproteins and glycolipids, two types of complex carbohydrates in which sugars are linked to proteins and lipids (fats), respectively. Several thousands of glycoprotein and glycholipid structures have been identified and their number grows almost daily. This diversity is surely significant: the repertoire of surface structures on a cell changes characteristically as it develops, differentiates or sickens. The array of carbohydrates on cancer cells is strikingly different from that on normal ones.

8. Why did most biologists dismiss the notion that carbohydrates played an important part in cellular recognition?
   A. The class of carbohydrates was large.
   B. Carbohydrates were thought to serve only as energy sources.
   C. Carbohydrates were too versatile.
   D. Carbohydrates were simple sugars and not sufficiently complex.

9. According to the passage, all of the following are characteristics of monosaccharide transmitted biological specificity EXCEPT
   A. carbohydrate words are spelled out by variations in the monosaccharides.
   B. carbohydrate words are spelled out by differences in links.
   C. carbohydrate words are spelled out by lipids.
   D. carbohydrate words are spelled out by the presence of branches.

10. The passage suggests that injected polysaccharides stimulating antibody production in animals provided evidence that
   A. carbohydrates could carry more information per unit weight than proteins.
   B. carbohydrates could define specificity.
   C. carbohydrates possessed structural diversity.
   D. lectins are rarely found on cells.

11. What discovery was crucial in the recognition of the significance of carbohydrates as carriers of information?
   A. That all cells carry a sugar coat.
   B. That the influenza virus binds to a red blood cell through sialic acid.
   C. That two amino acids can make one dipeptide.
   D. That chitin in the exoskeletons of insects was an important structural material.

12. What did Paul Ehrlich contribute to the lock-and-key hypothesis?
   A. Used it to account for highly specific immune system reactions.
   B. Used it to describe recognition between sperm and egg.
   C. Used it to recognize the value of carbohydrates as energy sources.
   D. Used it to prove the versatility of nucleic acids and proteins.

13. The passage suggests that discoveries about the involvement of carbohydrates in recognition may have practical applications in
   A. cancer treatment.
   B. determination of major ABO blood types.
   C. providing links between proteins and lipids.
   D. serving as markers for identifying and removing unwanted proteins.

14. Which of the following materials DOES NOT carry biological information in their structures?
   A. Carbohydrates
   B. Nucleic Acids
   C. Endothelial Venules
   D. Proteins

15. Why is the complexity of carbohydrate structures an issue in cell recognition?
   A. Amino acids can make one dipeptide.
   B. Monosaccharide units in oligosaccharides can attach to one another at multiple points.
   C. Monosaccharides create a large diversity of compounds which arc difficult to identify.
   D. Four different nucleotides can make 24 distinct tetranucleotides.

Passage 3:
Taken from book review of Before Writing, Volume 1: From Counting To Cuneiform,
Denise Schmandt-Besserat
Philip Morrison
Scientific American, November, 1992.
p. 133

Tokens were a common code. They are ideal symbols, save for their three-dimensional nature. They are discrete, recognizable, reputable, durable, cheap, yet open-ended enough to allow many new forms. They were a record-keeping device at village scale, one that "swept across the Near East on the coattails of agriculture" for 5,000 years, remarkably free of regional variations until cities began. At first there were at most a dozen or two simple forms. Then they entered a second, more complex phase, to dwindle once writing had come.

The first two hollow tablets reported have been followed by 115 more, most later than 4,000 B.C. Now these are recognized as envelopes of clay. Nearly all the envelopes are covered with repeated seal impressions, a signature—sometimes several—authenticating the security of the contents. Only a few have been opened to check the contents (x-ray techniques have not yet given good results). The number of tokens within is never very high; on the average there are about nine. These are no records of large-scale trade but rather of villagers' contributions to pooled grain or livestock surpluses, subject to some later redistribution. Step by step, such communities became "ranked societies," in which redistribution allows in the end for a tribute of offerings, fees and taxes.

16. By inference, why have so few hollow tablets been opened?
   - **A.** They are extremely rare and fragile.
   - **B.** X-ray techniques have not provided good results.
   - **C.** It is unclear whether they are authentic.
   - **D.** They contain few tokens.

17. The passage states that tokens were ideal symbols for each of the following EXCEPT
   - **A.** they were discreet.
   - **B.** they were three-dimensional.
   - **C.** they were durable.
   - **D.** they were cheap.

18. What constituted a signature on token envelopes?
   - **A.** Code symbols
   - **B.** Seal impressions
   - **C.** Tribute markings
   - **D.** Agricultural symbols

19. What material was used to make the tokens?
   - **A.** Carved stone
   - **B.** Carved wood
   - **C.** Inscribed clay
   - **D.** Metal

20. What ended the common use of tokens?
   - **A.** Cities began
   - **B.** Regional variations
   - **C.** Large-scale trade
   - **D.** Writing

21. What triggered the use of tokens?
   - **A.** Growth of small-scale trade
   - **B.** The advent of agriculture
   - **C.** Their low cost
   - **D.** Use of widely understood symbols

22. Tokens reflect the development of what kind of social system?
   - **A.** Egalitarian
   - **B.** Ranked
   - **C.** City centered
   - **D.** Free of taxes

Passage 4:
From "The Earliest History of the Earth"
Derek York
Scientific American, January, 1993. p. 90

To search for clues about the earth's youthful nature, geophysicists make use of an assortment of radioactive dating methods. These methods vary in their strengths and weaknesses, but they all rely on determining the relative abundance of a radioactive isotope and the subsequent isotope, or daughter nucleus, into which it decays. Every radioactive isotope eventually produces a final, stable decay product. Knowing the rate at which the nuclear transformation occurs (which can be measured to high precision in the laboratory) allows one to infer how long the decay products have been collecting in a rock. That information, taken with other evidence, reveals much about geologic history.

In the ongoing search for the oldest continental remnants, researchers primarily examine isotopes of uranium. Uranium ultimately decays into lead, so the relevant dating technique is called the uranium-lead method. That approach greatly benefits from the fact that samples of uranium and lead large enough to analyze can usually be extracted from zircon crystals. Such crystals are very commonly found in granite and metamorphic rocks, as well as in some volcanic rocks and sedimentary material derived from any of those rocks. Zircons also resist heat and weathering strongly, so they may survive intact in rocks that have experienced one or more metamorphic episodes.

23. What is the main idea of the passage?
- **A.** The nature of geological dating techniques
- **B.** The search for tools to measure radioactive decay in rocks
- **C.** The search for geological clues to the early earth
- **D.** The relative value of different dating techniques

24. What is the primary virtue of the uranium-lead method?
- **A.** Lead is a stable element.
- **B.** Sufficient samples can be found.
- **C.** Uranium decays very slowly.
- **D.** Scientists can precisely measure the decay rate of uranium.

25. All of the following are benefits of zircons EXCEPT
- **A.** they resist heat well.
- **B.** they resist weathering strongly.
- **C.** they are abundant.
- **D.** they always survive metamorphic episodes.

26. What do decay products allow scientist to infer?
- **A.** Geologic age
- **B.** Abundance of minerals
- **C.** Location and place of origin of rocks
- **D.** Determine the relative abundance of a radioactive isotope

27. What is the daughter nucleus of uranium isotopes?
- **A.** Zircon
- **B.** Lead
- **C.** Granite
- **D.** Volcanic rock

28. What is the importance of zircon crystals to the uranium-lead method?
- **A.** They are easily analyzed.
- **B.** They are very old.
- **C.** They contain large samples of uranium and lead.
- **D.** They are often found in metamorphic rocks.

29. Why do geophysicists use an assortment of radioactive dating techniques?
- **A.** Every radioactive isotope produces a decay product.
- **B.** The uranium-lead method is the most reliable technique.
- **C.** The methods vary in strengths and weaknesses.
- **D.** Rocks experience one or more metamorphic episodes.

Passage 5:
Taken from "Coral Bleaching"
Barbara E. Brown and John C. Ogden
Scientific American, January, 1993.
pp. 65–66

Tropical, shallow-water ecosystems, coral reefs are found around the world in the latitudes that generally fall between the southern tip of Florida and mid-Australia. They rank among the most biologically productive of all marine ecosystems. Because they harbor a vast array of animals and plants, coral reefs are often compared to tropical rain forests. Reefs also support life on land in several ways. They form and maintain the physical foundation for thousands of islands. By building a wall along the coast, they serve as a barrier against oceanic waves. And they sustain the fisheries and tourist diving industries that help to maintain the economies of many countries in the Caribbean and Pacific.

Although corals seem almost architectural in structure—some weigh many tons and stand between five and 10 meters high—they are composed of animals. Thousands of tiny creatures form enormous colonies: indeed, nearly 60 percent of the 220 living genera of corals do so. Each colony is made up of many individual coral animals, called polyps. Each polyp is essentially a hollow cylinder, closed at the base and interconnected to its neighbors by the gut cavity. The polyps have one or more rings of tentacles surrounding a central mouth. In this way, corals resemble sea anemones with skeletons. The soft external tissues of the polyps overlie a hard structure of calcium carbonate.

Many of the splendid colors of corals come from their symbionts, creatures that live in a mutually dependent relation with the coral. Symbiotic algae called zooxanthellae reside in the often transparent cells of the polyps. There are between one and two million algae cells per square centimeter of coral tissue. Through photosynthesis the algae produce carbon compounds, which help to nourish the coral—some species receive 60 percent of their food from their algae. Algal photosynthesis also accelerates the growth of the coral skeleton by causing more calcium carbonate to be produced. The corals provide algae with nutrients, such as nitrogen and phosphorus, essential for growth, as well as with housing. The association enables algae to obtain compounds that are scarce in the nutrient-poor waters of the tropics (where warm surface waters overlie and lock in cold, nutrient-rich waters—except in restricted areas of upwelling).

When corals bleach, the delicate balance among symbionts is destroyed. The corals lose algae, leaving their tissues so colorless that only the white, calcium carbonate skeleton is apparent. Other organisms such as anemones, sea whips and sponges—all of which harbor algae in their tissue—can also whiten in this fashion. Some of this loss is routine. A healthy coral or anemone continuously releases algae, but in very low numbers. Under natural conditions, less than 0.1 percent of the algae in a coral is lost during processes of regulation and replacement. When subject to adverse changes, such as temperature increases, however, the corals release increased number of algae. For example, transferring coral from a reef to a laboratory can cause a fivefold elevation in the numbers of algae expelled.

The mechanism of algae release is not fully understood. Even defining bleaching remains tricky. The current definition has its basis in laboratory measurements of the loss of algae and the reduction in algal pigments. The laboratory approach, however, is rarely, if ever, applied in the field. There judgement must rely on the naked eye's ability to detect loss of coloration. Although such methods may be reliable for instances of severe bleaching, a determination that pale colonies are bleached can be extremely arbitrary, given the natural variability of pigmentation.

30. What is the effect of algal photosynthesis on coral?
    A. They produce carbon compounds.
    B. They provide nourishment.
    C. They provide nitrogen nutrients.
    D. They can accelerate bleaching.

31. What is the definition of coral bleaching?
    A. Destruction of more than 0.1 percent of coral algae
    B. A fivefold increase above normal algae replacement
    C. Judgement of the naked eye
    D. No precise definition is provided in the passage

32. What provides the colors of many corals?
    A. Zooxanthellae
    B. Phosphorous
    C. Carbon compounds
    D. Warm surface waters

33. Corals provide algae with all of the following EXCEPT
    A. nitrogen.
    B. phosphorous.
    C. housing.
    D. carbon compounds.

34. According to the passage coral reefs are analogous to
    A. barriers against oceanic waves.
    B. marine ecosystems.
    C. tropical rain forests.
    D. elaborate architectural structures.

35. What happens when corals bleach?
    A. Polyps die
    B. Algal photosynthesis accelerates
    C. 0.1 percent of algae are lost
    D. Balance among symbionts is destroyed

36. Coral reefs provide all of the following EXCEPT
    A. warming of surface waters.
    B. barriers against waves.
    C. physical foundations for islands.
    D. fisheries.

37. According to the passage corals most resemble
    A. coastal walls.
    B. sea anemones with skeletons.
    C. a rich marine ecosystem.
    D. hollow cylinders.

Passage 6:
Taken from "Bacterial Endotoxins"
Ernst Theodor Rietschel and Helmut Brade
Scientific American, August, 1992.
pp. 59-60

...[Research] had begun to uncover many details of how endotoxins produce their effects.

It is now known, for instance, that endotoxins must be released from the bacterial surface in order to be effective. They are set free, as Pfeiffer recognized in 1892, when bacterial cells die, and also, it turns out, when the bacteria multiply. Some bacteria multiply within host cells, others without. Presumably, endotoxins made by the first group must additionally be released from infected cells in order to have an effect.

Once endotoxins are free to act, they do not, as might be expected, kill host cells or evoke other responses directly. They do not, for instance, produce fever by binding to cells in the temperature-regulating center of the brain. Instead,...they recruit particular host cells to secrete mediator molecules. These mediators then act locally or float through the blood, or both, to elicit a diversity of responses.

Studies...have since established that macrophages are the recruits most affected. These defensive cells normally take up and destroy any substance that might be harmful to a host. When they become activated, they secrete many different molecules that work in concert, sequentially or independently, to instigate or amplify both specific and nonspecific immune responses against an invader. (Nonspecific components of the immune system, such as macrophages, granulocytes and complement molecules, attack a broad range of invaders.) Some macrophages circulate in the blood; others reside in tissues.

Work in several laboratories has revealed that a small protein called tumor necrosis factor is one of the prime endotoxin mediators made by the macrophages. By itself, injected tumor necrosis factor mimics several of the responses attributed to endotoxins, including fever and, if doses are high enough, irreversible shock and death. On the positive side, as its name implies, tumor necrosis factor can also lure various defensive cells to sites of infection and destroy tumor cells.

More recently, endotoxin-stimulated macrophages have been shown to produce the proteins interleukin-1, interleukin-6 and interleukin-8, which exert many of the same effects as tumor necrosis factor. Activated macrophages also release a variety of lipids (some of which contribute to fever and regulate the activity of immune system cells), and they form highly reactive oxygenated compounds known as free radicals. Inside macrophages or on the surface, free radicals contribute to microbial destruction.

Thus, it seems that when a gram-negative bacterium invades tissues and releases moderate amounts of endotoxin there, this array of macrophage products can help eradicate the immediate infection by generating a localized and controlled immune response. The typical effects—mild fever, recruitment of both microbe-specific and less specialized immune components—usually serve recovery and help to protect against other microbial assaults.

But when infection is severe and a large amount of endotoxin accumulates in circulating blood, making contact with macrophages throughout the body, systemic release of potent mediators can produce life-threatening shock; as the circulation fails, cells everywhere malfunction and die. Endotoxins can enter the circulation on their own through damaged tissue. Generally, however, lethal effects occur when bacteria themselves gain access to the blood. They multiply rapidly in that medium and, in the process, can liberate huge supplies of toxin to act on macrophages.

Endotoxins, then, are not intrinsically poisonous; their effect depends on the host's response. As Lewis Thomas pointed out in The Lives of a Cell, it is the overwhelming, uncontrolled and self-destructive behavior of the host organism that makes endotoxins poisonous. Endotoxins, he wrote, "are read by our tissues as the very worst of bad news. When we sense lipopolysaccharide, we are likely to turn on every defense at our disposal; we will bomb, defoliate, blockade, seal off, destroy all tissues in the area.... All of this seems unnecessary, panic-driven."

38. Macrophages perform all of the following tasks EXCEPT
    A. secrete molecules.
    B. amplify immune responses.
    C. attack only specific endotoxins.
    D. circulate in the blood.

39. In the context of the passage what is the function of the quotation from Lewis Thomas?
    A. As a summary of reported findings
    B. As a restatement of the previously described process
    C. As a contrast to the process described previously
    D. As an elaborate metaphor

40. What is the effect of gram-negative bacterium with moderate release of endotoxin?
    A. Life-threatening shock
    B. Systemic release of potent mediators
    C. Recruitment of immune components
    D. High fever

41. What is tumor necrosis factor?
    A. An endoxic protein
    B. An endotoxin mediator
    C. A defensive cell
    D. A macrophage

42. Macrophages produce all of the following EXCEPT
    A. pyrotoxins.
    B. interleukin-6.
    C. lipids.
    D. proteins.

43. How to endotoxins act on host cells?
    A. Recruit them to secrete mediator molecules.
    B. Kill them.
    C. Bind to them.
    D. Evoke direct responses.

44. What is significant about experiments in which endotoxin-stimulated macrophages produce interleukin-1?
    A. The effects produced are not typical of endotoxin behavior.
    B. Endotoxin mediators can produce beneficial immune responses.
    C. Produced effects were unexpectedly toxic.
    D. Tumor necrosis factor was a byproduct.

45. Which of the following is most likely have lethal effects?
    A. Endotoxins entering the circulation through damaged tissue.
    B. Production of free radicals.
    C. Bacteria gain access to the blood.
    D. Presence of specialized immune components.

8.4 QUANTITATIVE ABILITY TEST

Each test item is a question or incomplete statement followed by suggested answers or completions. Read the item, decide which choice is the best, and circle only one answer per item.

Time Limit: 45 minutes

1. Find the largest of four consecutive even integers, which is two less than twice the smallest. Which of the following is the largest?
A. 8
B. 10
C. 6
D. 14

2. Which line is perpendicular to the Y-axis?
A. y = 3
B. x = 3
C. x = y
D. y = 1 – x

3. $\left(\frac{1}{x}\right)^6 + \left(\frac{2}{x^2}\right)^3 =$
A. $\frac{3}{x^2}$
B. $\frac{9}{x^6}$
C. $\frac{12}{x^6}$
D. $2x^6$

4. What is the probability of obtaining either tails or heads in five tosses of a fair coin?
A. $\frac{1}{2}$
B. $\frac{3}{5}$
C. $\frac{2}{5}$
D. $\frac{5}{8}$

5. What is the slope of a line containing the points (–2, 4) and (1, 3)?
A. 3
B. $\frac{1}{3}$
C. –3
D. $-\frac{1}{3}$

6. The value of $\frac{2}{3} + \frac{1}{4} - \frac{1}{2}$ is
A. $\frac{-1}{2}$
B. $\frac{1}{12}$
C. $\frac{1}{6}$
D. $\frac{5}{12}$

7. The value of $\frac{2}{3} \times \frac{3}{4} \times \frac{4}{5}$ is
A. $\frac{9}{12}$
B. $\frac{2}{5}$
C. $\frac{1}{4}$
D. $\frac{3}{8}$

8. If $ax^2 = 2y$, then $\frac{a}{y} =$
A. 2
B. $2x^2$
C. $\frac{2}{x^2}$
D. $\frac{x^2}{2}$

9. $\dfrac{\sqrt{15}\sqrt{3}}{\sqrt{10}} =$

A. $\dfrac{3}{2}$

B. $2\sqrt{5}$

C. $9\sqrt{5}$

D. $\dfrac{3\sqrt{2}}{2}$

10. If $2^{x/3} = 16$, then x =

A. –2

B. 4

C. 6

D. 12

11. If the perimeter of a square is 5.2, what is the area?

A. 1.3

B. 1.69

C. 52

D. 13

12. If an ordinary coin is tossed four times, what is the probability that all four tosses will be either all heads or all tails?

A. $\dfrac{1}{16}$

B. $\dfrac{1}{4}$

C. $\dfrac{1}{2}$

D. $\dfrac{1}{8}$

13. Which of the following is equal to (tan θ) (csc θ)?

A. sin θ

B. cos θ

C. sec θ

D. csc θ

14. Find the perimeter of the composite figure. Use 3.14 for π.

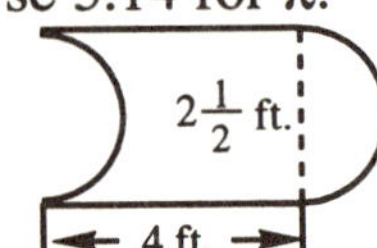

A. 15.85 ft.

B. 13.25 ft.

C. 10.5 ft.

D. 13 ft.

15. The angles of a triangle are in the ratio of 2:3:5. What is the measure of the smallest angle?

A. 48°

B. 36°

C. 90°

D. 45°

16. If the area of the triangle BCE is 32, what is the area of the square ABCD?

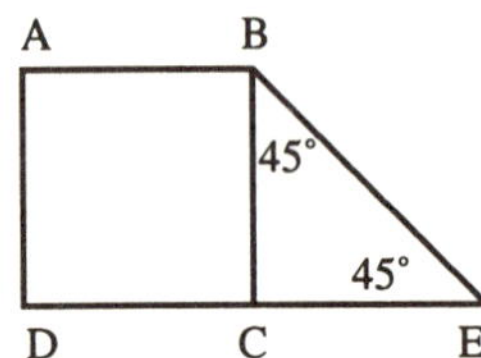

A. 64

B. 32

C. 16

D. 8

17. A child withdraws from his piggy bank 20% of the original sum in the bank. If he must add 80 cents to bring the amount in the bank back up to the original sum, what was the original sum in the bank?

A. $1.00

B. $1.80

C. $2.60

D. $4.00

18. $-4 - 3\{2 + 1[3 - (2 + 3) + 2] + 2\} + 4 =$

A. –12

B. 0

C. 2

D. 8

19. 0.01% of 10 =

A. 1

B. 0.1

C. 0.01

D. 0.001

20. If $2x - y = 7$ and $x + y = 2$, then $x - y =$
A. 6
B. 4
C. $\frac{3}{2}$
D. 0

21. The distance between Jimmy's house and the zoo is 12 miles. Jimmy rode his bicycle from his house to the zoo at an average speed of 12 miles per hour. He walked home from the zoo at an average speed of 6 miles per hour. Since he took the same route in both directions, what was his average speed?
A. 8 miles per hour
B. 12 miles per hour
C. 16 miles per hour
D. 20 miles per hour

22. Ned is three years older than Mike, who is twice as old as Linda. If the ages of the three total 28 years, how old is Mike?
A. 5 years old
B. 8 years old
C. 9 years old
D. 10 years old

23. Paul drove his car until the gas tank was 1/6 full. He stopped to refill the tank to capacity by putting in 20 gallons. What is the capacity of the gas tank?
A. 20
B. 21
C. 24
D. 28

24. In dentistry a mixture of gold and platinum is sometimes used to fabricate crowns (caps) for teeth, usually in the ratio 3:2 by weight. If the crowns made of these metals weigh 0.4 ounces, how many ounces of gold does the crown contain?
A. 0.20
B. 0.24
C. 0.32
D. 0.36

25. Simplify $\sqrt{\frac{3x^2}{9} + \frac{4x^2}{36}}$
A. $\frac{3x}{4}$
B. $\frac{2x}{3}$
C. $4x$
D. $\frac{2x^2}{3}$

26. Three times the first of three consecutive odd integers is five more than twice the third. Find the third integer.
A. 11
B. 13
C. 15
D. 17

27. Barbara invests $3,600 in the Security National Bank at 5%. How much additional money must she invest at 10% so that the total annual interest income will be equal to 8% of her entire investment?
A. $3,600
B. $1,200
D. $3,000
D. $5,400

28. A plane traveling 800 miles per hour is 40 miles from Kennedy Airport at 5:58 p.m. At what time will it arrive at the airport?
A. 6:00 p.m.
B. 6.01 p.m.
C. 6:02 p.m.
D. 6:03 p.m.

29. Mr. Bridges can wash his car in 30 minutes, while his son Dave takes twice as long to do the same job. If they work together, how many minutes will the job take them?
A. 5 min.
B. 10 min.
C. 20 min.
D. 28 min.

30. The sum of a number and eight equals four less than the product of four and the number. Find the number.
A. $x = 3$
B. $x = 2$
C. $x = 6$
D. $x = 4$

31. Sales decreases causes a department store to reduce its output by 25%. By what percent must the reduced sales be increased for production to be brought to normal?
A. 33.3%
B. 50%
C. 66.7%
D. 75%

32. Edward leaves home for work, driving at 24 miles per hour. Fifteen minutes later his wife notices he left his brief case. She decides to catch him on the road. If his wife drives 40 miles per hour, how far must she drive before she catches up with him?
A. 15 miles
B. 30 miles
C. 45 miles
D. 60 miles

33. There are three consecutive even integers such that the third of the three even integers is eight more than the sum of the first and second. Find the third even integer.
A. –8
B. –6
C. –4
D. –2

34. Elizabeth has $5.50 in nickels and dimes. She has five more nickels than dimes. How many dimes does she have?
A. 35
B. 30
C. 25
D. 20

35. If the ratio of P to Q is 3/4 and the ratio of Q to R is 12/19, what is the ratio of P to R?
A. 9/19
B. 1/4
C. 17/19
D. 3/19

36. Find the equation of the line that contains the point (– 1, 0) and has slope 2.
A. $y = 2x - 1$
B. $y = 2x + 2$
C. $y = 2x$
D. $y = 2x - 3$

37. The following right triangles ABC and DEF are similar. How long is DF?

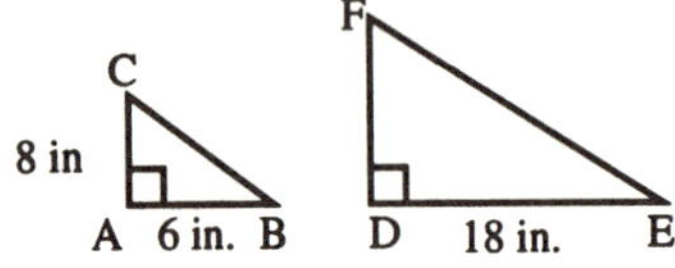

A. 24 in
B. 20 in
C. 16 in
D. 12 in

38. Which of the following is equal to $-2 < \frac{x}{3} \leq 2$?
A. $-3 < x \leq 3$
B. $-4 < x \leq 4$
C. $-9 < x \leq 9$
D. $-6 < x \leq 6$

39. $\sqrt{.64}\,(10^4) =$
A. 6400
B. 8000
C. 640
D. 800

40. Given log 2 = 0.3010, determine log 8.
A. 1.204
B. 0.602
C. 0.301
D. 0.903

8.5 VERBAL ABILITY

Each test item provides a word followed by suggested answers. Find the word opposite in meaning from the answer choices. Only one answer is correct for each question.

Antonyms

1. INTREPID
- **A.** fearful
- **B.** brave
- **C.** secretive
- **D.** unfit

2. CULPABLE
- **A.** liable
- **B.** greedy
- **C.** impeccable
- **D.** incoherent

3. OBSTREPEROUS
- **A.** lazy
- **B.** wasteful
- **C.** intimate
- **D.** docile

4. INDELIBLE
- **A.** vivid
- **B.** transient
- **C.** cryptic
- **D.** ambivalent

5. EXPEDIENT
- **A.** arbitrary
- **B.** efficient
- **C.** ludicrous
- **D.** intrinsic

6. IMPASSIVE
- **A.** banal
- **B.** stoic
- **C.** vibrant
- **D.** taciturn

7. HOARY
- **A.** youthful
- **B.** bald
- **C.** grizzled
- **D.** lavish

8. INDOLENT
- **A.** assiduous
- **B.** lazy
- **C.** redolent
- **D.** convivial

9. HETEROGENEOUS
- **A.** infused
- **B.** colored
- **C.** cloned
- **D.** mottled

10. ZEALOT
- **A.** pacifist
- **B.** fanatic
- **C.** abstainer
- **D.** mystic

11. CELERITY
- **A.** languor
- **B.** mystery
- **C.** clemency
- **D.** expedition

12. WHET
- **A.** curb
- **B.** dry
- **C.** pique
- **D.** satiate

13. RAREFIED
- **A.** prolific
- **B.** attenuated
- **C.** dense
- **D.** diluted

14. ODIOUS
- **A.** fragrant
- **B.** noxious
- **C.** repugnant
- **D.** pleasant

15. DILIGENT
A. circumspect
B. furtive
C. indolent
D. lethargic

16. INIMICAL
A. beneficial
B. malicious
C. flippant
D. surly

17. FORTUITOUS
A. inauspicious
B. serendipity
C. calculated
D. adventitious

18. EFFACE
A. harden
B. expunge
C. diminish
D. brand

19. ANTIPATHY
A. veneration
B. ennui
C. proclivity
D. malevolence

20. LATENT
A. dormant
B. overt
C. obscure
D. tardy

21. INNOCUOUS
A. naive
B. immune
C. vitriolic
D. devious

22. DICHOTOMY
A. cacophony
B. synergy
C. hierarchy
D. union

23. ECLECTIC
A. ordinary
B. catholic
C. exclusive
D. inflexible

24. SUCCINCT
A. loquacious
B. accomplished
C. reserved
D. moist

25. ABSTRACT
A. diffuse
B. coalescent
C. stylized
D. unrealistic

26. SURREPTITIOUS
A. overt
B. blatant
C. repetitious
D. intrinsic

27. RETICULATE
A. smooth
B. forward
C. circulate
D. dissipate

28. SUCCINCT
A. disparate
B. pithy
C. precocious
D. copious

29. FACTIOUS
A. conciliatory
B. truthful
C. unified
D. consensual

30. CONVERSANT
A. unacquainted
B. misleading
C. varietal
D. loquacious

31. ODIOUS
   A. endearing
   B. putrescent
   C. foreboding
   D. poetic

32. BELLICOSE
   A. musical
   B. conciliatory
   C. argumentative
   D. divergent

33. CATHARSIS
   A. refinement
   B. purification
   C. fulfillment
   D. sufficiency

34. COLLEGIAL
   A. autocratic
   B. educated
   C. elite
   D. inimical

35. INVECTIVE
   A. aggressive
   B. prayer
   C. acclamation
   D. conducive

36. IRASCIBLE
   A. unflappable
   B. irksome
   C. avaricious
   D. mischievous

37. SPURN
   A. tolerate
   B. engage
   C. demand
   D. overwhelm

38. STOLID
   A. upright
   B. stilted
   C. abusive
   D. emotional

39. INSIPID
   A. saporous
   B. spiteful
   C. ingenuous
   D. invalid

40. INSULAR
   A. temperate
   B. comprehensive
   C. inflated
   D. idealized

ANALOGIES

41. SNOW : DRIFT :: SAND :
   A. dune
   B. beach
   C. desert
   D. grain

42. POSSIBLE : PROBABLE :: HOPE :
   A. desire
   B. revert
   C. expect
   D. receive

43. QUILL : NIB :: AXE :
   A. temper
   B. hone
   C. chop
   D. blade

44. MNEMONIC : WORDS :: EUPHONIOUS :
   A. expressions
   B. sounds
   C. pictures
   D. vocabulary

45. INFANT : TODDLER :: CHILD :
   A. teen
   B. playful
   C. adult
   D. unsteady

46. STAR : GALAXY :: ISLAND :
   A. continent
   B. key
   C. archipelago
   D. atoll

47. GROUNDHOG : HIBERNATE :: SWALLOW :
   A. migrate
   B. dislocate
   C. perambulate
   D. procreate

48. YAWN : BOREDOM :: WINCE :
   A. pain
   B. amusement
   C. anger
   D. defiance

49. BUFFALO : PRAIRIE :: WILDEBEEST :
   A. pampas
   B. tundra
   C. steppes
   D. inlets

50. TEXT : ADDENDUM :: PLAY :
   A. epilogue
   B. prologue
   C. scene
   D. intermission

51. TRUNK : GNARLED :: JOURNEY :
   A. tortuous
   B. overt
   C. tedious
   D. solitary

52. WINTER : DORMANCY :: SPRING :
   A. rejuvenation
   B. fruition
   C. catalyst
   D. animation

53. SOLSTICE : HIBERNAL :: EQUINOX :
   A. bivalent
   B. diurnal
   C. vernal
   D. coincident

54. IMPASSE : HIATUS :: BRIDGE :
   A. link
   B. stalemate
   C. impediment
   D. union

55. MOROSE : PESSIMIST :: BUOYANT :
   A. pragmatic
   B. enthralling
   C. optimist
   D. evanescent

56. BREAD : LEAVEN :: SELTZER :
   A. carbonation
   B. bubbles
   C. mineral
   D. water

57. CYCLONE : DEBRIS :: MAELSTROM :
A. lava
B. ice
C. water
D. ghosts

58. SCALE : WEIGHT :: THERMOMETER :
A. mercury
B. degrees
C. heat
D. temperature

59. EXTRANEOUS : INTRINSIC :: PERIPHERY :
A. core
B. incline
C. centrifugal
D. fulcrum

60. MARINE : OCEAN :: ARBOREAL :
A. botany
B. forest
C. harbor
D. spring

61. EPHEMERAL : SNOWFLAKE :: BLOSSOM :
A. lily
B. evergreen
C. tuber
D. root

62. FRESCO : PAINTER :: OPERA :
A. corral
B. symphony
C. composer
D. soloist

63. MYOPIA : EYE :: TREE :
A. crown
B. sap
C. cicada
D. burl

64. BLUE : SAPPHIRE :: RED :
A. sanguine
B. garnet
C. crimson
D. chimera

65. LUSTER : TARNISH :: VERTICAL :
A. prone
B. precipitate
C. perpendicular
D. plumb

66. ALTRUISTIC : COMPENSATION :: FRACTIOUS :
A. union
B. whole
C. harmony
D. sum

67. HIEROGLYPH : WORD :: DELTA :
A. change
B. coda
C. letter
D. river

68. XANTHIC : PUSILLANIMOUS:: ERYTHEMA :
A. ire
B. panegyric
C. pallid
D. dastardly

69. PHONEME : SPEECH :: TESSELLATE :
A. hair
B. quatrefoil
C. mosaic
D. fringe

70. LEOPARD : LEAP :: LION :
A. pride
B. timorous
C. intrepid
D. feline

71. LACHRYMOSE : STOIC :: HIRSUTE :
A. glabrous
B. veracious
C. loquacious
D. efficacious

72. CARTOGRAPHER : SURVEY :: SURGEON :
A. anatomy
B. prognosis
C. patient
D. scalpel

73. LIMNOLOGY : LAKES :: HOROLOGY :
A. spring
B. bedrock
C. rhythm
D. dials

74. BRASS : BRONZE :: ZINC :
A. lead
B. copper
C. nickel
D. tin

75. ANADROMOUS : SALMON :: CATADROMOUS :
A. trout
B. pike
C. eel
D. squid

76. MAN : ATLAS :: WOMAN :
A. caryatid
B. telamon
C. doric
D. engendered

77. GRAINS : SCRUPLE :: SCRUPLES :
A. ounce
B. pound
C. dram
D. pennyweight

78. PENTIMENTO : SUPERIMPOSE :: PALIMPSEST :
A. redact
B. misappropriate
C. undermine
D. usurp

79. CRUCIATE : LENTICULAR :: RETICULAR :
A. discoid
B. pruritic
C. florid
D. granulomatous

80. CETACEAN : AMBERGRIS :: PACHYDERM :
A. emollient
B. eburnean
C. anemone
D. sibilant

8.6 PCAT SAMPLE TEST ANSWER KEYS

8.6.1 Biology

1. A
2. B
3. A
4. B
5. C
6. C
7. B
8. B
9. A
10. D
11. D
12. B
13. A
14. A
15. D
16. B
17. A
18. B
19. B
20. D
21. C
22. D
23. A
24. C
25. A
26. D
27. C
28. C
29. C
30. A
31. C
32. B
33. D
34. D
35. D
36. B
37. C
38. C
39. D
40. A
41. D
42. D
43. D
44. B
45. C
46. D
47. D
48. B
49. D
50. C
51. B
52. D
53. B

8.6.2 Chemistry

1. C
2. B
3. C
4. D
5. B
6. A
7. A
8. B
9. C
10. B
11. D
12. B
13. D
14. B
15. D
16. A
17. D
18. C
19. C
20. B
21. B
22. B
23. C
24. C
25. D
26. D
27. B
28. D
29. B
30. D
31. B
32. A
33. D
34. B
35. D
36. D
37. A
38. C
39. D
40. C
41. A
42. D
43. D
44. B
45. B
46. B
47. A
48. A
49. D
50. A
51. B
52. C
53. C
54. D
55. B
56. A
57. D
58. A
59. B
60. C

8.6.3 Reading Comprehension

1. A
2. B
3. B
4. D
5. C
6. C
7. C
8. B
9. C
10. B
11. A
12. A
13. A
14. C
15. C
16. A
17. B
18. B
19. C
20. D
21. B
22. B
23. C
24. B
25. D
26. A
27. B
28. C
29. C
30. B
31. D
32. A
33. D
34. C
35. D
36. A
37. B
38. C
39. B
40. C
41. A
42. A
43. A
44. B
45. C

8.6.4 Quantitative Ability

1. D
2. A
3. B
4. A
5. D
6. D
7. B
8. C
9. D
10. D
11. B
12. A
13. C
14. A
15. B
16. A
17. D
18. A
19. D
20. B
21. A
22. D
23. C
24. B
25. B
26. D
27. D
28. B
29. C
30. D
31. A
32. B
33. D
34. A
35. A
36. B
37. A
38. D
39. B
40. D

8.6.5 Verbal Ability (Antonyms and Analogies)

1. A. fearful
2. C. impeccable
3. D. docile
4. B. transient
5. A. arbitrary
6. C. vibrant
7. A. youthful
8. A. assiduous
9. C. cloned
10. A. pacifist
11. A. languor
12. A. curb
13. C. dense
14. D. pleasant
15. C. indolent
16. A. beneficial
17. C. calculated
18. D. brand
19. A. veneration
20. B. overt
21. C. vitriolic
22. D. union
23. C. exclusive
24. A. loquacious
25. B. coalescent
26. A. overt
27. A. smooth
28. D. copious
29. C. unified
30. A. unacquainted
31. A. endearing
32. B. conciliatory
33. C. fulfillment
34. D. inimical
35. C. acclamation
36. A. unflappable
37. C. demand
38. D. emotional
39. A. saporous
40. B. comprehensive
41. A. dune
42. C. expect
43. D. blade
44. B. sounds
45. A. teen
46. C. archipelago
47. A. migrate
48. A. pain
49. C. steppes
50. A. epilogue
51. A. tortuous
52. A. rejuvenation
53. C. vernal
54. D. union
55. C. optimist
56. A. carbonation
57. C. water
58. D. temperature
59. A. core
60. B. forest
61. A. lily
62. C. composer
63. D. burl
64. B. garnet
65. A. prone
66. C. harmony
67. A. change
68. A. ire
69. C. mosaic
70. A. pride
71. A. glabrous
72. A. anatomy
73. C. rhythm
74. D. tin
75. C. eel
76. A. caryatid
77. C. dram
78. D. usurp
79. A. discoid
80. B. eburnean

8.7 Explanatory Solutions For Reading Comprehension Problems

Question 1: The correct response (A) is found in the first paragraph and in particular with reference to Denmark.

Question 2: The correct response (B) is located in the first sentence of the second paragraph. Note that the correct response is phrased in the conditional using the term "potential" which is consistent with the author's tone.

Question 3: The first paragraph provides the basis for arriving at the correct response (B). Chip cards, writes the author, are increasingly replacing cash.

Question 4: The correct response (D) is located in the second paragraph since it is cited as a possible danger to personal privacy.

Question 5: The correct response (C) is contained in the final paragraph. It is important to recognize that individuals would not have any reason to gather data and that the author is concerned about the individual maintaining privacy.

Question 6: The correct response (C) can be either a vocabulary recognition problem or drawn from the context of "guaranteed records."

Question 7: The correct response (C) is based on contrasting information presented in the second and third paragraphs.

Question 8: The correct response (B) is contained in the third paragraph. It is worth noting that the passage as does the correct response both use the term "only."

Question 9: The correct response (C) does not jump off the page and may most easily identified by process of elimination. Another possibility is recognizing that response C does not deal with either sugars or structure.

Question 10: The correct response (B) depends on locating the relevant information in the sixth paragraph.

Question 11: The correct response (A) is contained in the final paragraph. It is also helpful to recognize that only response A mentions sugars, an essential component of carbohydrate.

Question 12: The correct response (A) is located in the first paragraph of the passage.

Question 13: The correct response (A) requires patience on the part of the reader since it does not appear until the end of the final paragraph of the passage.

Question 14: Endothelial venules (C) do not appear in the entire passage. Process of elimination might be the most efficient solution to this question.

Question 15: The correct response (C) should be triggered by recognition of the first sentence of the fourth paragraph.

Question 16: While response B is tempting it does not explain the why that is central to the question. Rather, the correct response (A) offers a reason why the inconclusive X-rays have not been simply bypassed and the envelopes opened.

Question 17: The passage explicitly mentions responses A, C, and D as virtues of tokens while the correct response (B) is refuted in the second sentence of the passage.

Question 18: The correct response (B) is contained in the third sentence of the second paragraph.

Question 19: The passage does not explicitly mention the material used to make the tokens but does explain that the envelopes were made of clay and that the material used was durable, cheap and easily formed thus leading to response C.

Question 20: The correct response (D) is contained in the last sentence of the first paragraph.

Question 21: The correct response is contained in the third sentence of the first paragraph.

Question 22: It is not until the final sentence of the passage that there is mention of social structure where the correct response (B) is then found.

Question 23: The last sentence of the first paragraph offers a vital clue as to the author's purpose in presenting information on dating methods and leads to the correct response (C).

Question 24: The second sentence of the passage contains the information necessary to arrive at the correct response (B).

Question 25: Use of the term "always" in response D should raise suspicions. A search through the paragraph reveals that there is no basis for assuming that zircons always survive metamorphic episodes and thus D is the correct response.

Question 26: The passage's first paragraph is essentially devoted to answering this question. A is the correct response.

Question 27: The correct response (B) is contained in the second sentence of the second paragraph.

Question 28: The correct response (C) is located in the third sentence of paragraph two.

Question 29: It can be presumed that the passage is an excerpt from a longer article and that while the uranium-lead method is the primary focus the first sentence of the passage suggests that other methods have value and might be discussed latter in the passage. Thus, response C is correct.

Question 30: The correct response (B) is located early in the third paragraph. While it is true that algal photosynthesis produces carbon compounds (response A) the question asks for the "effect" on coral.

Question 31: Test-takers dislike responses like D although it is the correct response. The last paragraph provides the necessary explanation when the authors write that the definition of bleaching is tricky and then proceed to explain why by detailing the shortcomings of current incomplete definitions. These definitions all lack precision.

Question 32: The correct response (A) is contained in the first two sentences of paragraph three.

Question 33: The relationship between corals and their algal symbionts is discussed in paragraph three. Response E is inverted; i.e. coral provide algae with carbon compounds and is thus the correct answer.

Question 34: This analogy, and the correct response (C) is contained in the first paragraph.

Question 35: The correct response (D) may seem too general but an examination of the fourth paragraph will reveal that the other responses are either too specific or simply incorrect.

Question 36: The first paragraph discusses this question and provides the correct response (A). The key term is "provide," and while coral reefs may exist in warm waters they do not cause them.

Question 37: The correct response (B) is contained in the second paragraph where corals are explicitly compared to sea anemones.

Question 38: In effect, this question asks what is the main idea of the passage? As the final paragraph argues, one of the key problems with the human immune response to endotoxins is that the host panics and can behave in a self-destructive fashion. Hence response C is correct.

Question 39: The quotation in the last paragraph restates the more technical and elaborate description which precedes it. Response B is correct.

Question 40: The correct response (C) is contained in the seventh paragraph. The paragraph is very technical and the question demands careful sorting through the information.

Question 41: This is a rather difficult question in that tumor necrosis can function both toxically and beneficially. The correct response (B) is located in the fifth paragraph.

Question 42: Information to arrive at the correct response (A) is scattered throughout the passage. Simply put, pyrotoxins are not mentioned. A process of elimination approach might be most appropriate.

Question 43: The correct response (A) is contained in the third paragraph.

Question 44: The correct response (B) is contained in the sixth paragraph but is arrived at indirectly. Endotoxin-stimulated production of interleukin-1 in turn form free radicals which contribute to the destruction of microbes.

Question 45: The correct response (C) is contained in the eighth paragraph. While response A could lead to lethal effects the question asks for the response that "is most likely" to have lethal effects and thus demands the choice of "the best" response.

8.8 REFERENCES

Psychological Corporation, The. *The Pharmacy College Admission Test* (candidate information booklet with application), latest ed. (San Antonio, Tex.)

Appendix A

Scope of Examinations

A.1 TEST CONTENT

The Pharmacy College Admission Test (PCAT) has approximately 300 multiple-choice questions and lasts for about four hours. Each question has four answer choices. Only one is correct. Each question and the corresponding answer is independent of the answers to any other questions.

The PCAT is divided into separate sections, each of which is timed separately. You will not be allowed to go back to earlier sections or on to later sections. Answer questions that are easy for you, skipping over those questions which require more time and calculations.

The **Verbal Ability** section measures general, nonscientific word knowledge using antonyms and analogies. There are approximately 50 questions in this section.

The **Quantitative Ability** section measures abilities to solve arithmetic problems including fractions, decimals, and percentages, and ability to reason through and understand quantitative concepts and relationships. Applications of algebra (but not of trigonometry or calculus) are included on the PCAT. There are approximately 65 questions in this section.

The **Biology** section measures knowledge of the principles and concepts of basic biology with major emphasis on human biology (both structure and function). There are approximately 50 questions in this section.

The **Chemistry** section measures knowledge of principles and concepts of inorganic and basic organic chemistry. There are more questions in inorganic chemistry than organic chemistry. There are approximately 60 questions in this section.

The **Reading Comprehension** section measures ability to comprehend, analyze, and interpret reading passages on scientific topics. There are approximately 45 questions in this section.

A.2 TOPIC OUTLINES

I. Biology and Chemistry Topics

A. Biology
1. origin of life
2. cell metabolism (including photosynthesis)
3. enzymology
4. thermodynamics
5. organelle structure and function (cell biology)
6. biological organization and relationship of major taxa using the five-kingdom system
   (a) Monera
   (b) angiosperms
   (c) arthropods
   (d) chordates

7. structure and function of human systems
    (a) integumentary
    (b) skeletal
    (c) muscular
    (d) circulatory
    (e) immunological
    (f) digestive
    (g) respiratory
    (h) urinary
    (i) nervous
    (j) endocrine
    (k) reproductive
8. fertilization, descriptive embryology, and developmental mechanics
9. Mendelian inheritance, chromosomal genetics, meiosis, molecular and human genetics
10. evolution, natural selection, population genetics, and speciation
11. microbiology
    (a) bacteria
    (b) viruses
12. plant biology

B. General Chemistry
1. stoichiometry
    (a) percent of composition
    (b) empirical formulas from percent of composition
    (c) balancing equations
    (d) weight/weight, weight/volume, and density problems
2. gases
    (a) kinetic molecular theory of gases
    (b) Graham's law
    (c) Dalton's law
    (d) Boyle's law
    (e) Charles's law
    (f) ideal gas law
3. liquids and solids
4. solutions
    (a) colligative properties
    (b) concentration calculations
5. acids and bases
6. chemical equilibrium
    (a) molecular
    (b) acid/base
    (c) precipitation and equilibria calculations
7. thermodynamics and thermochemistry
    (a) laws of thermodynamics
    (b) Hess's law
    (c) spontaneity prediction
8. chemical kinetics
    (a) rate laws
    (b) activation energy
    (c) half-life

9. oxidation-reduction reactions and electrochemistry
    (a) balancing equations
    (b) determinations of oxidation numbers
    (c) electro-chemical concepts and calculations
10. atomic and molecular structure
    (a) electron configuration
    (b) orbital types
    (c) Lewis-Dot diagrams
    (d) atomic theories
    (e) molecular geometry
    (f) bond types
    (g) quantum mechanics
11. periodic properties of elements
    (a) nonmetals
    (b) transition metals
    (c) nontransition metals
12. nuclear chemistry

C. Organic Chemistry
1. bonding
    (a) atomic orbitals
    (b) molecular orbitals
    (c) hybridization
    (d) Lewis structures
    (e) bond angles
    (f) bond lengths
2. chemical and physical properties of molecules
    (a) stability
    (b) solubility
    (c) polarity
    (d) inter- and intramolecular forces
3. stereochemistry
    (a) conformational analysis
    (b) optical activity
    (c) chirality
    (d) chiral centers
    (e) places of symmetry
    (f) enantiomers
    (g) diasteriomers
    (h) meso compounds
4. nomenclature (IUPAC rules identification of functional groups on molecules)
5. reaction of the major functional groups (prediction of reaction products and important mechanistic generalities
6. aromatic
    (a) concept of aromaticity
    (b) electrophilic aromatic substitution
7. synthesis (identification of the product of, or the reagents used in, a simple sequence of reactions)

II. **Reading Comprehension**

A. Ability to read, organize, and remember new information in basic sciences including pharmacy journals.

B. Ability to comprehend thoroughly when studying scientific information.
Note: Reading materials are typical of material encountered in the first year of pharmacy school and require no prior knowledge of the topic other than a basic undergraduate preparation in science.

III. **Quantitative Ability**

A. Algebraic equations

B. Fractions

C. Conversions
   1. ounces
   2. pounds
   3. inches
   4. feet
   5. liters

D. Percentages

E. Decimals and exponential notation

F. Probability and statistics

G. Geometry

H. Trigonometry

I. Applied mathematics problems